Systemic Autoinflammatory Diseases—Clinical Rheumatic Challenges Series 2

Systemic Autoinflammatory Diseases—Clinical Rheumatic Challenges Series 2

Editor

Eugen Feist

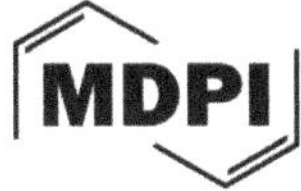

Basel • Beijing • Wuhan • Barcelona • Belgrade • Novi Sad • Cluj • Manchester

Editor
Eugen Feist
Department of
Rheumatology, Cooperation
Partner of the
Otto-von-Guericke University
Vogelsang-Gommern
Germany

Editorial Office
MDPI
St. Alban-Anlage 66
4052 Basel, Switzerland

This is a reprint of articles from the Special Issue published online in the open access journal *Journal of Clinical Medicine* (ISSN 2077-0383) (available at: https://www.mdpi.com/journal/jcm/special_issues/98BQ1KNK96).

For citation purposes, cite each article independently as indicated on the article page online and as indicated below:

Lastname, A.A.; Lastname, B.B. Article Title. *Journal Name* **Year**, *Volume Number*, Page Range.

ISBN 978-3-7258-1049-9 (Hbk)
ISBN 978-3-7258-1050-5 (PDF)
doi.org/10.3390/books978-3-7258-1050-5

Contents

About the Editor

Eugen Feist

Professor Eugen Feist studied medicine at the Institute of Medicine, Kiev, Ukraine, and the Charité Humboldt-University of Berlin, Germany, from 1989 to 1995. He worked at the Department of Rheumatology and Clinical immunology at the Charité-Universitätsmedizin as a board-certified internist and rheumatologist from 1995 to 2019. Professor Feist's clinical work and research activities are focused on systemic autoimmune and autoinflammatory diseases, with special interests in rheumatoid arthritis and adult-onset Still's disease. He has worked as an investigator in several phase I to IV clinical and investigator-initiated studies in the field of rheumatology. In 2009, he received a postdoctoral lecture qualification for his work on the topic of "Proteasomes and Autoimmunity" and in 2021, he became a board-certified immunologist. Since 2019, Professor Feist has worked as the medical director of the Helios Clinic for Rheumatology and Clinical Immunology in Vogelsang-Gommern with a university teaching position at the Otto-von-Guericke University Magdeburg.

Preface

Autoinflammatory diseases are not only of increasing interest for clinical immunologists as well as rheumatologists but fascinate researchers in other fields of medicine such as hematology, oncology and infectiology. Although related to different pathways, all autoinflammatory diseases share the prominent involvement of the innate immune system in their pathogenesis. This progress allows for a deeper understanding of closely linked diseases, such as inflammasomopathies, interferonopathies, relopathies, and proteasome-associated syndromes. These insights have not only improved their classification but have also helped us to identify new treatment targets of pro-inflammatory cytokines, including IL-1ß, IL-6, interferon-, and TNF-alpha. Nevertheless, there is still an urgent medical need, especially in the recognition of syndromes of undifferentiated recurrent fever and reliable outcome measures, for the confirmation of data from controlled clinical trials, in addition to data from registers regarding patients' long-term experiences.

The Special Issue entitled "Systemic Autoinflammatory Diseases—Clinical Rheumatic Challenges Series 2" of the *Journal of Clinical Medicine* includes articles on already established standards as well as remaining challenges in the management of certain complex and interdisciplinary conditions such as the recently described VEXAS. Special attention is also paid to patients' experience and the impact of COVID-19 vaccination. Of importance for clinicians, this Special Issue features an article that focuses on relevant differential diagnosis of fever of unknown origins, namely functional hyperthermia.

Since we have entered a new age in this complex field with a close link between rheumatology and immunology, it is our aim to raise awareness for autoinflammatory processes and to better understand their potential short- and long-term risks such as amyloidosis and fibrosis.

Eugen Feist
Editor

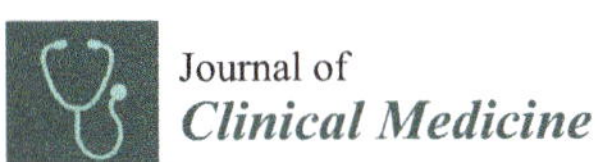

Journal of
Clinical Medicine

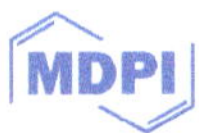

Article

Patient Experiences and Challenges in the Management of Autoinflammatory Diseases—Data from the International FMF & AID Global Association Survey

Jürgen Rech [1,2,3,*], Georg Schett [1,2,3], Abdurrahman Tufan [4], Jasmin B. Kuemmerle-Deschner [5], Seza Özen [6], Koray Tascilar [1,2,3], Leonie Geck [1,2,3], Tobias Krickau [2,3,7], Ellen Cohen [8], Tatjana Welzel [9], Marcus Kuehn [10] and Malena Vetterli [8]

[1] Department of Internal Medicine 3, Rheumatology and Immunology, Friedrich-Alexander University (FAU), Erlangen-Nürnberg and Universitätsklinikum Erlangen, 91054 Erlangen, Germany; georg.schett@uk-erlangen.de (G.S.); koray.tascilar@uk-erlangen.de (K.T.); leonie.geck@fau.de (L.G.)

[2] Deutsches Zentrum Immuntherapie, Friedrich-Alexander University (FAU), Erlangen-Nürnberg and Universitätsklinikum Erlangen, 91054 Erlangen, Germany; tobias.krickau@uk-erlangen.de

[3] Center for Rare Diseases Erlangen (ZSEER), Friedrich-Alexander University (FAU), Erlangen-Nürnberg and Universitätsklinikum Erlangen, 91054 Erlangen, Germany

[4] Division of Rheumatology, Department of Internal Medicine, Gazi University Ankara, 06560 Ankara, Turkey; atufan@gazi.edu.tr

[5] Division of Pediatric Rheumatology, Autoinflammation Reference Center Tübingen, Department of Pediatrics, University Hospital Tübingen, 72016 Tübingen, Germany; kuemmerle.deschner@uni-tuebingen.de

[6] Department of Pediatric Rheumatology, Hacettepe University, 06100 Ankara, Turkey; sezaozen@gmail.com

[7] Department of Paediatrics, Friedrich-Alexander University (FAU), Erlangen-Nürnberg and Universitätsklinikum Erlangen, 91054 Erlangen, Germany

[8] FMF & AID Global Association, 8306 Zurich, Switzerland; ecohen@verizon.net (E.C.); info@fmfandaid.org (M.V.)

[9] Pediatric Rheumatology, University Children's Hospital Basel (UKBB), University of Basel, 4001 Basel, Switzerland; tatjana.welzel@ukbb.ch

[10] Löwenpraxis, 6004 Luzern, Switzerland; kuehn.allergie@hin.ch

[*] Correspondence: juergen.rech@uk-erlangen.de

Citation: Rech, J.; Schett, G.; Tufan, A.; Kuemmerle-Deschner, J.B.; Özen, S.; Tascilar, K.; Geck, L.; Krickau, T.; Cohen, E.; Welzel, T.; et al. Patient Experiences and Challenges in the Management of Autoinflammatory Diseases—Data from the International FMF & AID Global Association Survey. *J. Clin. Med.* **2024**, *13*, 1199. https://doi.org/10.3390/jcm13051199

Academic Editor: Ferdinando Nicoletti

Received: 17 January 2024
Revised: 3 February 2024
Accepted: 13 February 2024
Published: 20 February 2024

Abstract: Background: Autoinflammatory diseases (AIDs) are rare, mostly genetic diseases that affect the innate immune system and are associated with inflammatory symptoms. Both paediatric and adult patients face daily challenges related to their disease, diagnosis and subsequent treatment. For this reason, a survey was developed in collaboration between the FMF & AID Global Association and the Erlangen Center for Periodic Systemic Autoinflammatory Diseases. Methods: The aim of the survey was to collect the personal assessment of affected patients with regard to their current status in terms of diagnostic timeframes, the interpretation of genetic tests, the number of misdiagnoses, and pain and fatigue despite treatment. Results: In total, data from 1043 AID patients (829 adults and 214 children/adolescents) from 52 countries were collected and analyzed. Familial Mediterranean fever (FMF) (521/50%) and Behçet's disease (311/30%) were the most frequently reported diseases. The average time to diagnosis was 3 years for children/adolescents and 14 years for adults. Prior to the diagnosis of autoinflammatory disease, patients received several misdiagnoses, including psychosomatic disorders. The vast majority of patients reported that genetic testing was available (92%), but only 69% were tested. A total of 217 patients reported that no increase in acute-phase reactants was detected during their disease episodes. The intensity of pain and fatigue was measured in AID patients and found to be high. A total of 88% of respondents received treatment again, while 8% reported no treatment. Conclusions: AID patients, particularly adults, suffer from significant delays in diagnosis, misdiagnosis, and a variety of symptoms, including pain and fatigue. Based on the results presented, raising awareness of these diseases in the wider medical community is crucial to improving patient care and quality of life.

Keywords: autoinflammatory diseases; familial Mediterranean fever (FMF); Behcet's disease; diagnosis; misdiagnoses; patient survey; pain; fatigue

1. Introduction

The term "autoinflammatory disease" was coined by McDermott et al. in 1999 and refers primarily to diseases of the innate immune system [1]. Most cases of autoinflammatory diseases are genetically classified as monogenic, while others are polygenic and multifactorial, caused by a variety of mutations. However, in more than half of individuals suspected of having an autoinflammatory disease, no causative gene was found [2]. Prior to genetic testing becoming widely available, patients were diagnosed solely on the basis of their clinical presentation. Many of these autoinflammatory diseases can mimic infectious, malignant, and rheumatic issues, resulting in a delayed diagnosis. Typically, medical survey data are collected by researchers for doctors. However, in this unique approach, patient experts (certified EUPATI—European Patients Academy on Therapeutic Innovation) and specialized physicians collaborated to develop this survey, aggregate the data, and collect the results. While participation was voluntary, respondents explicitly agreed to anonymized data analysis and the publication of results. The aim of this effort is to represent the value of the patients' voices by capturing their responses and experiences in managing their AIDs and related symptoms.

Autoinflammatory diseases often begin in childhood or early adulthood and are frequently diagnosed many years after their onset [3]. These diseases may also appear later in life and are often not recognized in adult patients. Diagnostic delays can be attributed to a variety of factors. For example, a common misconception is that patients with familial Mediterranean fever (FMF) must be of Mediterranean descent or that autoinflammatory patients must have homozygous mutations to develop symptoms [4,5]. In addition, although autoinflammatory diseases often present as periodic fever syndromes, patients do not always have a fever or elevated acute-phase reactants. Due to the rarity of these diseases, it is understandable that medical knowledge is limited, and therefore, effective treatments are often initiated late or are not available. Colchicine is widely used in AIDs, including Behçet's disease, as it reduces aphthous ulcers, controls inflammation, and reduces the intensity and frequency of relapses. Interleukin (IL)-1 inhibitors such as anakinra, canakinumab, and rilonacept are effective in the treatment of many different AIDs [6–10]. However, these biological drugs are not available in all countries, making effective disease control difficult [7–17].

Based upon these shortcomings and challenges, a survey was developed to investigate how these and other factors affect the diagnosis, treatment, and care of autoinflammatory disease patients.

2. Materials and Methods

2.1. Description of the Survey

A cross-sectional survey with 30 questions was developed by members of the patient organization FMF & AID Global Association (Executive Director, Malena Vetterli, and Research Officer, H. Ellen Cohen) under the guidance of Juergen Rech (MD, Head of the Centre for Periodic Systemic Autoinflammatory Diseases at the University of Erlangen-Nuremberg, Germany). For the purpose of the survey, the term uSAID (undifferentiated/undiagnosed systemic autoinflammatory diseases) is used when a patient has an unidentified autoinflammatory disease. The survey was first published at the beginning of 2021, was available for 6 weeks on the EU-Survey platform from the European Commission, and was shared on social media in Facebook closed groups. The survey was translated from English into German, French, Italian, Spanish, Portuguese, Turkish, Arabic, Greek, Hebrew, Russian, and Georgian. The objective of the survey was to collect data on the given diagnoses (FMF, periodic fever, aphthous stomatitis, pharyngitis, and adenitis (PFAPA) syndrome, familial cold autoinflammatory syndrome (FCAS), Muckle–Wells syndrome (MWS), neonatal-onset multisystem inflammatory disease and others). Chronic infantile neurological cutaneous and articular syndrome (NOMID/CINCA), TNF receptor-associated periodic syndrome (TRAPS), Mevalonate kinase deficiency (MKD), familial cold autoinflammatory syndrome-2 (FCAS2), NOD2-related systemic autoinflammatory granulomatosis (Blau Syndrome),

Yao syndrome (NOD2-associated autoinflammatory disease, presents with erythematous plaques and patches, periodic fevers, myalgia, gastrointestinal (GI), and sicca-like symptoms), deficiency of adenosine deaminase 2 (DADA2), Behçet's disease, unspecific systemic autoinflammatory disease (uSAID), patient access to specialists, genetic testing, diagnostic time frames, misdiagnoses, access to treatment, patient satisfaction, pain management, level of fatigue and patient wellbeing. In addition, it was shared with organizations affiliated with FMF & AID (see Acknowledgments section) and collaborating groups, with a total of approximately 100,000 patients worldwide. Participation in this survey was voluntary, and all those who took part agreed that the anonymized information from the survey could be analyzed and published. This study was approved by the International Review Board of the University Clinic Erlangen (#362_20 Bc).

2.2. Statistical Analysis

Statistical analyses were essentially descriptive and exploratory. Summary statistics were calculated based on the scales of the characteristics, i.e., categorical variables were summarized using counts and percentages, and scale variables were summarized using means and standard deviations. Data manipulation and visualization were undertaken using Excel.

3. Results

The survey dataset results indicated the average time to diagnosis in children/adolescents was 3 years and 14 years for adults. Patients received multiple misdiagnoses prior to a correct AID diagnosis, including psychosomatic disorders (210 patients), fibromyalgia (140 patients), osteoarthritis (69 patients), irritable bowel syndrome (200 patients), and asthma (78 patients). The vast majority of patients reported that genetic testing was available (92%), while only 69% were tested. A total of 217 patients reported that no elevation of acute-phase reactants was found during their flares. The intensity of pain and fatigue were measured among AID patients and found to be high. A total of 88% of respondents received treatment, while 8% reported no treatment.

3.1. Demographic Characteristics

FMF & AID received 1043 responses from patients who completed the survey (Figure 1). A total of 829 patients (79.48%) were adults (>18 years) and 214 children/adolescents (20.51%). AID patients from many different countries participated in this survey, with the majority of responses coming from patients in the USA, Turkey, and Germany. A wide spectrum of AID patients contributed to this survey, with FMF and Behcet's disease being the most frequent diagnoses. The average timeframe for a child/adolescent to be diagnosed with AID was 3 years, while the average timeframe for an adult patient was 14 years. While pediatric patients are diagnosed in a shorter timeframe than adults, parent and caregiver satisfaction was extremely low.

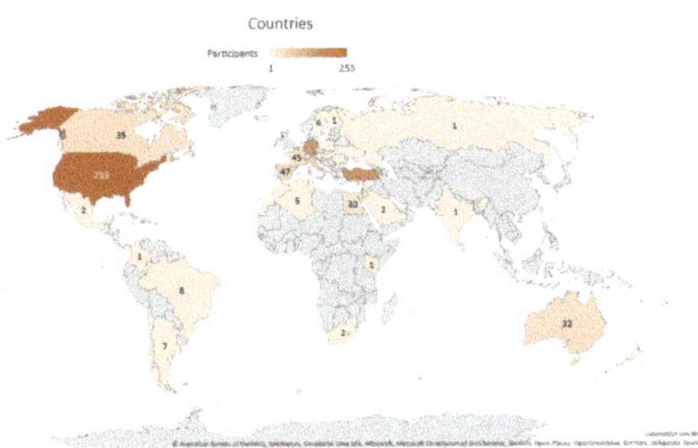

Figure 1. Indication of countries and the number of participants per country who completed the questionnaire.

3.2. Genetic Testing

The vast majority of patients reported that genetic testing was available (92%) and was carried out (69%) (Figures 2 and 3). Insurance paid for genetic testing in 56% of cases, while 19% required self-payment, and 6% reported a mixed payment model. Of note, not all tested patients had access to their genetic results, and other patients were denied genetic testing.

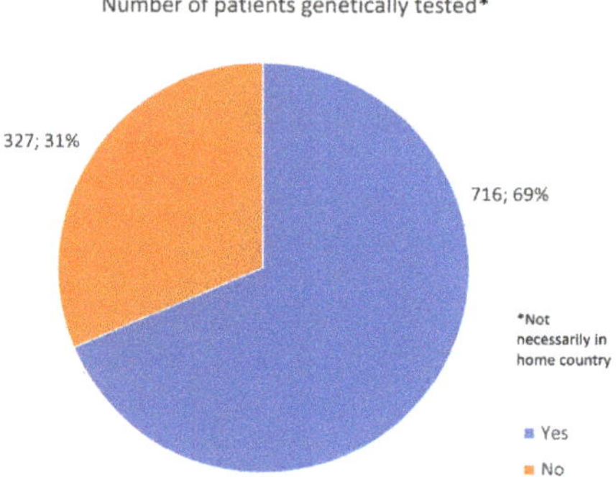

Figure 2. Percentage of participants who had or did not undergo genetic testing.

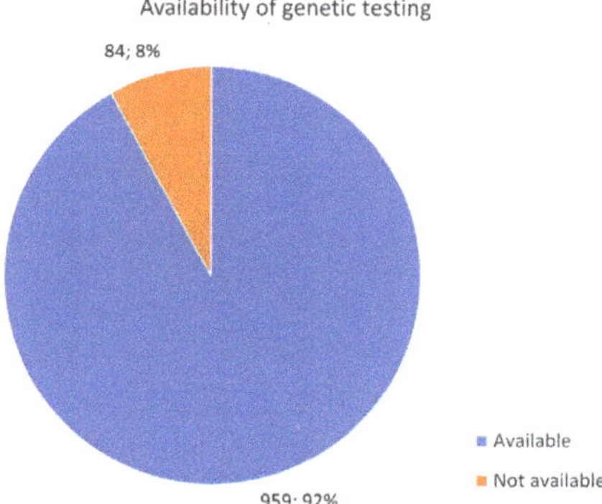

Figure 3. Basic availability of genetic testing overall across all countries of the participants in the survey.

3.3. Laboratory Changes

A total of 217 (20.81%) patients in this survey reported that inflammatory markers in blood tests, such as C-reactive protein (CRP), erythrocyte sedimentation rate (ESR), or serum amyloid A (SAA), were not elevated during a disease flare-up. Of note, SAA testing is not available in the United States.

3.4. Disease Impact on Pain and Fatigue

The intensity of pain associated with AID was measured using the standard visual analog scale (VAS 0–10). Patients were asked to rate their pain over the last 7 and 30 days. The patient feedback indicated substantial pain levels with a mean VAS of 4.2 (SD +/−3.0) during the last 7 days and 4.8 (SD +/−2.7) during the last 30 days (Figure 4).

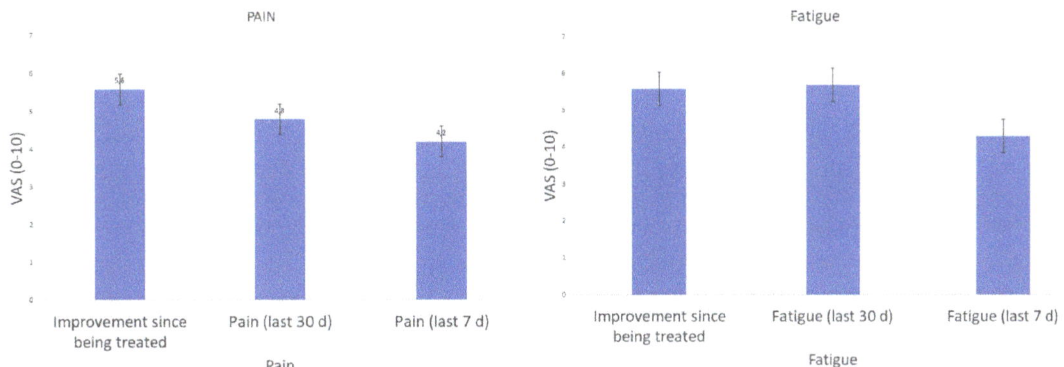

Figure 4. Display of pain and fatigue intensity 7 days (7 d) and 30 days (30 d) retrospectively, as well as the improvement in the entire period from the beginning of treatment to the present.

The intensity of fatigue was measured by VAS (VAS 0–10). Also, the fatigue burden was high, with a mean VAS of 5.3 (SD +/−3.0) during the last 7 days and 5.7 (SD +/−2.8) during the last 30 days (Figure 4).

Over-the-counter medications, such as acetaminophen, metamizole, and aspirin, as well as prescribed NSAIDs, such as ibuprofen, diclofenac, and naproxen, were used for pain control. Some patients also required opioids and neuropathic pain medications, such as pregabalin and gabapentin. A total of 88% of respondents received treatment, 8% did not receive treatment, and data were not available for 4% of participants.

3.5. Monogenic Patients Presenting with a Fever

A total of 690 patients with monogenic disease responded to the survey, and surprisingly, a marked difference should be noted between children and adults expressing fevers as a clinical symptom in their individual disease presentation.

Of the 547 adults identified, only 328 reported fevers as an initial disease presentation (Figure 5), whereas out of the 143 pediatric cases reported, 129 presented with a fever (Figure 6). While fevers are often an assumed factor in AID, they are not always present in all-age patients. Adults appear to present with fewer fevers than children. A total of 40% of adult respondents were absent from fevers, compared to only 9.8% of children.

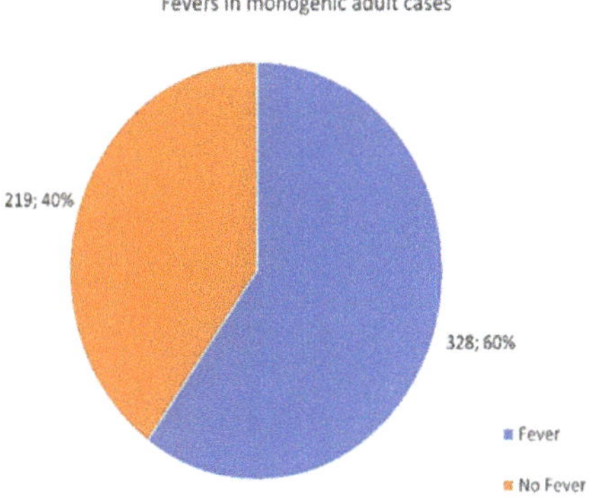

Figure 5. Number of adult patients who reported episodes of fever associated with their monogenic disease.

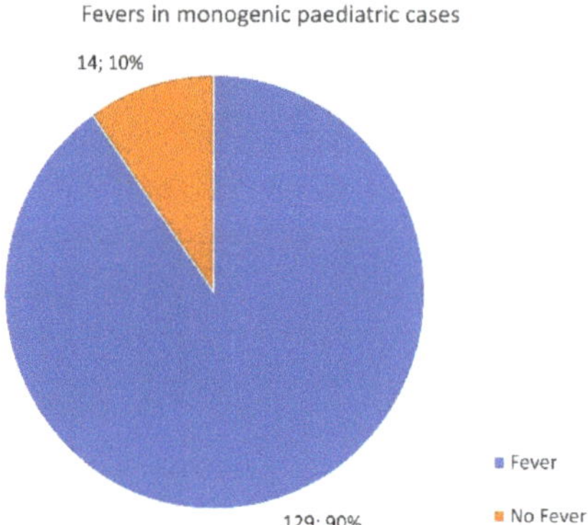

Figure 6. Number of pediatric patients who reported episodes of fever associated with their monogenic disease.

This significant difference raises issues as to how the aging process impacts body temperature in these innate immune responses over time and how unknown metabolic pathways or genetic variants alter the presentation of fevers from disease inception into adulthood.

It is important to note that 152 all-age patients indicated low or hypothermic temperatures (between 34 °C/93.2 °F and 36 °C/96.8 °F) present during flare times, and further medical investigation should be undertaken to not only better understand the mechanics of body temperature in these disorders but to also ensure that these patients are not incorrectly dismissed or ruled out of an AID diagnosis. Additionally, it is critical for adult AID-treating physicians to carefully review and note if childhood fevers in these older populations were a prior factor in their case work-up.

3.6. Monogenic Patients Presenting with Neurological Symptoms

Neurological impacts were also noted in 424 AID monogenic children and adults. Symptoms, including headaches, seizures, bad memory, brain fog, and lack of concentration, were reported by 356 adults (Figure 7) and 68 patients under the age of 18 (Figure 8).

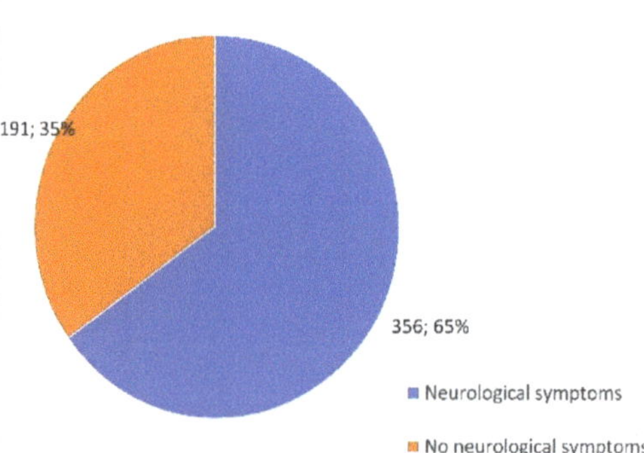

Figure 7. Number of adult patients who reported neurological problems related to their monogenic disease.

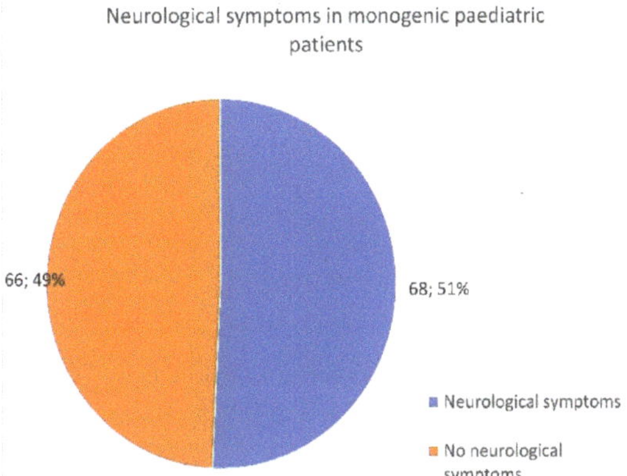

Figure 8. Number of child patients who reported neurological problems related to their monogenic disease.

While there is newfound awareness as to the importance of AID inflammation impacting the brain and central nervous system (CNS), it will be important for all age patients to be assessed and managed, as these neurological issues may change or emerge over time. A higher percentage of adults (65%) reported having problems per the survey as compared to 51% of children.

3.7. Issues in Diagnosis and Disease Management

A total of 669 AID patients (64.14%), 542 of whom were adults, and the remaining 127 children/adolescents considered that their medical team lacked specific knowledge and experience to appropriately diagnose, treat, and monitor AID (Figure 9). A total of 271 AID patients, among them 243 adults and 28 children/adolescents, reported being dismissed, contributing to a delay in care. Misdiagnosed conditions included psychosomatic disorder (210 patients), fibromyalgia (140 patients), osteoarthritis (69 patients), irritable bowel syndrome (200 patients), and asthma (78 patients) (Figure 10). The most important barriers patients experienced were not being taken seriously with regard to their symptoms, refusing appropriate and timely blood testing during flares, encountering physicians unwilling to consult with experts in the field, or rejecting the case outright.

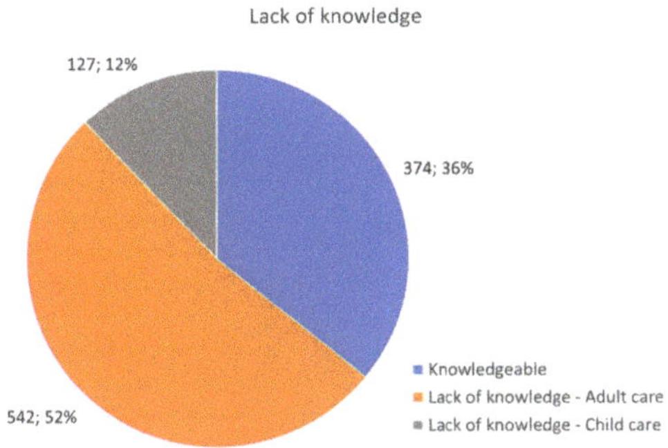

Figure 9. Lack of medical knowledge and experience was reported by patients.

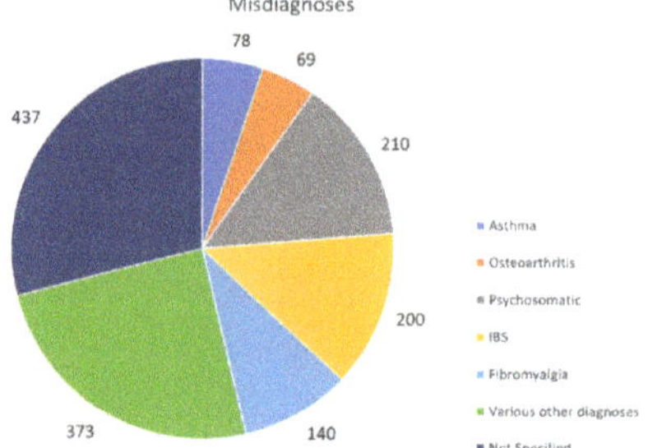

Figure 10. Frequency and designation of incorrect diagnoses.

3.8. Medical Treatment in AID

The majority of patients (921 patients; 88%) responded that their AID was treated after being diagnosed (Figure 11). A total of 697 (66%) patients were put on drug treatment. Colchicine, which is the first line of treatment for FMF, is also widely used for PFAPA, Behcet's, uSAID, CAPS, TRAPS, and HIDS. It was the most frequently used drug cited in this survey (Figure 12).

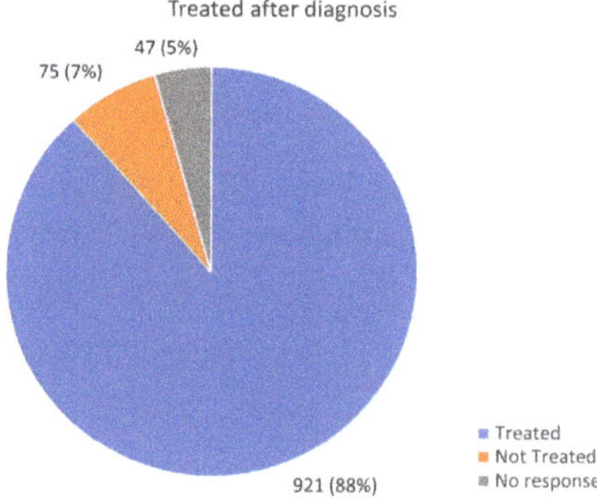

Figure 11. Number of patients treated after diagnosis.

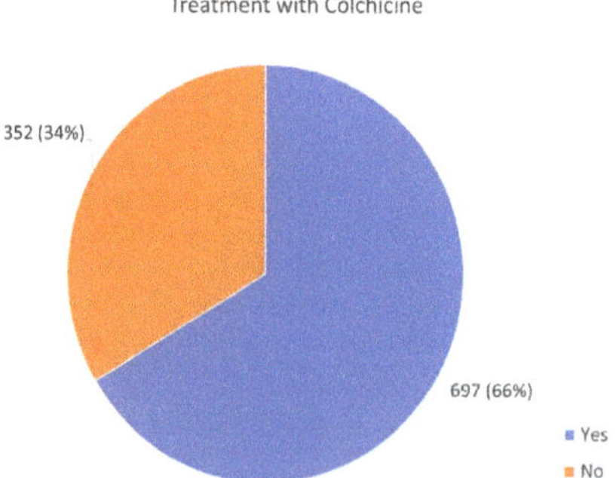

Figure 12. Number of patients treated with colchicine.

Biological drugs such as IL-1 inhibitors (anakinra, canakinumab, and rilonacept), IL-6 inhibitors (tocilizumab), and TNF-alpha blockers (i.e., infliximab, adalimumab, and etanercept) are also used for AID treatment. Conventional immune-modulating medications such as prednisolone, azathioprine, methotrexate, and hydroxychloroquine were also reportedly used.

3.9. IL-1 Biologic Use in Pediatrics and Adults—Quality of Life Improvement

According to survey responses, IL-1 inhibitors had different quality of life (QoL) success rates between children and adults. While 55% of pediatric patients reported QoL improvement on IL-1 biologic treatment, a surprising 39% only had a partial resolution, which did not translate into a robust and symptom-free QoL. A total of 6% reported no QoL improvement on IL-1 medications (Figure 13). Whereas 53 percent of adult patients reported that using IL-1 biologics did not provide enough efficacy for full QoL, only 34% regained full functionality. A total of 13% reported no improvement with medication use (Figure 14).

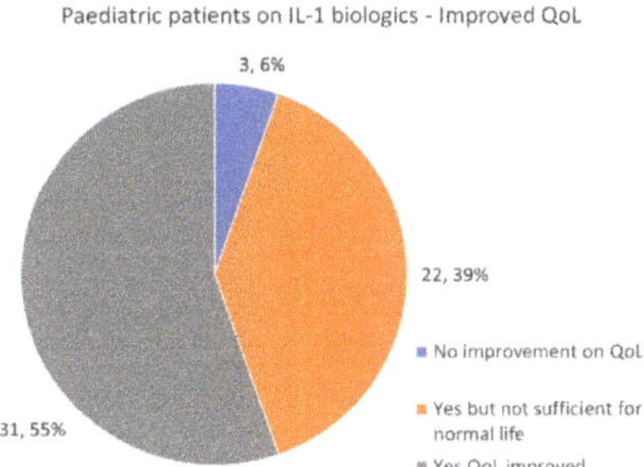

Figure 13. Number of pediatric patients receiving IL-1 biological therapy and Quality of Life (QoL) response.

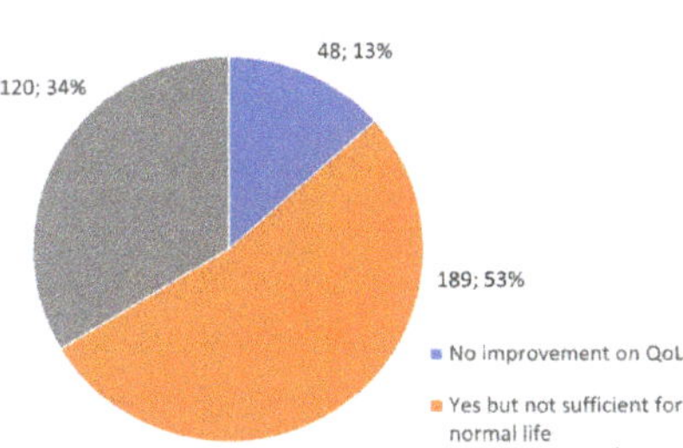

Figure 14. Number of adult patients receiving IL-1 biological therapy and Quality of Life (QoL) response.

These data raise a variety of concerns related to the overall efficacy of IL-1 inhibitors, implications from the medical literature reporting full symptom resolution based on small samples of rare patients, and equal tolerability of these medications in all age populations.

Patients who do not make a full resolution on these IL-1 inhibitors should be considered for an increased dose of medication or for prescribing a secondary biologic for better symptom control. Despite the use of biologics, even at higher doses, patients may present with infrequent breakthrough flares and require additional medications, including steroids and pain control.

3.10. Treated Patients Recording a 5+ Pain Score

Despite treatment, 468 out of 1043 respondents reported having a mean pain score of 5+ or above in the last 30 days (pain score: 0 "no pain"—10 "as bad as it could possibly be"). Out of these 468 patients, 288 diagnosed with a monogenic disease (240 adults (Figure 15) and 48 children (Figure 16)) experienced a pain score of 6 or above despite being treated with colchicine, biologics, or a combination of both.

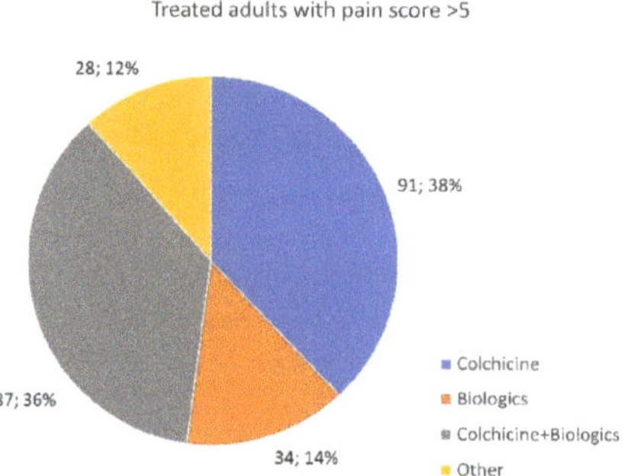

Figure 15. Distribution of applied therapies in adult patients with a monogenic disease and a pain score assessment according to the visual analogue scale > 5 (norm 0–10).

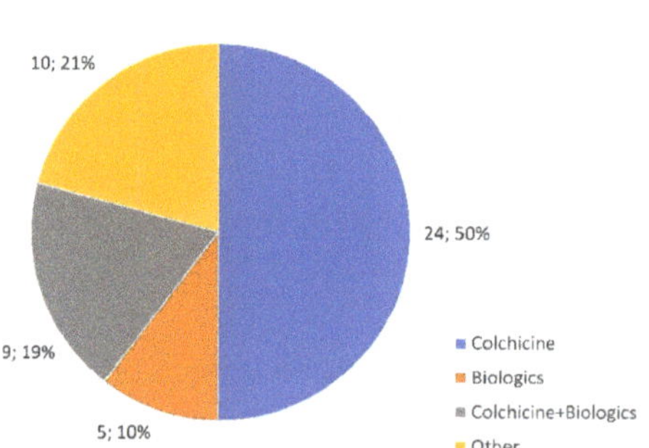

Figure 16. Distribution of applied therapies in pediatric patients with a monogenic disease and a pain score assessment according to the visual analogue scale > 5 (norm 0–10).

The survey data indicate that 44.9% of treated patients have high levels of pain, which must be taken seriously by treating physicians. With almost half of patients reporting elevated pain scores, treatment protocols should be revised and further researched. Dosing adjustments of both colchicine and biologic medications should be reconsidered based on patient symptoms and pain response, despite negative APR results. Patients on colchicine, experiencing pain, or those on the highest safe doses should be considered for a biological drug addition if medication is available, regardless of cost.

Finally, it is important to change the perception that colchicine and/or biologics provide complete resolution of all disease symptoms, as there is no cure for autoinflammatory diseases. Additional medication options must be incorporated based on the treated patient's lived experience. It should be recognized that pain management in autoinflammatory diseases may not always be effective, as some patients do not respond to or tolerate NSAIDs and may require opioids or corticosteroids to control breakthrough symptoms and pain. These add-on treatments should be considered the standard of care for all those managing uncontrolled symptoms.

3.11. Global Distribution of Familial Mediterranean Fever Cases

Familial Mediterranean fever (FMF) is a monogenic disorder and the most common inherited autoinflammatory disease. The disease presentation is more prevalent in people of Mediterranean descent. However, patients with FMF have been identified globally. It equally affects males and females, usually presenting before 20 years of age. Symptoms include abdominal pain, recurring fevers, joint pain and swelling, headaches, pharyngitis, ankle swelling, monoarthritis, chest pain, pericarditis, leg pain, myalgia, cutaneous manifestations (erysipelas-like erythema, non-specific purpuric rash, Henoch–Schönlein purpura), orchitis, fatigue and others.

The survey was completed by 415 patients who were diagnosed with FMF and without other co-existing autoinflammatory diseases. Patients with FMF included 70 children/adolescents and 345 adult cases. Respondents from 31 countries diagnosed with FMF were noted in the survey, with Turkey having the highest number with 95 cases, followed by the United States with 71 cases, and Germany with 69 cases (Figure 17). FMF is diagnosed worldwide.

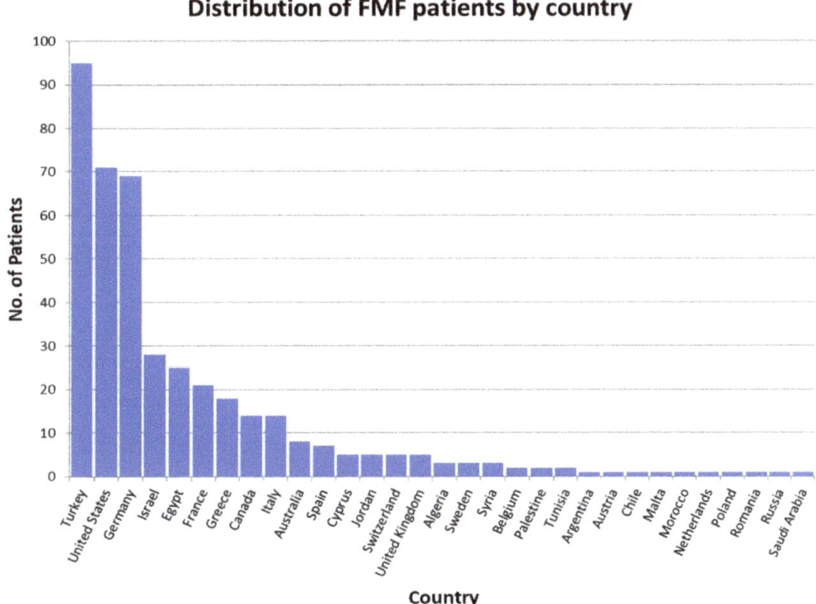

Figure 17. Worldwide distribution of Familial Mediterranean fever (FMF) patients per country who participated in the survey.

3.12. FMF Patients QoL Improvement after Treatment

A total of 415 all-age FMF patients reported on QoL after treatments were used, including colchicine, anakinra, canakinumab, Humira, Enbrel, and tocilizumab.

Despite treatment, only 206 patients reported an improved QoL, while 164 reported that, although medicated, their QoL was still compromised. A total of 45 patients reported that, with treatment, QoL had not improved (Figure 18). FMF is a complex autoinflammatory disease, and despite the global use of colchicine, it does not provide 100% symptom relief for all patients. Additionally, IL-1 inhibitors, used with or without colchicine, do not always provide symptom resolution.

QoL for FMF patients remains challenging, and survey responses raise important questions with regard to the dosing of medications and the overall efficacy of limited treatments. It is critical in the future for medications to be developed targeting the inflammatory pathways unique to FMF patients.

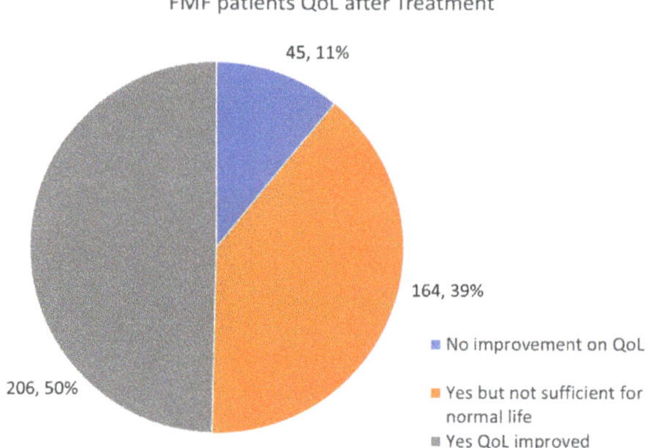

Figure 18. Assessment of the response to therapy and improvement of QoL in FMF patients.

3.13. Global Distribution of Behçet's Cases

Behçet's disease is a polygenic disorder that likely developed along the ancient "silk road" and impacted people of Mediterranean and Asian descent. This vascular-driven autoinflammatory disease typically presents more severely in males and involves a constellation of symptoms, including mouth/genital ulcers, uveitis/inflammatory eye issues, skin pustules, GI ulcerations, neurological problems, joint pain, and various-size vessel vasculitis.

The survey was completed by 278 Behçet patients (8 children/adolescents and 270 adults). The location of patients responding suggests that the disease manifests perhaps more globally than current medical literature suggests (Figure 19). Respondents from 32 countries diagnosed with Behçet's were noted in the survey, with the USA having the highest number with 113 cases, followed by Turkey with 46 patients. Further research is needed to determine the actual prevalence of Behçet in all countries and all sections of the population.

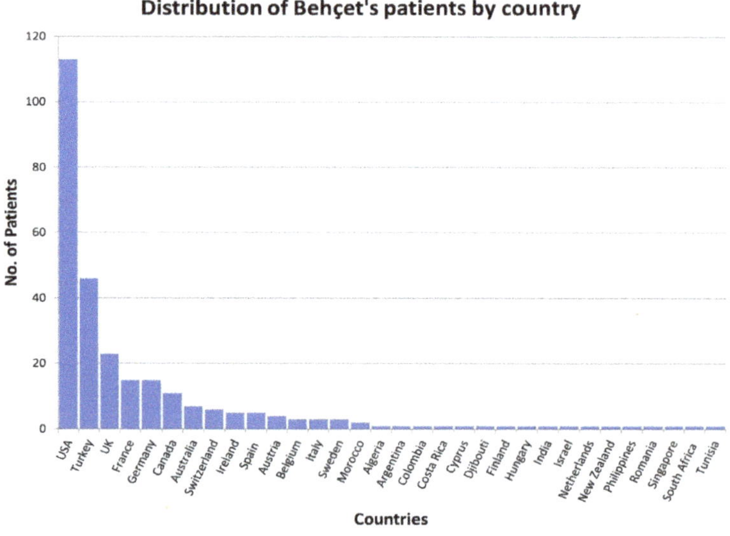

Figure 19. Worldwide distribution of the number of Behçet patients per country.

Despite the country of origin where the symptomatic patient resides, it is important that treating physicians do not dismiss these cases with the incorrect assumption that the location of the patient is the overarching criteria for a Behçet's diagnosis. Cases continue to be identified in Europe, Australia, the United States, South America, and others beyond the Middle East and Asian regions.

3.14. Improving the Quality of Life of Behcet Patients after Treatment

A total of 278 all-age Behçet (polygenic) patients reported on QoL after treatments including colchicine, apremilast, baricitinib, tofacitinib, cyclosporine, azathioprine/Imuran, methotrexate, infliximab, etanercept, adalimumab, secukinumab, tocilizumab, ustekinumab, anakinra, rituxan, interferon, golimumab, certolizumab pegol, and IVIG replacement.

Despite a wide variety of treatments utilized, QoL was reported to be compromised in 69% of these patients (Figure 20). Behçet's is a complex multi-organ disease that impacts a wide variety of body systems and presents differently in each case. Treatment decisions are often made based on affected organs and tissues. For this reason, the list of possible drugs is larger.

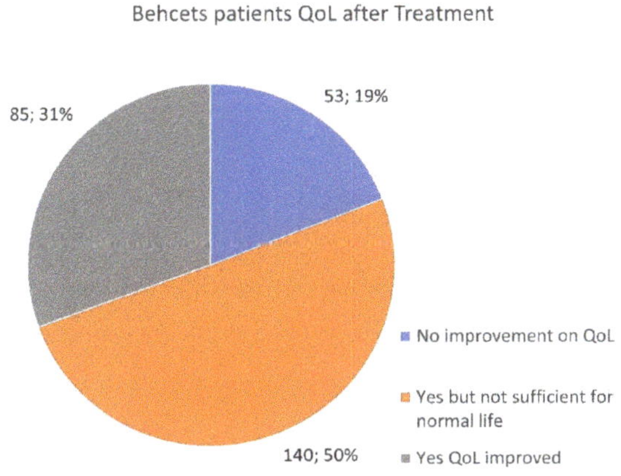

Figure 20. Assessment of the response to therapy and improvement of QoL in Behçet patients.

Regardless of the various treatments used, concerns about QoL remain challenging and raise issues as to the dosing efficacy of listed medications, unknown genetic factors impacting symptom control, and other physiologically affected pathways that have yet to be acknowledged or discovered.

4. Discussion

Autoinflammatory diseases are genetically based disorders associated with a dysregulation of the innate immune system, resulting in uncontrolled inflammation [17]. Variants associated with AIDs are included in the 2022 classification of human inborn errors of immunity [18], many of them caused by monogenic germline or somatic mutations, and include 485 distinct disorders categorized into autoimmune, autoinflammatory, allergic, and malignant phenotypes [19]. The most well-known AID is familial Mediterranean fever (FMF), which is caused by variants in the MEFV gene [20]. It is known to be highly prevalent in the eastern Mediterranean region. However, with advances in genetic screening and migration, the diagnosis of FMF patients has markedly increased across all countries [21–37]. AIDs are often severe conditions that require specialized care but are not readily recognized. They usually affect patients early in their lives and will accompany them for a lifetime. Proper management is of paramount importance. This survey, with over a thousand responses, provides an overview of patients' experiences related to the diagnosis and management of AID.

Familial Mediterranean fever and Behcet's disease were the most common diseases reported in the survey. While both may present in higher population numbers within the Mediterranean and Asian regions, it is critical that medical professionals globally recognize that each disease is prevalent across numerous countries and affects all age patients [20,38,39]. The survey responses also highlight the poor QoL in FMF and Behcet's patients despite treatment, which can be attributed to the complexity of these rare diseases and the lack of specialized medical knowledge.

While diagnosis in pediatric patients is relatively timely, adults with AID are often misdiagnosed and not treated. This is due to overlapping symptoms mimicking infections, skin diseases, malignancies, gastrointestinal diseases, allergic conditions, and immune deficiencies. It is also common for AID patients to be diagnosed with autoimmune diseases such as Sjögren's syndrome, rheumatoid arthritis, and systemic lupus erythematosus, with detrimental impacts on the patient's health due to a delayed diagnosis and incorrect treatment. Additionally, since AIDs are rare diseases that are not routinely included in medical curricula, physicians may not be aware of them. As a consequence, patients are often not listened to, not taken seriously, and even ignored, which requires them to seek several consultations until they can locate a provider who has the necessary experience, knowledge, and expertise to diagnose and manage their AID [31,32].

Recent advancements in molecular research on these diseases have resulted in a more accurate classification that will continue to grow as new genetic mutations are identified. In 2002, Infevers [40] was developed as a database tool for doctors and clinicians to verify genetic data for AIDs. The aim of this international registry is to collect and report demographic, genetic, and clinical data for all currently known monogenic autoinflammatory disorders. Nevertheless, there is a high percentage of patients who have symptoms but have not yet received a proper diagnosis. These patients may be overlooked due to being uSAID, lacking specific inflammatory markers, or having unclassified genetic variants. The survey revealed that although genetic testing is performed frequently, patient access to full results (all mutations found, including benign) is still suboptimal, and inadequate interpretation may be an obstacle. Additionally, reimbursement or insurance coverage for genetic testing remains challenging.

The survey also reveals that pain is one of the predominant causes of disability in AID [41–45]. Only 10% of patients reported they were pain-free. Half of the survey respondents indicated a pain score of more than 4 on a 0–10 scale, reflecting inadequate pain control despite the use of medication. Pain is often poorly understood in AID, although there is increasing evidence that the immune system may play a role in the development of pain.

Additionally, fatigue is a major component of AID and is described by patients as profoundly debilitating, impacting every aspect of their lives [38,39,45–49]. Consequently, fatigue may severely affect wellbeing, causing a financial burden for the individual, family, and society. In childhood/adolescence, it affects school attendance and performance, socialization, and participation in sports or physical activities. In adults, the fatigue may be disabling and impacting the overall quality of life, including career/work, relationships, family/parenting, and self-esteem.

Moreover, it is vital for each age group to be appropriately assessed and treated by neurologists for the medical impacts of headaches and seizures. However, it is also important to consider that all-age patients expressing symptoms be cognitively evaluated by a neuropsychology specialist for executive function deficiencies, short/long-term memory retrieval, educational disabilities, ADHD, etc. These types of evaluations and findings will ensure that learning and workplace productivity can be optimized by incorporating accommodations and treatments as needed, thus allowing for robust patient functionality [45,47–49].

It is also relevant to ensure that cognitive issues in children are addressed by caregivers, as pediatric patients often do not have the language abilities to express struggles with complex processing issues. Assessment and capture of each individual's problems will be important to allow for necessary support in schools and other educational environments.

In rheumatic diseases, the association between fatigue and pain has been well documented. Fatigue is often associated with increased pain, and both can be synchronous [38,39,46–51]. Inflammatory mechanisms related to the etiology of fatigue implicate a significant involvement of cytokines. Interleukin (IL)-1 beta (IL-1β), tumor necrosis factor alpha (TNF-α), IL-6, and interferon gamma (IFN-γ) are mediators that can induce fatigue. Cytokines regulate normal physiological functions, including mood, cognition, and sleep, and their expression varies over the course of the day and in response to local activity. Consequently, it is likely that dysregulation of inflammatory cytokines in AIDs can contribute to fatigue [46,52–62].

Autoinflammatory diseases often present with recurring attacks of fever, abdominal pain, arthritis, and skin rashes. These symptoms are often tied to elevated acute-phase reactants [50]. This survey also revealed that testing for the elevation of inflammatory markers is not often attainable for patients during flare periods. Testing for serum markers of inflammation is not always available or ordered by physicians. Isolated CRP testing may not reveal the entire molecular spectrum of inflammation in AID patients. Additionally, expectations of having extremely elevated inflammatory markers while ignoring mild elevations or subclinical changes, including symptoms, may lead to misconceptions about the presence of an AID [35]. Also, acute-phase reactants may not be present in each individual AID entity [35].

Colchicine is the first-line treatment for FMF [3,62]. It is often used in other AIDs such as PFAPA, Behcet's disease, and uSAID. This medication is particularly useful for treating oral and/or genital lesions and significantly reduces inflammation while increasing the symptom-free interval between flares [20]. Colchicine is an inexpensive and safe drug and the most frequently used medication cited in this survey. There are differences among the colchicine brands. Individual patients may tolerate or respond differently to the various preparations [7–11]. However, certain patients may not tolerate or respond effectively to colchicine and, therefore, require alternative treatments such as IL-1 targeting agents [13–16]. Patients requiring biological drugs often encounter accessibility challenges, such as physicians refusing to prescribe medications due to high costs, insurance companies not approving biological medications, limited approval (only a small number of patients are allocated to receive medication), or the drugs not being available in the patient's country of residence.

Beyond prescribing issues, in some cases, patients may refuse biological treatment due to a fear of not understanding how the medication works, concern about lifelong medication use, and possible adverse reactions. Thus, doctors may require extended time with patients to explain why the medication is being prescribed, common side effects, and how to manage potential reactions. These issues may change in the future due to new and promising therapeutic approaches, which are currently in either study phases or in development. These include inhibiting the NLRP3 inflammasome and small-molecule inhibitors that impact signaling pathways either upstream or downstream of the inflammasome [57].

Doses of biologics for controlling AID may vary. For example, CAPS (Cryopyrin-associated periodic syndrome) patients may require higher or more frequent doses of IL-1 biologic medications [13]. Inadequate or suboptimal dosing of IL-1 drugs for autoinflammation may lead to underreporting of medication efficacy.

There were limitations in this study. Respondents were not required to submit laboratory reports or medical records. Additionally, both monogenic and polygenic autoinflammatory diseases were included. Although the diagnosis of these participants could not be confirmed via medical records, there would be little purpose for patients or their parents to allot time to respond to the survey questions, as the link was only shared with those in autoinflammatory-specific and private social media groups.

This study had the largest global response of pediatric and adult patients providing feedback regarding their disease status. Over a thousand responses support the data presented in this paper.

5. Conclusions

The survey results ascertain that autoinflammatory patients of all ages are burdened in many ways by not receiving a timely or correct diagnosis. Patients, per their survey responses, often struggle through multiple misdiagnoses, incorrect treatments, and a lack of specialized medical care, as well as contend with a compromised quality of life. The most common misdiagnoses reported included asthma, osteoarthritis, psychosomatic, IBS, fibromyalgia, etc. The patient ordeal is reflected as adults are noted to have longer diagnostic delays of, on average, 14 years vs. 3 years for most pediatric cases.

These delays are attributed to a lack of both medical knowledge and specialized autoinflammatory care. Genetic testing is an important tool for AID diagnosis. Unfortunately, it is not available in every country. Additionally, genetic criteria may be absent despite symptoms, emphasizing the importance of patients receiving a clinical diagnosis of uSAID to access treatment.

Biomarkers for these diseases require further discovery, as many patients in our survey reported having negative acute-phase reactants (APR) during disease flare-ups, which are considered a hallmark of AID. Lack of elevations in APR delays diagnosis and treatment, prolonging the patient's pain and suffering. Worldwide availability and low cost make colchicine a commonly prescribed drug for the initial treatment of AID, while biological agents were also used, according to the survey results. However, treatment with either colchicine or IL-1 biologics does not guarantee that patients will be asymptomatic and have full disease resolution. As our survey indicates, patients' pain is a common finding, and medications used include NSAIDs, opioids, and others.

This unique collaboration between FMF & AID Global Association and their medical partners in Erlangen enabled the development and execution of this study. This model of relationship-building between patient organizations and dedicated autoinflammatory centers is unique and allows for the identification of critical patient diagnostic shortfalls, gaps in treatment efficacy, and quality-of-life issues impacting all-age patients. These important factors are key to guiding therapy and developing new drugs. In the future, it will be critical to include the voice, experience, and expertise of these rare autoinflammatory patients prior to planning research initiatives and clinical trials. Patients and their families living with AID carry a significant social, financial, and medical burden that requires comprehensive support and care. Efforts must be made to strengthen physicians' and medical professionals' knowledge by providing continuing medical education opportunities, specialized training courses from AID expert centers, and an early interventional curriculum on AID for medical students. Collectively, patient organizations, treating physicians, researchers, health authorities, and medical institutions need to work together in partnership to improve the lives of AID patients.

Author Contributions: M.V., E.C. and J.R. initiated the survey concept and design. M.V. and E.C. contributed to the recruitment of patients. M.V., E.C. and J.R. contributed to data acquisition. M.V., E.C. and J.R. wrote the first draft of the manuscript, M.V., E.C., J.R. and K.T. analyzed the data. M.V., E.C., J.R. and G.S. drafted the final manuscript. K.T., A.T., L.G., J.B.K.-D., S.Ö., T.W., M.K. and T.K. co-wrote the manuscript and contributed to the interpretation of the data. All authors have read and agreed to the published version of the manuscript.

Funding: This research received no external funding.

Institutional Review Board Statement: Based on ethics approval #20-362-Br., the approval date is 20 September 2020.

Informed Consent Statement: Informed consent was obtained from all subjects involved in the study.

Data Availability Statement: Raw data were generated at FMF & AID Global Association, www.fmfandaid.org, Zurich, Switzerland. Derived data supporting the findings of this study are available from the corresponding author (JR) upon request.

Acknowledgments: We would like to thank all participating patients, caregivers, physicians, partner Facebook groups (Behcet's Disease: You are not alone, Global pericarditis support group, Greek

FMF groups) and the patient organizations worldwide affiliated to FMF & AID Global Association: AIFP Associazione Italiana Febbri Periodiche (Italy), AMRI Malattie autoinfiammatorie (Italy), Associazione IRIS Onlus (Italy), Associazione Leoncini Coraggiosi ODV (Italy), FMF de Argentina (Argentina), Asociación Española de CAPS (Spain), FMF España (Spain), Asociación Autoinflamatorias Chile (Chile), Behçet ve Ailevi Akdeniz Ateşi Hastaları Derneği BEFEMDER (Turkey), AADAG Autoinflammatory & Autoimmune Assoc. of Georgia (Georgia), INBAR Israel (Israel), RACC-UK Rare Autoinflammatory Conditions Community- UK (United Kingdom), FMF et MAI France (France), FMF u. AIE Deutschland e. V. (Germany), FMF & AID Australia, FMF Maroc (Morocco), Associação Nacional de Doenças Autoinflamatórias (Brazil), Autoinflammatory Syndromes Patients' Club (Thailand), FMF & AID Middle East and North Africa and EAI El Salvador (El Salvador).

Conflicts of Interest: Author J.R. has received research grants from Novartis Pharma GmbH and Swedish Orphan Biovitrium GmbH. The other authors state that there is no potential conflict of interest with respect to the manuscript and the results contained.

References

1. McDermott, M.F.; Aksentijevich, I.; Galon, J.; McDermott, E.M.; Ogunkolade, B.; Centola, M.; Mansfield, E.; Gadina, M.; Karenko, L.; Pettersson, T.; et al. Germline mutations in the extracellular domains of the 55 kDa TNF receptor, TNFR1, define a family of dominantly inherited autoinflammatory syndromes. *Cell* **1999**, *97*, 133–144. [CrossRef] [PubMed]
2. Booty, M.G.; Chae, J.J.; Masters, S.L.; Remmers, E.F.; Barham, B.; Le, J.M.; Barron, K.S.; Holland, S.M.; Kastner, D.L.; Aksentijevich, I. Familial Mediterranean fever with a single MEFV mutation: Where is the second hit? *Arthritis Rheum.* **2009**, *60*, 1851–1861. [CrossRef]
3. Alpsoy, E.; Leccese, P.; Emmi, G.; Ohno, S. Treatment of Behçet's Disease: An Algorithmic Multidisciplinary Approach. *Front. Med.* **2021**, *8*, 624795. [CrossRef]
4. Marek-Yagel, D.; Berkun, Y.; Padch, S.; Abu, A.; Reznik-Wolf, H.; Livneh, A.; Pras, M.; Pras, E. Clinical disease among patients heterozygous for familial mediterranean fever. *Arthritis Rheum.* **2009**, *60*, 1862–1866. [CrossRef]
5. Gedik, K.C.; Lamot, L.; Romano, M.; Demirkaya, E.; Piskin, D.; Torreggiani, S.; Adang, L.A.; Armangue, T.; Barchus, K.; Cordova, D.R.; et al. The 2021 European Alliance of Associations for Rheumatology/American College of Rheumatology points to consider for diagnosis and management of autoinflammatory type I interferonopathies: CANDLE/PRAAS, SAVI and AGS. *Ann. Rheum. Dis.* **2022**, *81*, 601–613. [CrossRef] [PubMed]
6. Yeh, T.C.; Chen, W.S.; Chang, Y.S.; Lin, Y.C.; Huang, Y.H.; Tsai, C.Y.; Chen, J.H.; Chang, C.C. Risk of obstructive sleep apnea in patients with Sjögren syndrome and Behçet's disease: A nationwide, population-based cohort study. *Sleep Breath* **2020**, *24*, 1199–1205. [CrossRef] [PubMed]
7. Ozen, S.; Demirkaya, E.; Erer, B.; Livneh, A.; Ben-Chetrit, E.; Giancane, G.; Ozdogan, H.; Abu, I.; Gattorno, M.; Hawkins, P.N.; et al. EULAR recommendations for the management of familial Mediterranean fever. *Ann. Rheum. Dis.* **2016**, *75*, 644–651. [CrossRef]
8. Ozen, S.; Kone-Paut, I.; Gül, A. Colchicine resistance and intolerance in familial mediterranean fever: Definition, causes, and alternative treatments. *Semin. Arthritis Rheum.* **2017**, *47*, 115–120. [CrossRef]
9. Baglan, E.; Ozdel, S.; Bulbul, M. Do all colchicine preparations have the same effectiveness in patients with familial Mediterranean fever? *Mod. Rheumatol.* **2021**, *31*, 481–484. [CrossRef]
10. Emmungil, H.; Ilgen, U.; Turan, S.; Yaman, S.; Küçükşahin, O. Different pharmaceutical preparations of colchicine for Familial Mediterranean Fever: Are they the same? *Rheumatol. Int.* **2020**, *40*, 129–135. [CrossRef]
11. Tufan, A.; Babaoglu, M.O.; Akdogan, A.; Yasar, U.; Calguneri, M.; Kalyoncu, U.; Karadag, O.; Hayran, M.; Ertenli, A.I.; Bozkurt, A.; et al. Association of drug transporter gene ABCB1 (MDR1) 3435C to T polymorphism with colchicine response in familial Mediterranean fever. *J. Rheumatol.* **2007**, *34*, 1540–1544. [PubMed]
12. Broderick, L.; Hoffman, H.M. IL-1 and autoinflammatory disease: Biology, pathogenesis and therapeutic targeting. *Nat. Rev. Rheumatol.* **2022**, *18*, 448–463. [CrossRef] [PubMed]
13. Vana, D.R. Canakinumab (ILARIS®) in cryopyrin-associated periodic syndrome (CAPS) patients below 2 years of age: Review of four cases and literature. *Curr. Pediatr. Res.* **2017**, *21*, 646–651.
14. Sibley, C.H.; Chioato, A.; Felix, S.; Colin, L.; Chakraborty, A.; Plass, N.; Rodriguez-Smith, J.; Brewer, C.; King, K.; Zalewski, C.; et al. A 24-month open-label study of canakinumab in neonatal-onset multisystem inflammatory disease. *Ann. Rheum. Dis.* **2015**, *74*, 1714–1719. [CrossRef]
15. Fingerhutová, Š.; Jančová, E.; Doležalová, P. Anakinra in Paediatric Rheumatology and Periodic Fever Clinics: Is the Higher Dose Safe? *Front. Pediatr.* **2022**, *10*, 823847. [CrossRef]
16. Savic, S.; Coe, J.; Laws, P. Autoinflammation: Interferonopathies and Other Autoinflammatory Diseases. *J. Investig. Dermatol.* **2022**, *142*, 781–792. [CrossRef]
17. Tangye, S.G.; Al-Herz, W.; Bousfiha, A.; Cunningham-Rundles, C.; Franco, J.L.; Holland, S.M.; Klein, C.; Morio, T.; Oksenhendler, E.; Picard, C.; et al. Human Inborn Errors of Immunity: 2022 Update on the Classification from the International Union of Immunological Societies Expert Committee. *J. Clin. Immunol.* **2022**, *42*, 1473–1507. [CrossRef]
18. Poulter, J.A.; Savic, S. Genetics of somatic auto-inflammatory disorders. *Semin. Hematol.* **2021**, *58*, 212–217. [CrossRef]

19. Sharma, P.; Jain, A.; Scaria, V. Genetic Landscape of Rare Autoinflammatory Disease Variants in Qatar and Middle Eastern Populations Through the Integration of Whole-Genome and Exome Datasets. *Front. Genet.* **2021**, *12*, 631340. [CrossRef] [PubMed]
20. Hammam, N.; Li, J.; Evans, M.; Kay, J.L.; Izadi, Z.; Anastasiou, C.; Gianfrancesco, M.A.; Yazdany, J.; Schmajuk, G. Epidemiology and treatment of Behçet's disease in the USA: Insights from the Rheumatology Informatics System for Effectiveness (RISE) Registry with a comparison with other published cohorts from endemic regions. *Arthritis Res. Ther.* **2021**, *23*, 1–9. [CrossRef] [PubMed]
21. Yepiskoposyan, L.; Harutyunyan, A. Population genetics of familial Mediterranean fever: A review. *Eur. J. Hum. Genet.* **2007**, *15*, 911–916. [CrossRef] [PubMed]
22. Krainer, J.; Siebenhandl, S.; Weinhäusel, A. Systemic autoinflammatory diseases. *J. Autoimmun.* **2020**, *109*, 102421. [CrossRef] [PubMed]
23. Shen, X.; Song, S.; Li, C.; Zhang, J. Synonymous mutations in representative yeast genes are mostly strongly non-neutral. *Nature* **2022**, *606*, 725–731. [CrossRef] [PubMed]
24. Arpacı, A.; Doğan, S.; Erdoğan, H.F.; El, Ç.; Cura, S.E. Presentation of a new mutation in FMF and evaluating the frequency of distribution of the MEFV gene mutation in our region with clinical findings. *Mol. Biol. Rep.* **2021**, *48*, 2025–2033. [CrossRef]
25. Çankaya, T.; Bora, E.; Bayram, M.T.; Ülgenalp, A.; Kavukçu, S.; Türkmen, M.A.; Soylu, A. Clinical Significance of R202Q Alteration of MEFV Gene in Children With Familial Mediterranean Fever. *Arch. Rheumatol.* **2015**, *30*, 51–56. [CrossRef]
26. Faulk, T.; Carroll, M.B. Case Report: A Patient Helps Diagnose Familial Mediterranean Fever. *The Rheumatologist*, 16 August 2019.
27. Topaloglu, R.; Ozaltin, F.; Yilmaz, E.; Ozen, S.; Balci, B.; Besbas, N.; Bakkaloglu, A. E148Q is a disease-causing MEFV mutation: A phenotypic evaluation in patients with familial Mediterranean fever. *Ann. Rheum. Dis.* **2005**, *64*, 750–752. [CrossRef]
28. El Roz, A.; Ghssein, G.; Khalaf, B.; Fardoun, T.; Ibrahim, J.-N. Spectrum of *MEFV* Variants and Genotypes among Clinically Diagnosed FMF Patients from Southern Lebanon. *Med. Sci.* **2020**, *8*, 35. [CrossRef]
29. Sohar, E.; Gafni, J.; Pras, M.; Heller, H. Familial Mediterranean fever. A survey of 470 cases and review of the literature. *Am. J. Med.* **1967**, *43*, 227–253. [CrossRef]
30. Yoshida, S.; Sumichika, Y.; Saito, K.; Matsumoto, H.; Temmoku, J.; Fujita, Y.; Matsuoka, N.; Asano, T.; Sato, S.; Migita, K. Effectiveness of Colchicine or Canakinumab in Japanese Patients with Familial Mediterranean Fever: A Single-Center Study. *J. Clin. Med.* **2023**, *12*, 6272. [CrossRef] [PubMed]
31. Özen, S.; Batu, E.D.; Demir, S. Familial Mediterranean Fever: Recent Developments in Pathogenesis and New Recommendations for Management. *Front. Immunol.* **2017**, *8*, 253. [CrossRef] [PubMed]
32. Ozdogan, H.; Ugurlu, S. Familial Mediterranean Fever. *La Presse Médicale* **2019**, *48*, e61–e76. [CrossRef] [PubMed]
33. Kuemmerle-Deschner, J.B.; Verma, D.; Endres, T.; Broderick, L.; de Jesus, A.A.; Hofer, F.; Blank, N.; Krause, K.; Rietschel, C.; Horneff, G.; et al. Clinical and Molecular Phenotypes of Low-Penetrance Variants of *NLRP3*: Diagnostic and Therapeutic Challenges. *Arthritis Rheumatol.* **2017**, *69*, 2233–2240. [CrossRef] [PubMed]
34. Verma, D.; Särndahl, E.; Andersson, H.; Eriksson, P.; Fredrikson, M.; Jönsson, J.-I.; Lerm, M.; Söderkvist, P. The Q705K polymorphism in NLRP3 is a gain-of-function alteration leading to excessive interleukin-1β and IL-18 production. *PLoS ONE* **2012**, *7*, e34977. [CrossRef] [PubMed]
35. Theodoropoulou, K.; Wittkowski, H.; Busso, N.; Von Scheven-Gête, A.; Moix, I.; Vanoni, F.; Hengten, V.; Horneff, G.; Haas, J.P.; Fischer, N.; et al. Increased Prevalence of NLRP3 Q703K Variant Among Patients With Autoinflammatory Diseases: An In-ternational Multicentric Study. *Front. Immunol.* **2020**, *11*, 877. [CrossRef] [PubMed]
36. von Mühlenen, I.; Gabay, C.; Finckh, A.; Kuemmerle-Deschner, J. NLRP3 Q703K and TNFRSF1A R92Q mutations in a patient with auto inflammatory disease. *Pediatr. Rheumatol.* **2015**, *13*, P47. [CrossRef]
37. E Saper, V.; Ombrello, M.J.; Tremoulet, A.H.; Montero-Martin, G.; Prahalad, S.; Canna, S.; Shimizu, C.; Deutsch, G.; Tan, S.Y.; Remmers, E.F.; et al. Severe delayed hypersensitivity reactions to IL-1 and IL-6 inhibitors link to common HLA-DRB1*15 alleles. *Ann. Rheum. Dis.* **2022**, *81*, 406–415. [CrossRef]
38. Sezgin, E.; Kaplan, E. Diverse selection pressures shaping the genetic architecture of behçet disease susceptibility. *Front. Genet.* **2022**, *13*, 983646. [CrossRef]
39. Sazzini, M.; Garagnani, P.; Sarno, S.; De Fanti, S.; Lazzano, T.; Yang Yao, D.; Boattini, A.; Pazzola, G.; Maramotti, S.; Boiardi, L.; et al. Tracing Behçet's disease origins along the Silk Road: An anthropological evolu-tionary genetics perspective. *Clin. Exp. Rheumatol.* **2015**, *33* (Suppl. 94), S60–S66.
40. Touitou, I.; Lesage, S.; McDermott, M.; Cuisset, L.; Hoffman, H.; Dode, C.; Shoham, N.; Aganna, E.; Hugot, J.P.; Wise, C.; et al. Infevers: An evolving mutation database for auto-inflammatory syndromes. *Hum Mutat.* **2004**, *24*, 194–198. [CrossRef]
41. Price, T.J.; Gold, M.S. From Mechanism to Cure: Renewing the Goal to Eliminate the Disease of Pain. *Pain Med.* **2018**, *19*, 1525–1549. [CrossRef]
42. Moens, M.; Jansen, J.; De Smedt, A.; Roulaud, M.; Billot, M.; Laton, J.; Rigoard, P.; Goudman, L. Acceptance and Commitment Therapy to Increase Resilience in Chronic Pain Patients: A Clinical Guideline. *Medicina* **2022**, *58*, 499. [CrossRef] [PubMed]
43. Totsch, S.K.; Sorge, R.E. Immune System Involvement in Specific Pain Conditions. *Mol. Pain* **2017**, *13*, 1744806917724559. [CrossRef] [PubMed]
44. Chen, M.C.; Meckfessel, M.H. Autoinflammatory disorders, pain, and neural regulation of inflammation. *Dermatol. Clin.* **2013**, *31*, 461–470. [CrossRef] [PubMed]

45. de Moraes, M.P.M.; Nascimento, R.R.N.R.D.; Abrantes, F.F.; Pedroso, J.L.; Perazzio, S.F.; Barsottini, O.G.P. What General Neurologists Should Know about Autoinflammatory Syndromes? *Brain Sci.* **2023**, *13*, 1351. [CrossRef] [PubMed]

46. Gok, I.; Huseyinoglu, N.; Ilhan, D. Genetic polymorphisms variants in interleukin-6 and interleukin- 1beta patients with obstructive sleep apnea syndrome in East Northern Turkey. *Med. Glas.* **2015**, *12*, 216–222. [CrossRef]

47. Renson, T.; Hamiwka, L.; Benseler, S. Central nervous system manifestations of monogenic autoinflammatory disorders and the neurotropic features of SARS-CoV-2: Drawing the parallels. *Front. Pediatr.* **2022**, *10*, 931179. [CrossRef] [PubMed]

48. Uccelli, A.; Gattorno, M. Neurological manifestations in autoinflammatory diseases. *Clin. Exp. Rheumatol.* **2018**, *36* (Suppl. 110), 61–67.

49. Pisanti, S.; Rimondi, E.; Pozza, E.; Melloni, E.; Zauli, E.; Bifulco, M.; Martinelli, R.; Marcuzzi, A. Prenylation Defects and Oxidative Stress Trigger the Main Consequences of Neuroinflammation Linked to Mevalonate Pathway Deregulation. *Int. J. Environ. Res. Public Heal.* **2022**, *19*, 9061. [CrossRef]

50. Ben-Chetrit, E.; Gattorno, M.; Gul, A.; Kastner, D.L.; Lachmann, H.J.; Touitou, I.; Ruperto, N. Consensus proposal for taxonomy and definition of the autoinflammatory diseases (AIDs): A Delphi study. *Ann. Rheum. Dis.* **2018**, *77*, 1558–1565. [CrossRef]

51. Senusi, A.; Seoudi, N.; Bergmeier, L.A.; Fortune, F. Genital ulcer severity score and genital health quality of life in Behçet's disease. *Orphanet. J. Rare Dis.* **2015**, *10*, 117. [CrossRef]

52. Irwin, M.R. Sleep and inflammation: Partners in sickness and in health. *Nat. Rev. Immunol.* **2019**, *19*, 702–715. [CrossRef] [PubMed]

53. Jewett, K.A.; Krueger, J.M. Humoral sleep regulation; interleukin-1 and tumor necrosis factor. *Vitam. Horm.* **2012**, *89*, 241–257. [CrossRef] [PubMed]

54. American Autoimmune Related Diseases Association (AARDA). Profound, Debilitating Fatigue Found to Be a Major Issue for Autoimmune Disease Patients in New National Survey. *ScienceDaily*, 23 March 2015.

55. Nikolaus, S.; Bode, C.; Taal, E.; van de Laar, M.A.F.J. Fatigue and factors related to fatigue in rheumatoid arthritis: A systematic review. *Arthritis Care Res.* **2013**, *65*, 1128–1146. [CrossRef] [PubMed]

56. Bergman, M.J.; Shahouri, S.S.; Shaver, T.S.; Anderson, J.D.; Weidensaul, D.N.; Busch, R.E.; Wang, S.; Wolfe, F. Is fatigue an inflammatory variable in rheumatoid arthritis (RA)? Analyses of fatigue in RA, osteoarthritis, and fibromyalgia. *J. Rheumatol.* **2009**, *36*, 2788–2794. [CrossRef] [PubMed]

57. Pollard, L.C.; Choy, E.H.; Gonzalez, J.; Khoshaba, B.; Scott, D.L. Fatigue in rheumatoid arthritis reflects pain, not disease activity. *Rheumatology* **2006**, *45*, 885–889. [CrossRef]

58. van Dartel, S.A.; Repping-Wuts, J.W.; van Hoogmoed, D.; Bleijenberg, G.; van Riel, P.L.; Fransen, J. Association between fatigue and pain in rheumatoid arthritis: Does pain precede fatigue or does fatigue precede pain? *Arthritis Care Res.* **2013**, *65*, 862–869. [CrossRef]

59. Dantzer, R.; Heijnen, C.J.; Kavelaars, A.; Laye, S.; Capuron, L. The neuroimmune basis of fatigue. *Trends Neurosci.* **2013**, *37*, 39–46. [CrossRef]

60. Morris, G.; Berk, M.; Walder, K.; Maes, M. Central pathways causing fatigue in neuro-inflammatory and autoimmune illnesses. *BMC Med.* **2015**, *13*, 1–23. [CrossRef]

61. Zielinski, M.R.; McKenna, J.T.; McCarley, R.W. Functions and Mechanisms of Sleep. *AIMS Neurosci.* **2016**, *3*, 67–104. [CrossRef]

62. Kelesoglu, F.M.; Aygun, E.; Okumus, N.K.; Ersoy, A.; Karapınar, E.; Saglam, N.; Aydın, N.G.; Senay, B.B.; Gonultas, S.; Sarisik, E.; et al. Evaluation of subclinical inflammation in familial Mediterranean fever patients: Relations with mutation types and attack status: A retrospective study. *Clin. Rheumatol.* **2016**, *35*, 2757–2763. [CrossRef]

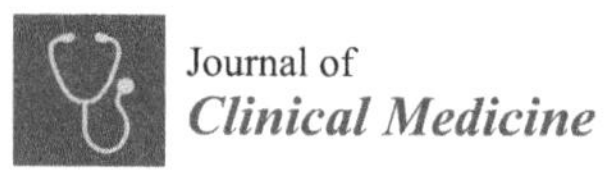

Journal of
Clinical Medicine

VEXAS and Myelodysplastic Syndrome: An Interdisciplinary Challenge

Virginie Kreutzinger [1], Anne Pankow [2], Zhivana Boyadzhieva [2], Udo Schneider [2], Katharina Ziegeler [3], Lars Uwe Stephan [3], Jan Carl Kübke [3], Sebastian Schröder [3], Christian Oberender [3], Philipp le Coutre [3], Sebastian Stintzing [3] and Ivan Jelas [3,*]

[1] Department of Radiology, Vivantes Klinikum im Friedrichshain, 10249 Berlin, Germany
[2] Department of Rheumatology and Clinical Immunology, Campus Charité Mitte, Charitéplatz 1, 10117 Berlin, Germany
[3] Department of Hematology, Oncology, and Cancer Immunology, Campus Charité Mitte, Charitéplatz 1, 10117 Berlin, Germany
*   Correspondence: ivan.jelas@charite.de

Abstract: VEXAS (vacuoles, E1 enzyme, X-linked, autoinflammatory, somatic) syndrome is a recently recognized systemic autoinflammatory disease caused by somatic mutations in hematopoietic progenitor cells. This case series of four patients with VEXAS syndrome and comorbid myelodysplastic syndrome (MDS) aims to describe clinical, imaging, and hematologic disease presentations as well as response to therapy. Four patients with VEXAS syndrome and MDS are described. A detailed analysis of imaging features, hemato-oncological presentation including bone marrow microscopy and clinical–rheumatological disease features and treatment outcomes is given. All patients were male; ages ranged between 64 and 81 years; all were diagnosed with MDS. CT imaging was available for three patients, all of whom exhibited pulmonary infiltrates of varying severity, resembling COVID-19 or hypersensitivity pneumonitis without traces of scarring. Bone marrow microscopy showed maturation-disordered erythropoiesis and pathognomonic vacuolation. Somatic mutation in the *UBA1* codon 41 were found in all patients by next-generation sequencing. Therapy regimes included glucocorticoids, JAK1/2-inhibitors, nucleoside analogues, as well as IL-1 and IL-6 receptor antagonists. No fatalities occurred (observation period from symptom onset: 18–68 months). Given the potential underreporting of VEXAS syndrome, we highly recommend contemporary screening for *UBA1* mutations in patients presenting with ambiguous signs of systemic autoinflammatory symptoms which persist over 18 months despite treatment. The emergence of cytopenia, especially macrocytic hyperchromic anemia, should prompt early testing for *UBA1* mutations. Notably conspicuous, pulmonary alterations in CT imaging of patients with therapy-resistant systemic autoinflammatory symptoms should be discussed in interdisciplinary medical teams (Rheumatology, Hematology, Radiology and further specialist departments) to facilitate timely diagnosis during the clinical course of the disease.

Keywords: autoinflammation; imaging; myelodysplastic syndrome; VEXAS syndrome

Citation: Kreutzinger, V.; Pankow, A.; Boyadzhieva, Z.; Schneider, U.; Ziegeler, K.; Stephan, L.U.; Kübke, J.C.; Schröder, S.; Oberender, C.; le Coutre, P.; et al. VEXAS and Myelodysplastic Syndrome: An Interdisciplinary Challenge. *J. Clin. Med.* **2024**, *13*, 1049. https://doi.org/10.3390/jcm13041049

Academic Editor: Alicia Rovó

Received: 7 January 2024
Revised: 6 February 2024
Accepted: 9 February 2024
Published: 12 February 2024

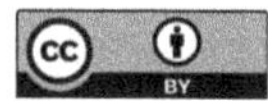

1. Introduction

The VEXAS syndrome is an autoinflammatory systemic disease first described in 2020 [1]; the acronym stands for vacuoles, E1 enzyme, X-linked, autoinflammation and somatic (mutation). The majority of affected patients are men in their fifties to seventies, presenting with a severe inflammatory syndrome and hematologic abnormalities [2–4]. Diagnosis is made by confirmation of alterations in the *UBA1* gene, which is typically performed using genomic DNA from peripheral blood leukocytes or bone marrow tissue [5–7]. The disease is characterized by a somatically acquired mutation affecting methionine 41 of the E1-ubiquitin ligase *UBA1*, resulting in the expression of a catalytically impaired isoform that drives inflammation processes in the body. Common clinical features observed in VEXAS syndrome patients include skin lesions (83%), non-infectious fever (64%), weight loss (62%), lung involvement (50%), ocular symptoms (39%), relapsing chondritis (36%), venous thrombosis (35%), lymphadenopathy (34%), and arthralgia (27%) [3]. Additionally, patients with VEXAS syndrome experience progressive hematologic abnormalities such as macrocytic anemia, thrombocytopenia, and myeloid dyspoiesis [8–10]. In a substantial number of cases, the disease may progress to an overt hematologic malignant condition [11–13]. Bone marrow aspirates typically show characteristic vacuoles restricted to myeloid and erythroid precursor cells [6,9]. Due to the novelty of the disease, there are currently no evidence-based recommendations for treatment. Treatment options include the use of glucocorticoids, conventional disease-modifying antirheumatic drugs (DMARDs), biologically targeted drugs, and allogeneic hematopoietic stem cell transplantation [14–17]. The literature reflects the difficulty of diagnosing VEXAS syndrome patients during their lifetime with many publications being retrospective in nature.

Our case series aims to demonstrate that the diagnosis of VEXAS syndrome can be made during the course of the illness if clinical characteristics are carefully documented, discussed in an interdisciplinary manner, and if patients receive the necessary diagnostic evaluations. Furthermore, we illustrate the management and response to therapy in four patients with VEXAS syndrome who also have concurrent MDS, and we explain why a comprehensive investigation of the disease's imaging features could be helpful in identifying these very rare patients.

2. Materials and Methods

2.1. Imaging

All available imaging datasets were reviewed and discussed in consensus by two radiologists with deep clinical expertise in rheumatological imaging (K.Z. and V.K.). Special consideration was given to previously described imaging features of VEXAS syndrome, including pleuro-pulmonary manifestations, polychondritis, and lymphadenopathy as well as signs of vasculitis. Special consideration was given to imaging manifestations in the skeletal system including bone marrow changes associated with MDS and patterns of arthritis, which could not be attributed to typical aging.

2.2. Bone Marrow Smear

Approximately 5 mL of semi-liquid bone marrow content was immediately processed on pre-prepared glass slides and stained with Wright–Giemsa and iron staining.

2.3. Next-Generation-Sequencing

Genomic DNA was extracted from bone marrow (n = 4) and samples were analyzed by next-generation sequencing using a 68- and a 98-gene panel to detect mutations of *UBA1* and further somatic mutations (e.g., *U2AF1*, *DNMT3A* and *TET2*).

2.4. Ethical Approval, Data Availability and Patient and Public Involvement

All patients provided written informed consent for the use of their data for scientific purposes. This investigation was overseen by the ethics committee of Charité Universitätsmedizin Berlin (EA4/053/21). All data and materials from this study are available upon reasonable request to the corresponding author. There was no specific patient or public involvement in this investigation.

3. Results

3.1. Clinical Features, Treatment and Outcome

Patient 1: A male patient in his late 60 s presented with a history of peripheral deep vein thromboses, dyspnea, muscle weakness, Raynaud-like symptoms, and persistent fever. The patient was over 35 months under rheumatological outpatient and inpatient care and received during this time DMARDs (methotrexate, leflunomide) and glucocorticoids intermittently with more than 20 mg prednisolone per day. Over time, the patient developed persistent macrocytic hyperchromic anemia, which could not be explained by a deficiency in folic acid, vitamin B12, side effects of present medication, or other diagnosed diseases. The patient was referred to the divisions of rheumatology and hematology at Charité—Universitätsmedizin Berlin for further care. After a comprehensive interdisciplinary evaluation of the patient's clinical course so far, an investigation into macrocytic hyperchromic anemia was initiated, ultimately leading to a bone marrow aspiration. The bone marrow aspirate smears from the patient demonstrated signs of dysplasia, including nuclear abnormalities in erythroid precursor cells and multinucleated micro-megakaryocytes. Furthermore, cytoplasmic vacuolation of myeloid and erythroid precursors was particularly noticeable during the cytological examination. Next-generation sequencing (NGS) detected mutations in DNMT3A and UBA1, leading to a diagnosis of low-risk MDS (IPSS-R of 2) and VEXAS syndrome.

Due to the mild cytopenia, a "watch and wait" strategy was initially pursued for MDS, since symptoms of autoinflammation persisted and led to an overall deterioration in his health. Due to the limited data available on treatment options in VEXAS syndrome, an off-label use of the JAK1/2 inhibitor ruxolitinib was initiated at 20 mg twice daily, and glucocorticoids were discontinued [18].

During the treatment, the dose of ruxolitinib was adjusted due to side effects such as dizziness, headache, fever, and constipation. The first dose reduction in ruxolitinib was to 15 mg, which was followed by adjustments to 10 mg and finally to 5 mg twice daily. Additionally, despite these those adjustments, muscle weakness and fever persisted, leading to the initiation of concurrent treatment with glucocorticoids (15 mg Prednisolon once daily).

Simultaneously, blood tests over six months consistently indicated a worsening of anemia. Consequently, a repeat bone marrow aspiration was performed, revealing a progressive maturation disorder, particularly in erythropoiesis, while the blast cell count remained normal. In the context of persistently limited data regarding further alternative treatment options, we decided to initiate a treatment with 5-azacytidine (75 mg/m^2 daily for 7 days, followed by a rest period of 21 days) [14].

After the switch to 5-azacytidine, rapid improvement in autoinflammatory symptoms and anemia was observed. However, continued treatment with 7.5 mg of prednisolone once daily was necessary to control clinical symptoms like muscle weakness and fever. The patient received six cycles of 5-azacytidine (28-day treatment cycle). The tolerability of the therapy over the six cycles was good. Clinically relevant signs of toxicity were not observed. As of now, blood results and autoinflammatory symptoms have further stabilized, but long-term effects are yet to be determined and need to be followed up closely

Patient 2: A male in his mid-70s presented with recurrent episodes of fever, dyspnea, and unexplained pulmonary inflammation (no detected pathogen, no elevation of procalcitonin), one episode of pleuritis, recurrent sterile parotitis, and deep venous thrombosis. Furthermore, he experienced arthralgia in the wrists and had elevated rheumatoid factors. Imaging findings were suggestive of interstitial lung disease, with peripheral consolidations and mild ground glass opacities prompted pronchoalveolar lavage, which revealed a CD4/CD8 ratio of 0.9; antigen testing for hypersensitivity pneumonitis (which was initially suspected) was negative. Pulmonary symptoms responded to prednisolone, but withdrawal attempts resulted in a recurrence of dyspnea, requiring a continued dose of 20 mg prednisolone. Insufficient control of autoinflammatory symptoms over 26 months and worsening of hematopoiesis over 4 months prompted the transfer of the patient to the divisions of rheumatology and hematology at Charité—Universitätsmedizin Berlin for further diagnostics and clinical care. Following a thorough interdisciplinary assessment in both divisions, considering the patient's clinical history and the progressing inefficacy of hematopoiesis, a bone marrow biopsy was performed.

In the bone marrow aspirate smears of the patient, signs of dysplasia and cytoplasmic vacuolation of myeloid and erythroid precursors were detected. NGS testing revealed mutations in TET2, U2AF1, and UBA1, leading to the diagnosis of low-risk MDS (IPSS-R of 2.5) and VEXAS syndrome.

The initiated treatment with prednisolone (20 mg) was quickly escalated to 5-azacytidine due to persistent anemia and thrombocytopenia. Under the combination treatment of prednisolone and 5-azacytidine, complete recovery of blood cell counts was achieved, but only limited improvement in autoinflammation (fever) was observed. A dose reduction in prednisolone resulted in an immediate recurrence of severe arthralgia and more frequent fever episodes. Therefore, we transitioned to ruxolitinib (JAK1/2 inhibitor) at a dose of 20 mg twice daily.

With ruxolitinib, there was a slight decrease in hemoglobin levels, while platelet and leukocyte counts remained stable. However, there was a significant improvement in autoinflammatory symptoms (no episodes of fever and/or arthralgia) and also a substantial clinical improvement in pulmonary symptoms as well as pulmonary imaging findings. The tolerability was excellent, and no side effects occurred, allowing ruxolitinib therapy to continue without complications for 12 months up to the current point. However, the long-term effects remain undetermined, and the patient is currently under close medical care and follow-up.

Patient 3: A male in his early 80s presented with intermittent fever, unintentional weight loss, and a history of skin rashes and polyarthritis. Biopsy of affected skin showed neutrophilic dermatosis, raising suspicion of a paraneoplastic origin. Based on imaging, a diagnosis of polyarticular CPPD was made, and treatment with systemic prednisolone and an interleukin-1 antagonist (anakinra, starting dosage 2 mg/kg daily) was initiated but with limited clinical response. The patient underwent rheumatological outpatient and inpatient care for over 18 months, since the patients develop gradual pancytopenia (macrocytic hyperchromic anemia) referral to the divisions of hematology at Charité—Universitätsmedizin Berlin for further diagnostics. After intensive interdisciplinary examination of the patient's case by the departments of Hematology and Rheumatology, due to a suspected diagnosis of MDS and VEXAS syndrome, a bone marrow biopsy was performed. The bone marrow analysis revealed hypercellularity with increases in two lineages. Furthermore, there were prominent signs of dysplasia, megaloblastoid changes, and nuclear abnormalities in erythroid precursor cells along with typical cytoplasmic vacuolation in myeloid and erythroid precursor cells. NGS testing did not reveal any MDS-specific mutations but did identify a UBA1 mutation. Consequently, the patient was diagnosed with very-low-risk MDS (IPSS-R of 1) and VEXAS syndrome.

Due to ongoing clinical signs of autoinflammation, an off-label treatment with ruxolitinib (20 mg twice daily) in combination with prednisolone (20 mg) was initiated. Repeated attempts to taper off prednisolone failed during the course of treatment because, at a dose below 5 mg, the autoinflammatory symptoms, especially arthritis, worsened significantly. The combination therapy was well-tolerated, and there were no significant toxicities or side effects that necessitated a modification of the treatment with ruxolitinib. Blood counts, especially anemia, recovered quickly after initiating the treatment. The patient is presently receiving attentive medical supervision and ongoing follow-up.

Patient 4: A male patient in his mid-60s presented with intermittent fever, night sweats, and a history of dermatosis and chronic polyarthritis. Chronic neutrophilic urticarial dermatosis and adult-onset Still's disease were suspected. Sequential treatments with DMARD (methotrexate), anakinra (an interleukin-1 antagonist), and canakinumab (an interleukin-1β blocker) were attempted but terminated due to suspicion of therapy-induced pancytopenia and interstitial lung disease.

Due to inadequate control of autoinflammatory symptoms over 68 months, along with an existing and progressively worsening macrocytic hyperchromic anemia, as well as mild thrombocytopenia, the patient sought a second opinion at Charité—Universitätsmedizin Berlin for further diagnostics and clinical care. Following an interdisciplinary presentation and discussion of the case, a suspected diagnosis of MDS and VEXAS Syndrome was made. An extended hematological–oncological diagnostic evaluation was initiated. Subsequently, a bone marrow biopsy was performed, revealing binuclearity in erythroid cell precursors as well as noticeable cytoplasmic vacuolation of myeloid and erythroid precursors. No pathological increase in blast cells was observed. Subsequent NGS examination identified a mutation in the EZH2 gene with unclear significance and a UBA1 mutation, leading to a diagnosis of very low-risk MDS (IPSS-R of 1) and VEXAS syndrome.

Therapy with 5-azacytidine (daily for 7 days, followed by a rest period of 21 days) in combination with prednisolone (7.5 mg) was initiated. Blood improved over time, particularly the macrocytic hyperchromic anemia, as did the clinical signs of autoinflammation. Prednisolone was completely discontinued, and the therapy with 5-azacytidine was dose-reduced from 7 to 4 days per cycle (28-day treatment cycle) starting from cycle 16. Cumulatively, the patient received 30 cycles of 5-azacytidine with clinically well-controlled VEXAS syndrome and hematologically stable MDS. The patient is currently undergoing treatment with 5-azacytidine and is under careful medical monitoring.

Further patient characteristics are given in Tables 1 and 2

Table 1. Laboratory findings and observation periods. Values upon initial presentation at our center. * = both patients received high-dose oral prednisolone (>50 mg/d). Observation periods: from first patient reported systemic autoinflammatory symptoms until time of manuscript preparation.

	Patient 1	**Patient 2**	**Patient 3**	**Patient 4**
Hemoglobin (g/dL)	10.3	8.2	8.1	8.0
Mean corpuscular volume (fL)	109.1	124.1	95.0	111.0
White blood count (/nL)	6.54	6.60	6.67	4.70
Platelet count (/nL)	195	38	212	82
C-reactive protein at initial presentation (mg/L)	98.3	26.5 *	139.3	10.5 *
Observation period (months)	35	26	18	68

Table 2. Next-generation sequencing.

	UBA1	**Further Somatic Mutations**
Patient 1	*UBA1* codon 41 (p.Met41Val (NM_003334.4:c.121A>G))	*DNMT3A* (p.Arg882Cys (NM_022552.5:c.2644C>T))
Patient 2	*UBA1* codon 41 (p.Met41Val (NM_003334.4:c.121A>G))	*TET2* (p.M633I (c.1899G>A)), *U2AF1* (p.Q157P (c.470A>C))
Patient 3	*UBA1* codon 41 (p.Met41Leu (NM_003334.4:c.121A>C))	none
Patient 4	*UBA1* codon 41 (p.Met41Leu (NM_003334.4:c.121A>C))	*EZH2* gene: intronic, non-coding region 2-base deletion near a splice site, with unclear significance

3.2. Imaging

3.2.1. Chest

Three of the patients received CT imaging of the lungs at different time points. In all these patients, a pattern of almost exclusively peripherally located consolidations, without upper- or lower lobe predominance was observed—one of the cases (patient 2) is depicted in Figure 1. In this patient, consolidations resolved over a course of two months with still clearly visible ground glass opacities in areas of previous consolidations yet no evident fibrosis or scarring. Hilar lymphadenopathy was seen in two out of four (patients 2 and 3) patients; both symmetric and asymmetric manifestations were seen in the same patient (patient 2) over the course of the disease. No bronchial wall abnormalities indicating relapsing chondritis were observed.

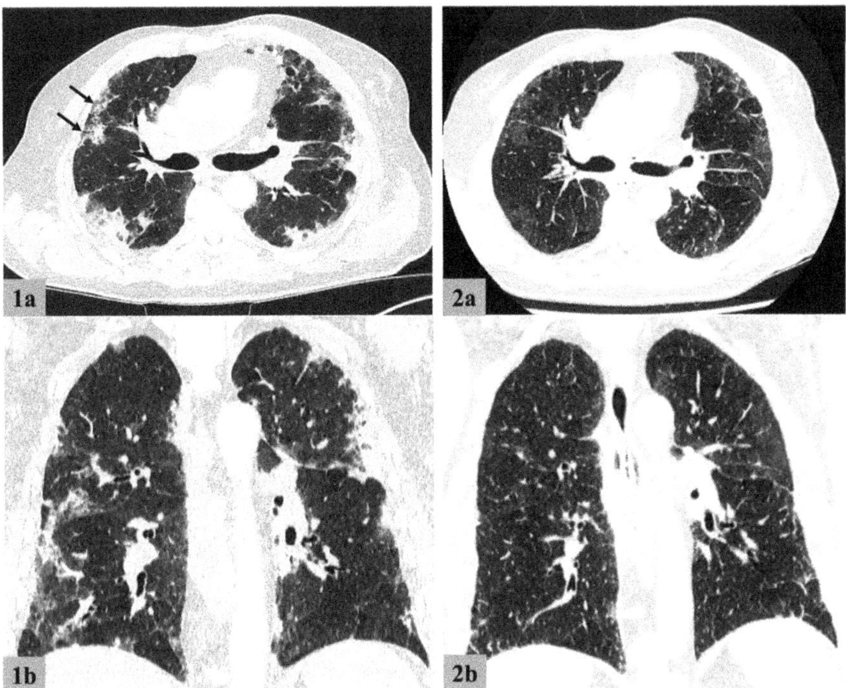

Figure 1. Pulmonary findings on computed tomography (Patient 2). 1 = time of initial diagnosis; 2 = two months later. a = axial reconstructions; b = coronal reconstructions. Marked subpleural consolidations without topographical predominance are seen (marked with arrows). After two months, patchy ground glass opacities remain without notable scarring.

3.2.2. Joints and Bones

Spinal imaging was only available for two patients, one of whom exhibited extensive bone marrow reconversion, which was consistent with MDS. Two patients (2 and 3) reported symmetric arthralgia of the wrists, prompting imaging investigations of arthritis. One patient received MR imaging, showing non-specific patchy bone marrow edema of the carpalia without synovitis, erosion, or tendon involvement. Patient 3 received a whole-body PET-CT which showed symmetrically increased tracer uptake in both wrists; in this patient, radiography showed degenerative lesions and calcifications of the triangular fibrocartilage of the wrists, but no erosions, resulting the diagnosis of CPPD.

3.3. Bone Marrow Microscopy

All patients exhibited an increase in cellularity (ranging between 50% and 80%) with maturation-disordered erythropoiesis (megaloblastic precursors, binucleation, nuclear rounding) and pathognomonic vacuolation (Figure 2)—the latter in three out of four patients.

The granulopoiesis to erythropoiesis (G:E) ratio shifted in favor of granulopoiesis to ratios of 3–6:1. No pathological increases in blasts were observed. Next-generation sequencing (NGS) revealed somatic mutations in the UBA1 codon in all patients—results are given in Table 2.

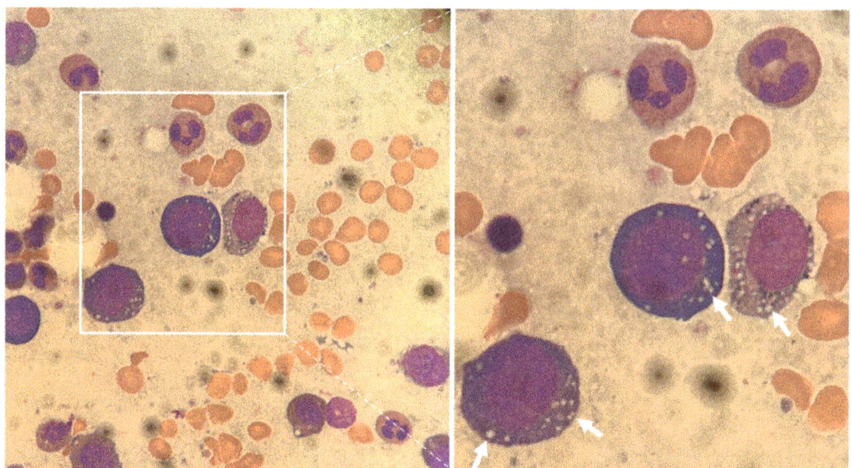

Figure 2. Bone marrow aspirate smear (Patient 1). Left: microscopic magnification 100×. Characteristic cytoplasmic vacuolation of myeloid and erythroid precursors is indicated by white arrows.

4. Discussion

In this report, we present a detailed account of four patients diagnosed with VEXAS syndrome and comorbid MDS from a single center in Germany (Charité—Universitätsmedizin Berlin). All patients exhibited systemic autoinflammatory symptoms that progressed over an extended time period (18 to 68 months). None of the four patients showed significant responsiveness to various immunosuppressive treatments throughout their clinical course, having either no response or only partial responsiveness. Despite receiving outpatient and intermittently inpatient rheumatological care, a definitive diagnosis could not be established based on their clinical progression.

The decision to refer these patients to our specialized clinical departments was prompted by uncontrolled systemic autoinflammatory symptoms and discrete worsening of blood counts, particularly progressive macrocytic hyperchromic anemia. The comprehensive interdisciplinary evaluation of these patients, involving the Departments of Rheumatology, Hematology, and Radiology, led to the diagnosis of MDS-VEXAS syndrome within six weeks after the initial consultation. Based on our observations and experiences, the prolonged time to diagnose represents one of the main challenges for MDS-VEXAS syndrome patients. This fact is underscored but not prominently highlighted in the existing literature. In addition to the absence of evidence-based treatment options, the extended time to diagnosis is, from our perspective, one of the key medical needs that should be addressed in the future. This becomes particularly evident when considering the findings of Huang et al., who reported in their series that 10 out of 25 patients died from disease-related causes such as progressive anemia or therapy-related complications [5]. The delayed diagnosis also explains why many comprehensive reports are of a retrospective nature [1,2].

Therefore, we suggest that a basic standardized diagnostic criteria classifier should be developed to simplify the identification of these patients in clinical routine. This MDS-VEXAS syndrome classifier should include patient characteristics, key clinical features, the number of prior therapies, duration of symptoms, laboratory findings, and radiological alterations.

The clinical courses of the four reported MDS-VEXAS syndrome patients reflect the current medical situation in routine patient care and align with previously published series [1,2,5]. Patients with VEXAS syndrome have a lengthy medical history, spanning months to years, characterized by ambiguous autoinflammatory symptoms.

The clinical phenotype and autoinflammatory symptoms of patients with VEXAS syndrome, with or without MDS, have already been well described by other working groups in the literature [1,2,5,19]. Our four patients showed no new clinical features and insights. All of our patients presented with systemic autoinflammatory symptoms, especially fever, which was in line with publications by Beck et al. and Georgin-Lavialle. Arthralgia and arthritis were observed in three out of four patients, which was consistent with previous descriptions in the literature [2,20]. The chest images of our MDS-VEXAS syndrome patients demonstrated lung involvement, as previously described in the literature. The radiologically identified consolidations transitioning to ground glass opacity, with no discernible parenchymal scarring, are consistent with previous publications [6,21–23]. Notably, there was a radiological overlap with COVID-19, which was characterized by predominantly peripheral/subpleural infiltrates. Interestingly, this manifested in a reversed order compared to early COVID-19, where ground glass opacity is typically seen [7]. As described for patient 2, these imaging findings have limited specificity and show substantial overlap to interstitial lung diseases; thus, a radiologist with limited clinical background information may misdirect clinical diagnosis, which further highlights the need for a truly interdisciplinary approach. Imaging findings in MDS, especially the loss of the typical fat signal of bone marrow in T1-weighted sequences, should not be mistaken for bone marrow edema. In such investigations, supplying the diagnosing radiologist with information about comorbid MDS, rather than just inquiring about the presence of arthritis or other inflammatory skeletal findings, will safeguard against overdiagnosis of arthritis. One of our patients was diagnosed with CPPD on imaging; the interplay of systemic autoinflammation and symptomatic crystal deposition disease may be of interest in future research. Overall, radiological findings must be considered in an interdisciplinary context, alongside other clinical parameters and symptoms, and could be implemented in the basic standardized diagnostic criteria classifier mentioned above.

Limited but promising results have been achieved with the JAK1/2 inhibitor ruxolitinib or the hypomethylating agent 5-azacytidine [8–10,18,24]. Due to this fact and the absence of evidence-based recommendations, we treated our patients with these two substances.

Fortunately, all four of our patients responded to the selected systemic therapy. However, in the cases of patients 1 and 2, insufficient clinical and laboratory therapeutic responses were initially observed, leading to a change in treatment. The mechanistic reasons for treatment response or the lack of response to ruxolitinib or 5-azacytidine in some VEXAS syndrome and MDS patients are currently unclear and cannot be explained by previously published works [8–10,14,18,24]

Despite ruxolitinib or 5-azacytidine demonstrating a good treatment response, all four of our patients required intermittent or permanent high doses of systemic glucocorticoids (7.5–50 mg/day prednisolone). This fact underscores the clinical need to develop further targeted therapy options for the autoinflammatory spectrum of the disease. In particular, the JAK1/2 inhibitor ruxolitinib appears to be a suitable candidate for reducing the concurrent need for glucocorticoids in VEXAS syndrome patients, whether or not they have myeloid neoplasia [9].

Our clinical experience supports the effectiveness of ruxolitinib and 5-azacytidine, as described in the literature. Furthermore, we see the potential for both agents to be used in combination treatment for MDS-VEXAS syndrome and MDS patients. Phase II data of ruxolitinib in combination with 5-azacytidine in myelodysplastic syndrome/myeloproliferative neoplasms demonstrated a tolerable safety profile with a good response rate [21]. Therefore, a prospective study will be required to explore the potential of this combination in the future.

The only known treatment that leads to a cure for MDS-VEXAS syndrome patients is allogeneic hematopoietic stem cell transplantation (AHSCT). Currently, an ongoing phase II study for patients with VEXAS syndrome aims to evaluate the impact of AHSCT for this condition (NCT05027945)

In summary, our report emphasizes the challenges posed by overlapping symptoms in rheumatological and hematological conditions, compounded by the rarity of the disease, making it difficult to identify these patients in routine clinical care. Based on our clinical observations and experience, this study identifies prolonged diagnosis as one of the main problems for MDS-VEXAS syndrome patients. Therefore, we see an opportunity for the development of a basic standardized diagnostic criteria classifier for clinical routine to prevent delayed diagnosis in their clinical course. This future MDS-VEXAS syndrome classifier should include patient characteristics, key clinical features, the number of prior therapies, duration of symptoms, laboratory findings, and radiological alterations. Moreover, we recommend that patients with prolonged therapy-resistant autoinflammatory symptoms undergo a comprehensive interdisciplinary evaluation and discussion. This should involve at least the Departments of Rheumatology, Hematology, and Radiology. Only an early and accurate diagnosis, including molecular genetic analyses, allows for the early treatment of these patients and their inclusion in current and future clinical studies.

Author Contributions: Conceptualization, V.K., P.l.C. and I.J.; Data curation, C.O., P.l.C., S.S. (Sebastian Stintzing) and I.J.; Investigation, V.K., A.P., Z.B., U.S., K.Z., J.C.K., C.O. and I.J.; Methodology, V.K., K.Z. and P.l.C.; Project administration, I.J.; Resources, L.U.S., J.C.K., S.S. (Sebastian Schroeder), I.J.; Supervision, C.O., P.l.C. and S.S. (Sebastian Stintzing); Visualization, V.K., K.Z. and L.U.S.; Writing—original draft, V.K. and I.J.; Writing—review and editing, V.K., A.P., Z.B., U.S., K.Z., L.U.S., J.C.K., S.S. (Sebastian Schroeder), C.O., P.l.C., S.S. (Sebastian Stintzing) and I.J. All authors have read and agreed to the published version of the manuscript.

Funding: We acknowledge support from the German Research Foundation (DFG) and the Open Access Publication Fund of Charité—Universitätsmedizin Berlin.

Institutional Review Board Statement: The study was conducted in accordance with the Declaration of Helsinki, and approved by the Institutional Review Board Ethics Committee of Charité—Universitätsmedizin Berlin (no. EA4/053/21, date: 04 September 2021).

Informed Consent Statement: Informed consent was obtained from all subjects involved in the study.

Data Availability Statement: All data and materials presented in this study are available on reasonable request from the corresponding author upon reasonable request.

Conflicts of Interest: Sebastian Stintzing declares advisory roles for AMGEN, AstraZeneca, Bayer, BMS, ESAI, Jansen, Lily, Merck KGaA Darmstadt, Germany, MSD, Pierre-Fabre, Roche, Sanofi, Servier, Taiho, Takeda, honoraria from AMGEN, AstraZeneca, Bayer, BMS, ESAI, Leo-Pharma, Lilly, Merck KGaA, Darmstadt, Germany, MSD, Pierre-Fabre, Roche, Sanofi, Servier, Talho, Takeda and research funding from Merck KGaA, Darmstadt, Germany, Pierre-Fabre, Servier, Roche outside the submitted work. Ivan Jelas declares advisory roles/Honoraria for talks/travel expenses for Roche, BMS, Merck KGaA, Pierre-Fabre, Roche, Servier, Taiho Pharma, Takeda Pharmaceutical. All other others declare no conflicts of interest.

References

1. Beck, D.B.; Ferrada, M.A.; Sikora, K.A.; Ombrello, A.K.; Collins, J.C.; Pei, W.; Balanda, N.; Ross, D.L.; Ospina Cardona, D.; Wu, Z.; et al. Somatic Mutations in UBA1 and Severe Adult-Onset Autoinflammatory Disease. *N. Engl. J. Med.* **2020**, *383*, 2628–2638. [CrossRef]
2. Georgin-Lavialle, S.; Terrier, B.; Guedon, A.F.; Heiblig, M.; Comont, T.; Lazaro, E.; Lacombe, V.; Terriou, L.; Ardois, S.; Bouaziz, J.D.; et al. Further characterization of clinical and laboratory features in VEXAS syndrome: Large-scale analysis of a multicentre case series of 116 French patients. *Br. J. Dermatol.* **2022**, *186*, 564–574. [CrossRef]
3. Koster, M.J.; Kourelis, T.; Reichard, K.K.; Kermani, T.A.; Beck, D.B.; Cardona, D.O.; Samec, M.J.; Mangaonkar, A.A.; Begna, K.H.; Hook, C.C.; et al. Clinical Heterogeneity of the VEXAS Syndrome: A Case Series. *Mayo Clin. Proc.* **2021**, *96*, 2653–2659. [CrossRef]
4. Ruffer, N.; Krusche, M. VEXAS syndrome: A diagnostic puzzle. *RMD Open* **2023**, *9*, e003332. [CrossRef]
5. Huang, H.; Zhang, W.; Cai, W.; Liu, J.; Wang, H.; Qin, T.; Xu, Z.; Li, B.; Qu, S.; Pan, L.; et al. VEXAS syndrome in myelodysplastic syndrome with autoimmune disorder. *Exp. Hematol. Oncol.* **2021**, *10*, 23. [CrossRef]
6. Patel, N.; Dulau-Florea, A.; Calvo, K.R. Characteristic bone marrow findings in patients with UBA1 somatic mutations and VEXAS syndrome. *Semin. Hematol.* **2021**, *58*, 204–211. [CrossRef]

7. Poulter, J.A.; Collins, J.C.; Cargo, C.; De Tute, R.M.; Evans, P.; Ospina Cardona, D.; Bowen, D.T.; Cunnington, J.R.; Baguley, E.; Quinn, M.; et al. Novel somatic mutations in UBA1 as a cause of VEXAS syndrome. *Blood* **2021**, *137*, 3676–3681. [CrossRef] [PubMed]
8. Austestad, J.; Madland, T.M.; Sandnes, M.; Haslerud, T.M.; Benneche, A.; Reikvam, H. VEXAS Syndrome in a Patient with Myeloproliferative Neoplasia. *Case Rep. Hematol.* **2023**, *2023*, 6551544. [CrossRef] [PubMed]
9. Cherniawsky, H.; Friedmann, J.; Nicolson, H.; Dehghan, N.; Stubbins, R.J.; Foltz, L.M.; Leitch, H.A.; Sreenivasan, G.M.; Ambler, K.L.S.; Nevill, T.J.; et al. VEXAS syndrome: A review of bone marrow aspirate and biopsies reporting myeloid and erythroid precursor vacuolation. *Eur. J. Haematol.* **2023**, *110*, 633–638. [CrossRef] [PubMed]
10. Himmelmann, A.; Brucker, R. The VEXAS Syndrome: Uncontrolled Inflammation and Macrocytic Anaemia in a 77-Year-Old Male Patient. *Eur. J. Case Rep. Intern. Med.* **2021**, *8*, 002484. [CrossRef] [PubMed]
11. Lotscher, F.; Seitz, L.; Simeunovic, H.; Sarbu, A.C.; Porret, N.A.; Feldmeyer, L.; Borradori, L.; Bonadies, N.; Maurer, B. Case Report: Genetic Double Strike: VEXAS and TET2-Positive Myelodysplastic Syndrome in a Patient with Long-Standing Refractory Autoinflammatory Disease. *Front. Immunol.* **2021**, *12*, 800149. [CrossRef]
12. Obiorah, I.E.; Patel, B.A.; Groarke, E.M.; Wang, W.; Trick, M.; Ombrello, A.K.; Ferrada, M.A.; Wu, Z.; Gutierrez-Rodrigues, F.; Lotter, J.; et al. Benign and malignant hematologic manifestations in patients with VEXAS syndrome due to somatic mutations in UBA1. *Blood Adv.* **2021**, *5*, 3203–3215. [CrossRef]
13. Oganesyan, A.; Hakobyan, Y.; Terrier, B.; Georgin-Lavialle, S.; Mekinian, A. Looking beyond VEXAS: Coexistence of undifferentiated systemic autoinflammatory disease and myelodysplastic syndrome. *Semin. Hematol.* **2021**, *58*, 247–253. [CrossRef]
14. Comont, T.; Heiblig, M.; Riviere, E.; Terriou, L.; Rossignol, J.; Bouscary, D.; Rieu, V.; Le Guenno, G.; Mathian, A.; Aouba, A.; et al. Azacitidine for patients with Vacuoles, E1 Enzyme, X-linked, Autoinflammatory, Somatic syndrome (VEXAS) and myelodysplastic syndrome: Data from the French VEXAS registry. *Br. J. Haematol.* **2022**, *196*, 969–974. [CrossRef] [PubMed]
15. Diarra, A.; Duployez, N.; Fournier, E.; Preudhomme, C.; Coiteux, V.; Magro, L.; Quesnel, B.; Heiblig, M.; Sujobert, P.; Barraco, F.; et al. Successful allogeneic hematopoietic stem cell transplantation in patients with VEXAS syndrome: A 2-center experience. *Blood Adv.* **2022**, *6*, 998–1003. [CrossRef] [PubMed]
16. Kunishita, Y.; Kirino, Y.; Tsuchida, N.; Maeda, A.; Sato, Y.; Takase-Minegishi, K.; Yoshimi, R.; Nakajima, H. Case Report: Tocilizumab Treatment for VEXAS Syndrome With Relapsing Polychondritis: A Single-Center, 1-Year Longitudinal Observational Study In Japan. *Front. Immunol.* **2022**, *13*, 901063. [CrossRef] [PubMed]
17. Raaijmakers, M.; Hermans, M.; Aalbers, A.; Rijken, M.; Dalm, V.; van Daele, P.; Valk, P.J.M. Azacytidine Treatment for VEXAS Syndrome. *Hemasphere* **2021**, *5*, e661. [CrossRef] [PubMed]
18. Heiblig, M.; Ferrada, M.A.; Koster, M.J.; Barba, T.; Gerfaud-Valentin, M.; Mekinian, A.; Coelho, H.; Fossard, G.; Barraco, F.; Galicier, L.; et al. Ruxolitinib is more effective than other JAK inhibitors to treat VEXAS syndrome: A retrospective multicenter study. *Blood* **2022**, *140*, 927–931. [CrossRef] [PubMed]
19. Kipfer, B.; Daikeler, T.; Kuchen, S.; Hallal, M.; Andina, N.; Allam, R.; Bonadies, N. Increased cardiovascular comorbidities in patients with myelodysplastic syndromes and chronic myelomonocytic leukemia presenting with systemic inflammatory and autoimmune manifestations. *Semin. Hematol.* **2018**, *55*, 242–247. [CrossRef] [PubMed]
20. Ferrada, M.A.; Sikora, K.A.; Luo, Y.; Wells, K.V.; Patel, B.; Groarke, E.M.; Ospina Cardona, D.; Rominger, E.; Hoffmann, P.; Le, M.T.; et al. Somatic Mutations in UBA1 Define a Distinct Subset of Relapsing Polychondritis Patients With VEXAS. *Arthritis Rheumatol.* **2021**, *73*, 1886–1895. [CrossRef]
21. Assi, R.; Kantarjian, H.M.; Garcia-Manero, G.; Cortes, J.E.; Pemmaraju, N.; Wang, X.; Nogueras-Gonzalez, G.; Jabbour, E.; Bose, P.; Kadia, T.; et al. A phase II trial of ruxolitinib in combination with azacytidine in myelodysplastic syndrome/myeloproliferative neoplasms. *Am. J. Hematol.* **2018**, *93*, 277–285. [CrossRef] [PubMed]
22. Kouranloo, K.; Ashley, A.; Zhao, S.S.; Dey, M. Pulmonary manifestations in VEXAS (vacuoles, E1 enzyme, X-linked, autoinflammatory, somatic) syndrome: A systematic review. *Rheumatol. Int.* **2023**, *43*, 1023–1032. [CrossRef] [PubMed]
23. Lohaus, N.; Schaab, J.; Schaer, D.; Balabanov, S.; Huellner, M.W. VEXAS Syndrome With Tracheal Involvement but Absence of Vasculitis in FDG PET/CT. *Clin. Nucl. Med.* **2023**, *48*, e444–e445. [CrossRef] [PubMed]
24. Mekinian, A.; Zhao, L.P.; Chevret, S.; Desseaux, K.; Pascal, L.; Comont, T.; Maria, A.; Peterlin, P.; Terriou, L.; D'Aveni Piney, M.; et al. A Phase II prospective trial of azacitidine in steroid-dependent or refractory systemic autoimmune/inflammatory disorders and VEXAS syndrome associated with MDS and CMML. *Leukemia* **2022**, *36*, 2739–2742. [CrossRef]

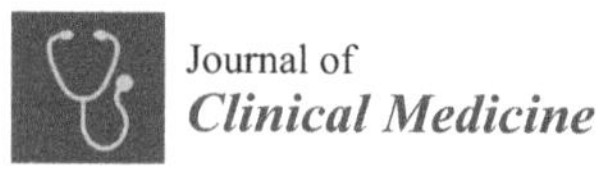

Journal of
Clinical Medicine

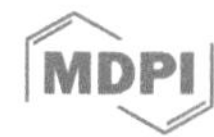

Article

Characteristics of Functional Hyperthermia Detected in an Outpatient Clinic for Fever of Unknown Origin

Kosuke Oka [1,*], Kazuki Tokumasu [1], Hideharu Hagiya [2] and Fumio Otsuka [1,2]

[1] Department of General Medicine, Okayama University Graduate School of Medicine, Dentistry and Pharmaceutical Sciences, Okayama 700-8558, Japan; tokumasu@okayama-u.ac.jp (K.T.); fumiotsu@md.okayama-u.ac.jp (F.O.)
[2] Department of Infectious Diseases, Okayama University Hospital, Okayama 700-8558, Japan; hagiya@okayama-u.ac.jp
* Correspondence: me20014@s.okayama-u.ac.jp; Tel.: +81-86-235-7342; Fax: +81-86-235-7345

Abstract: Background: Functional hyperthermia (FH) is characterized by hyperthermia resulting from sympathetic hyperactivity rather than inflammation, and it is frequently overlooked by medical practitioners due to the absence of abnormalities in a medical examination. Although FH is an important differential diagnosis for fever of unknown origin (FUO), the literature on FUO cases in Japan lacks information on FH. In this study, we aimed to uncover the population of FH patients hidden in FUO cases. **Methods:** An outpatient clinic for FUO was established at Okayama University Hospital, and 132 patients were examined during the period from May 2019 to February 2022. **Results:** A diagnosis of FH was made in 31.1% of the FUO cases, and FH predominantly affected individuals in their third and fourth decades of life with a higher incidence in females (68.3%). The frequency of a history of psychiatric illness was higher in patients with FH than in patients with other febrile illnesses. Although the C-reactive protein (CRP) is generally negative in FH cases, some obese patients, with a body mass index ≥ 25 had slightly elevated levels of CRP but were diagnosed with FH. **Conclusions:** The results showed the importance of identifying FH when encountering patients with FUO without any organic etiology.

Keywords: C-reactive protein (CRP); fever of unknown origin (FUO); functional hyperthermia (FH); psychiatric disorder; psychogenic fever

Citation: Oka, K.; Tokumasu, K.; Hagiya, H.; Otsuka, F. Characteristics of Functional Hyperthermia Detected in an Outpatient Clinic for Fever of Unknown Origin. *J. Clin. Med.* **2024**, *13*, 889. https://doi.org/10.3390/jcm13030889

Academic Editor: Eugen Feist

Received: 12 January 2024
Revised: 31 January 2024
Accepted: 1 February 2024
Published: 3 February 2024

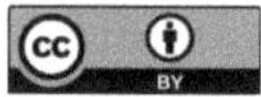

1. Introduction

Functional hyperthermia (FH), also known as psychogenic fever, manifests as an elevation in body temperature that is not orchestrated by inflammatory cytokines but is a result of sympathetic hyperactivity [1,2]. Increased body temperature secondary to various types of stress has been studied in animal models, and various acute psychological stresses have been reported to increase body temperature [3–20]. Of interest, such a stress-induced increase in body temperature was also observed in many species of animals other than rats and mice [21–30]. Since the publication of a report in 1977 showing that prostaglandins act on the preoptic area of the hypothalamus to cause fever, the mechanism of the control of body temperature has been gradually unveiled [31]. It has been suggested that both inflammatory diseases and FH result in elevated body temperature due to increased heat production via adrenergic β3 receptors and due to the suppression of heat release by vasoconstriction via α1 receptors stimulated by the dorsomedial hypothalamus (DMH) [32,33].

In cases of infectious fever, temperature elevation is caused by the prostaglandin E2 deinhibition of inhibitory inputs from the hypothalamic preoptic area to the DMH [34–36]. On the other hand, in cases of FH, temperature elevation is caused during stress through input signals from the dorsal peduncular cortex/dorsal tenia tecta (DP/DTT) in the medial prefrontal cortex area [37,38], wherein stress signals from multiple brain regions can be accumulated and connected to the induction of stress responses. Hence, a single stress stimulus causes transient hyperthermia, and continued chronic exposure to a stressor can lead to a habitually elevated body temperature without exposure to the stressor [39–41].

In humans, FH occurs mainly in young individuals and adolescents, and it is characterized by an absence of elevated inflammatory markers and the ineffectiveness of non-steroidal anti-inflammatory drugs (NSAIDs) [42–45]. Individuals afflicted with FH frequently complain of fatigue, headache, insomnia, and other symptoms. Even a temperature marginally surpassing 37 °C becomes distressing because it exacerbates fatigue [46]. Since the main symptom of FH is prolonged fever, patients often visit a department of internal medicine for the diagnosis and treatment of fever of unknown origin (FUO). However, FH is inadequately recognized among internists, and it frequently escapes notice due to the dearth of specific clinical findings or biomarkers. The confirmation of diagnosis hinges on the elevation of body temperature in response to psychological stress or the normalization of body temperature after the removal of the stressor. Explicit diagnostic criteria for FH have not yet been established, and diagnosis depends on the subjective clinical discernment of the attending clinician.

In general, FUO is one of the most challenging medical conditions, with causative diseases exhibiting diversity and variance contingent upon regional characteristics and practice settings. Since Petersdorf and Beeson reported their seminal study on FUO in 1961, a plethora of investigations on FUO have been reported [47]. Concerning the epidemiology of FUO cases in Japan, prevailing reports suggest relatively high incidences of autoimmune and malignant diseases as causative factors, which are attributable to improved diagnostic capabilities and an aging population [48,49]. Goto's study indicated the importance of encompassing a broad spectrum of febrile patients in studies for patients with temperatures surpassing 37 °C, challenging the conventional definition of FUO, which stipulates a fever of 38.3 °C or higher [50]. Previous studies, including our previous study, have shown the diagnostic utility of disease classification in febrile patients, the potential association between subclinical thyrotoxicosis and tachycardia during fever, and the efficacy of procalcitonin in febrile patients [51–53].

Although the significance of FH as a pivotal differential diagnosis in the domain of FUO has been proposed in several reports, there has been no study in which FH is incorporated into an investigation of the breakdown of final diagnoses in cases of FUO. Earlier reports suggest that approximately 20–30% of febrile cases remain undiagnosed, and we suspect that FH may account for some of these undiagnosed cases. We established an Outpatient Clinic for Fever of Unknown Origin at the Department of General Medicine of Okayama University Hospital. Through comprehensive analysis of FUO cases, we aimed to elucidate the prevalence of FH in cases of FUO, delineate the patient cohort for which the cause remained elusive in previous reports, and scrutinize trends and pathological conditions among patients presenting with FH.

2. Patients and Methods

2.1. Inclusion of Patients

Of the 146 patients who were referred to the Outpatient Clinic for FUO at Okayama University Hospital during the period from May 2019 to February 2022, 132 patients (47 males and 85 females) were included in this study after the exclusion of patients under 20 years of age. The Outpatient Clinic for FUO accepts patients with persistent temperatures of 37 °C or higher without being bound by the classic definition of FUO, for which the diagnosis is difficult. Their diagnostic breakdown and characteristics were systematically analyzed. The study protocol (#K-2308035) received approval from the Institutional Review Board (IRB) of Okayama University Graduate School of Medicine, Dentistry, and Pharmaceutical Sciences.

2.2. Definition of FH

In this study, the definition of FH was based on the following conditions according to previous reports [1,2,50]: (1) prolonged hyperthermia of 37 °C or higher for two months or longer, (2) the exclusion of organic febrile illness (through various tests, such as blood tests, endocrine tests, CT scans, etc.), (3) the history of a definitive stressor and the ensuing onset of prolonged fever, and (4) reproducible temperature increases with the stressor or return to normal temperature when the stressor is resolved. FH was diagnosed when criteria 1 + 2 + (3 and/or 4) were met.

2.3. Laboratory Examination

All the blood tests, including blood chemistry tests, were performed using an auto-analyzer system at the central laboratory of Okayama University Hospital for the differential diagnosis of FUO. The main system in our central laboratory was as follows: assays for complete blood count were performed using an electrical resistance method and a cyanmethemoglobin method using ADVIA2120 (Bayer AG, Leverkusen, Germany), and assays for serum CRP were performed using the latex agglutination turbidimetric immunoassay and BM8040 (JEOL, Tokyo, Japan). Assays for serum lactate dehydrogenase were also performed using BM8040. Assays for serum ferritin, plasma adrenocorticotropin, serum cortisol, serum-free thyroxin, and thyrotropin were performed using an electro-chemiluminescence immunoassay (ECLIA) and Cobas 8000 (F. Hoffmann-La Roche AG, Basel, Switzerland).

Specifically, the assay for the serum soluble interleukin-2 receptor was an enzyme immunoassay (EIA) using LUMIPULSE L2400 (Fujirebio, Tokyo, Japan). The assay for the serum anti-nuclear antibody was performed using a fluorescent antibody method in the laboratory. The assay for serum rheumatoid factor was a latex immunoturbidimetric assay using BM6050 (JEOL). The assay for serum anti-cyclic citrullinated peptide antibodies was a chemiluminescent enzyme immunoassay (CLEIA) using ARCHITECT i2000SR (Abbott, Chicago, IL, USA). The assay for serum anti-neutrophil antibodies was a fluorescence enzyme immunoassay (FEIA) using ImmunoCAP250 Phadia (Thermo Fisher Scientific, Waltham, MA, USA). Assays for serum cytomegalovirus antibodies were FEIAs using VIDAS (bioMerieux, Craponne, France). The assay for Epstein–Barr (EB) viral nucleic acid quantification was performed by a real-time polymerase chain reaction in the laboratory.

2.4. Statistical Analysis

The Mann–Whitney U test, Kruskal–Wallis test, and Fisher's exact probability test were used to analyze each group of data. In cases where there were discrepancies in the Kruskal–Wallis test, Steel–Dwass's post hoc test was used to ascertain which means exhibited differentiation. All statistical analyses were performed using EZR version 4. 2. 2; a p-value less than 0.05 was deemed indicative of a statistically significant difference. EZR (Saitama Medical Center, Jichi Medical University, Saitama, Japan) was used as the interface for R (The R Foundation for Statistical Computing, Vienna, Austria). To be precise, it is a modified version of the R commander curated to integrate statistical functions frequently employed in biostatistics [54].

3. Results

3.1. Clinical Backgrounds of the Patients with FUO

Table 1 shows the clinical backgrounds of the patients. The median age of the patients was 44 years. The majority of the patients were between the ages of 20 and 59 years. The patients included 85 females (64.4%) and 47 males (35.6%). The median axillary body temperature of the patients at the initial visit was 36.9 °C. The median duration of fever before the first visit to our clinic was 63 days. The median body mass index (BMI) of the patients was 21.1. In addition, 43 patients (32.6%) had a history of smoking.

Table 1. Background of patients who visited the Outpatient Clinic for Fever of Unknown Origin.

Patients' Background		
Age	**Case Number (Total 132 Patients)**	**Male/Female**
Median [IQR], years	44 [28–61.5]	47/85
20–29 years	42 (31.8%)	16/26
30–39 years	16 (12.1%)	4/12
40–49 years	20 (15.2%)	5/15
50–59 years	18 (13.6%)	9/9
60–69 years	11 (8.3%)	3/8
70–79 years	16 (12.1%)	7/9
80–89 years	9 (6.8%)	3/6
Body temperature Median [IQR] (°C)	36.9 [36.6–37.2]	
Fever duration Median [IQR] (days)	63 [30–240]	
BMI Median [IQR] (kg/m^2)	21.1 [18.5–26.1]	

IQR: Interquartile range.

3.2. Breakdown of the Final Diagnosis of FUO

Figure 1 shows a breakdown of the final diagnosis in individuals with FUO. A diagnosis of FH was made in 41 (31.1%) of the patients. There were 17 FH cases that met only the criteria of (3), 3 FH cases that met only the criteria of (4), and 21 FH cases that met the criteria of (3) and (4). Of the 41 patients with FH, 11 patients developed FH secondary to some physical event, such as an upper respiratory tract infection. Thirteen patients had joint pain, and four patients had skin rashes. Other diagnoses were familial Mediterranean fever in 8 patients (6.0%), microscopic polyangiitis in 3 patients (2.2%), polymyalgia rheumatica in 2 patients (1.5%), a chronic active EB virus infection in 2 patients (1.5%), and other identified diseases in 22 patients (16.7%). There were 54 unidentified febrile cases (40.9%). For the process of diagnosing FUO, 130 patients (85.6%) underwent a CT scan of their whole body, and 10 patients (7.6%) underwent a PET-CT scan. In addition, 5 patients received genetic testing in order to detect familial Mediterranean fever. As shown in Table 2, other identified diseases included myelodysplastic syndromes, adult-onset Still's disease, miliary tuberculosis, HIV infection, rheumatoid arthritis, dermatomyositis, cytomegalovirus infection, Graves' disease, and Fitzhugh–Curtis syndrome.

3.3. Distributions of Ages and Genders of Patients with FH

Figure 2 shows the distribution of ages and genders in the patients diagnosed with FH. Patients with FH were predominantly women in their 20 s to 40 s. Males accounted for 31.7% of the cases, and females accounted for 68.3% of the cases.

3.4. Past Psychiatric Disorders in the Patients with FH

Figure 3 shows the percentage of patients diagnosed with FH who previously attended a psychiatrist for any reason. FH patients with a psychiatric history accounted for about half (48.8%) of the FH patients, and this percentage was significantly higher than that in the organic disease group (10.8%; $p < 0.01$).

3.5. Interrelationship between Serum CRP Level and BMI in Patients with FH

Figure 4A shows the serum CRP levels in FH patients in two BMI-dependent groups, and Figure 4B shows the serum CRP levels in patients with a diagnosis other than FH in the two BMI-dependent groups. Obese patients with BMI $\geq$ 25 showed significantly higher serum CRP levels than those in patients with BMI < 25 ($p < 0.01$). There were no significant differences between the two BMI groups for patients with a diagnosis other than FH.

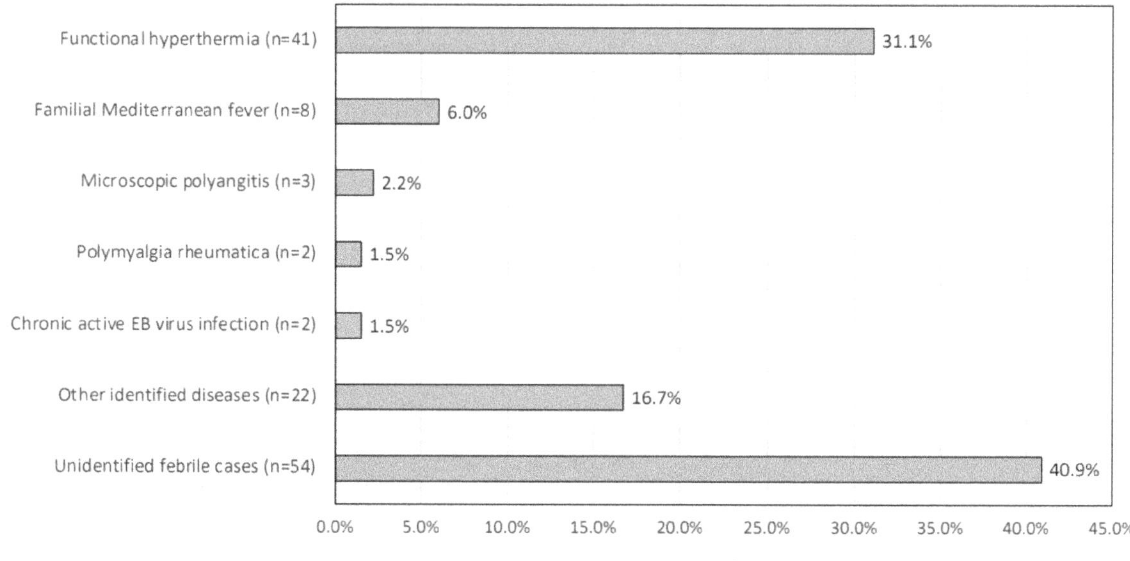

Figure 1. Final diagnosis of the patients with FUO. The diagnostic breakdown of patients who visited the Outpatient Clinic for Fever of Unknown Origin is shown.

Table 2. List of final diagnoses included in other identified diseases.

Final Diagnosis
Adult-onset Still's disease
Aseptic meningitis
Aspiration pneumonia
Carcinomatous pleurisy
Clostridium difficile-associated diarrhea
Cytomegalovirus infection
Dermatomyositis
Drug allergy
Fitz–Hugh–Curtis syndrome
Graves' disease
Human immunodeficiency virus infection
Inflammatory lymphadenitis
Lung abscess
Miliary tuberculosis
Myelodysplastic syndromes
Neurogenic fever
PFAPA syndrome
Pharyngeal carcinoma
Post-vaccination reaction to coronavirus vaccine
Pseudogout
Rheumatoid arthritis
Ureteral obstruction

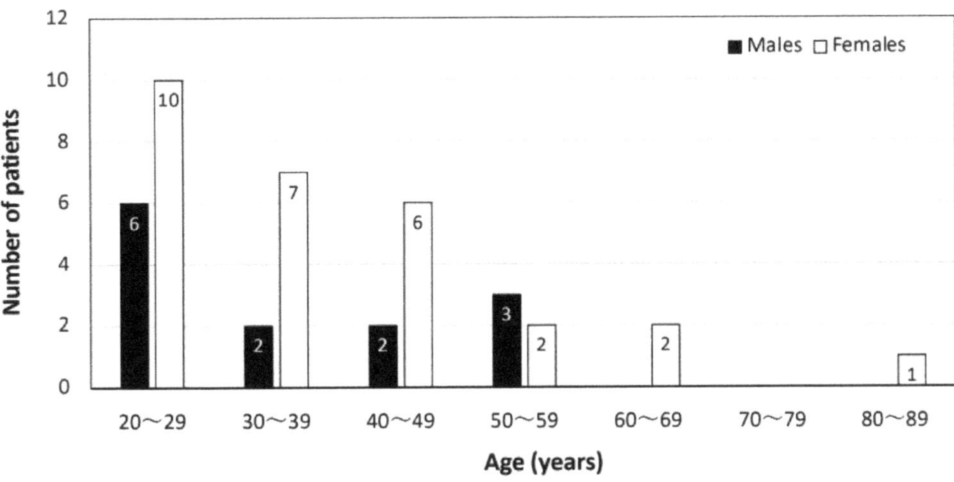

Figure 2. Characteristics of patients with FH. The age and gender distributions of patients diagnosed with FH in the Outpatient Clinic for Fever of Unknown Origin are shown.

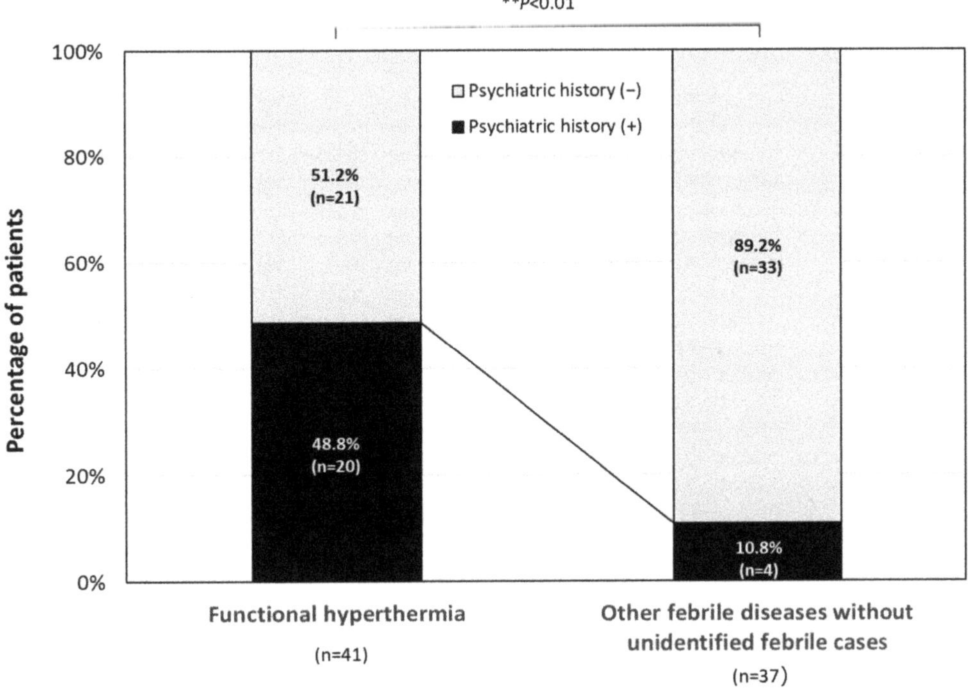

Figure 3. Past psychiatric disorders in patients with FH. The psychiatric histories of patients with FH are shown. Data were analyzed using Fisher's exact probability test. ** $p < 0.01$ between the indicated groups.

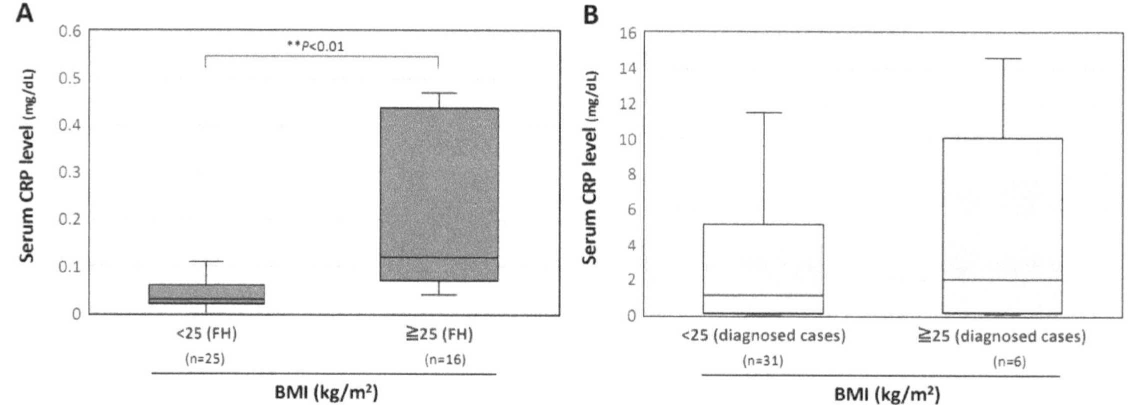

Figure 4. Relationships between the serum CRP level and obesity in patients with FH. Serum CRP levels are shown in two BMI groups (<25 and ≥25) (**A**) for patients with FH and (**B**) for patients with a diagnosis other than FH. The median is shown by the horizontal bar within the box, and the IQR is shown by the upper and lower horizontal bars of the box. The upper and lower horizontal bars outside the box represent the maximum and minimum values within 1.5 times the interquartile range. Data were analyzed using the Kruskal–Wallis test. If differences were detected, Steel–Dwass's post hoc test was used to determine divergent means. ** $p < 0.01$ between the indicated groups.

4. Discussion

In the present study, we show the proportion of FH cases in FUO cases and the clinical characteristics of FH. FH cases accounted for about 30% of the FUO cases examined in our outpatient clinic for FUO. Although there have been reports on cases of FUO in Japan, including reports from Okayama University Hospital, those reports predominantly focused on inflammatory diseases such as infectious diseases, malignant diseases, and collagen diseases with no mention of FH [46,48,49,51,53]. The reason why FH has not been described in previous reports on FUO may be that FH has been relegated to the unidentified category of fever cases because there are no abnormalities that can be identified in a medical examination, and its presence is relatively unfamiliar to physicians. However, our study suggests that FH is a crucial differential diagnosis and that FH cases account for the majority of FUO cases.

The majority of patients with persistent FUO have a favorable prognosis, the characteristics of which align well with those of FH [50,55]. In cases of FUO examined in departments other than internal medicine, FH was reported to be diagnosed in 18.3%, 5.2%, and 4.4% of outpatients in pediatrics, child psychiatry, and obstetrics and gynecology departments, respectively [43]. Consequently, FH is not uncommon in clinical practice and is likely to be diagnosed in various medical departments. Internists, who play a pivotal role in fever treatment, need to be aware of FH.

In this study, familial Mediterranean fever was the second most prevalent cause of fever after FH. Familial Mediterranean fever, categorized as an autoinflammatory disease, belongs to a category that is different from infectious diseases, collagen diseases, and malignant diseases, which historically served as representative causes of FUO. It is imperative to adopt a flexible approach in the identification of the cause of FUO that is not subjected to constraints imposed by antecedent reports. The causative diseases of FUO other than FH and the familial Mediterranean fever in the present study were similar to those previously reported. Patients diagnosed with FH were predominantly women in their 20 s to 40 s, with a male-to-female ratio of 1:2.15. Although patients aged 19 years or younger were excluded from the present study, making direct comparisons with other studies difficult, the results of this study suggest that FH occurs more frequently in relatively young women, in accordance with the results of previous studies.

The results of the present study also suggest that patients with a history of psychiatric consultation are a high-risk group for FH. Since FH is characterized by an elevation in body temperature under stressful mental conditions, a history of psychiatric visits may be helpful in diagnosing FH in febrile patients without organic disease. It is also considered to be important to resolve the backgrounds of psychiatric disorders for the treatment of patients with FH [56]. In the present study, FH in approximately one-quarter of the patients with FH was possibly triggered by their preceding physical stress. Chronic fatigue syndrome (CFS), similarly triggered by physical stress events, is known to be complicated by hyperthermia [1,57–59]. The similarity between the modes of onset of FH and CFS and the fact that FH and CFS can merge with each other suggest that FH and CFS may have a common pathogenesis [60]. Further investigation is needed to determine whether patients with FH concurrently manifest CFS.

In the FH group, obese patients with a BMI $\geq 25 \text{ kg/m}^2$ showed a significantly higher CRP level than that in patients with a BMI $< 25 \text{ kg/m}^2$. Previous studies showed that there is a marginal elevation of CRP in obese patients, and a similar trend was observed in the present study [61–63]. While CRP is generally negative in patients without inflammatory disease, including those with FH, obese patients may show a slightly heightened inflammatory response even in the absence of inflammatory disease. Consequently, in obese patients with FUO, FH should remain within the differential diagnosis, even if they have a slightly increased level of CRP.

The present study has several limitations. This study was a single-center study and only included patients who visited the Outpatient Clinic for Fever of Unknown Origin, not a general outpatient clinic. The high prevalence of FH in comparison with the prevalence of infectious diseases, collagen diseases, and malignant diseases, historically reported as the primary pathogenesis of FUO, may be due to the single-center nature of this study, in which only patients visiting an outpatient clinic for FUO were included. Correspondingly, data from another outpatient clinic for FUO in the National Center for Global Health and Medicine indicated that FH accounted for 23.5% of FUO cases [64]. These findings imply that the high prevalence of FH in the FUO cases in this study, unlike in previous studies, may merely indicate that FH is more likely to be encountered in an outpatient clinic for FUO.

In conclusion, this study shows that FH may account for a substantial proportion of FUO cases and that FH occurs predominantly in women in their 20 s to 40 s. This study also shows that patients with a history of psychiatric visits are at high risk for FH and that the possibility of FH cannot be excluded even if serum CRP levels are slightly elevated in FUO cases among obese patients. Recognizing that FH is an important differential disease in FUO practice could help medical practitioners to accurately diagnose and guide FUO patients to a resolution.

Author Contributions: K.O. and F.O. conceived and designed the study; K.O. and K.T. performed data collection; K.O. and H.H. analyzed the data; K.O. and K.T. wrote the paper; H.H. and F.O. revised the paper. All authors have read and agreed to the published version of the manuscript.

Funding: This research was supported by a Research Grant from the Japanese Society of Hospital General Medicine (K.O.).

Institutional Review Board Statement: This study was conducted in accordance with the Declaration of Helsinki and was approved by the Ethics Committee of Okayama University Hospital (#K-2308035, approved on 21 July 2023).

Informed Consent Statement: Obtaining informed consent from the patients was not necessary due to the anonymization of the data. Information regarding the present study was provided on our hospital wall and the website of our hospital, and patients who wished to opt out were offered that opportunity.

Data Availability Statement: Detailed data are available if requested from the corresponding author.

Acknowledgments: We are sincerely grateful to the clinical and office staff at the Department of General Medicine who contributed to the present work.

Conflicts of Interest: The authors declare no conflicts of interest.

Abbreviations

Chronic fatigue syndrome (CFS), C-reactive protein (CRP), Epstein-Barr (EB), fever of unknown origin (FUO), functional hyperthermia (FH), and non-steroidal anti-inflammatory drugs (NSAIDs).

References

1. Oka, T. Stress-induced hyperthermia and hypothermia. *Handb. Clin. Neurol.* **2018**, *157*, 599–621.
2. Oka, T. Psychogenic fever: How psychological stress affects body temperature in the clinical population. *Temperature* **2015**, *2*, 368–378. [CrossRef]
3. Singer, R.; Harker, C.T.; Vander, A.J.; Kluger, M.J. Hyperthermia induced by open-field stress is blocked by salicylate. *Physiol. Behav.* **1986**, *36*, 1179–1182. [CrossRef] [PubMed]
4. Soszynski, D.; Kozak, W.; Kluger, M.J. Endotoxin tolerance does not alter open field-induced fever in rats. *Physiol. Behav.* **1998**, *63*, 689–692. [CrossRef] [PubMed]
5. Butterweck, V.; Prinz, S.; Schwaninger, M. The role of interleukin-6 in stress-induced hyperthermia and emotional behaviour in mice. *Behav. Brain Res.* **2003**, *144*, 49–56. [CrossRef] [PubMed]
6. Long, N.C.; Vander, A.J.; Kunkel, S.L.; Kluger, M.J. Antiserum against tumor necrosis factor increases stress hyperthermia in rats. *Am. J. Physiol.* **1990**, *258 Pt 2*, R591–R595. [CrossRef] [PubMed]
7. Morimoto, A.; Nakamori, T.; Morimoto, K.; Tan, N.; Murakami, N. The central role of corticotrophin-releasing factor (CRF-41) in psychological stress in rats. *J. Physiol.* **1993**, *460*, 221–229. [CrossRef] [PubMed]
8. Oka, T.; Oka, K.; Kobayashi, T.; Sugimoto, Y.; Ichikawa, A.; Ushikubi, F.; Narumiya, S.; Saper, C.B. Characteristics of thermoregulatory and febrile responses in mice deficient in prostaglandin EP1 and EP3 receptors. *J. Physiol.* **2003**, *551 Pt 3*, 945–954. [CrossRef] [PubMed]
9. Shibata, H.; Nagasaka, T. Contribution of nonshivering thermogenesis to stress-induced hyperthermia in rats. *Jpn. J. Physiol.* **1982**, *32*, 991–995. [CrossRef] [PubMed]
10. Shibata, H.; Nagasaka, T. Role of sympathetic nervous system in immobilization- and cold-induced brown adipose tissue thermogenesis in rats. *Jpn. J. Physiol.* **1984**, *34*, 103–111. [CrossRef]
11. Gao, B.; Kikuchi-Utsumi, K.; Ohinata, H.; Hashimoto, M.; Kuroshima, A. Repeated immobilization stress increases uncoupling protein 1 expression and activity in Wistar rats. *Jpn. J. Physiol.* **2003**, *53*, 205–213. [CrossRef]
12. Ootsuka, Y.; Blessing, W.W.; Nalivaiko, E. Selective blockade of 5-HT2A receptors attenuates the increased temperature response in brown adipose tissue to restraint stress in rats. *Stress* **2008**, *11*, 125–133. [CrossRef]
13. Borsini, F.; Lecci, A.; Volterra, G.; Meli, A. A model to measure anticipatory anxiety in mice? *Psychopharmacology* **1989**, *98*, 207–211. [CrossRef] [PubMed]
14. Zethof, T.J.J.; Van Der Heyden, J.A.M.; Tolboom, J.T.B.M.; Olivier, B. Stress-induced hyperthermia as a putative anxiety model. *Eur. J. Pharmacol.* **1995**, *294*, 125–135. [CrossRef] [PubMed]
15. Vinkers, C.H.; van Bogaert, M.J.V.; Klanker, M.; Korte, S.M.; Oosting, R.; Hanania, T.; Hopkins, S.C.; Olivier, B.; Groenink, L. Translational aspects of pharmacological research into anxiety disorders: The stress-induced hyperthermia (SIH) paradigm. *Eur. J. Pharmacol.* **2008**, *585*, 407–425. [CrossRef] [PubMed]
16. Beig, M.I.; Baumert, M.; Walker, F.R.; Day, T.A.; Nalivaiko, E. Blockade of 5-HT2A receptors suppresses hyperthermic but not cardiovascular responses to psychosocial stress in rats. *Neuroscience* **2009**, *159*, 1185–1191. [CrossRef] [PubMed]
17. Hayashida, S.; Oka, T.; Mera, T.; Tsuji, S. Repeated social defeat stress induces chronic hyperthermia in rats. *Physiol. Behav.* **2010**, *101*, 124–131. [CrossRef] [PubMed]
18. Lkhagvasuren, B.; Nakamura, Y.; Oka, T.; Sudo, N.; Nakamura, K. Social defeat stress induces hyperthermia through activation of thermoregulatory sympathetic premotor neurons in the medullary raphe region. *Eur. J. Neurosci.* **2011**, *34*, 1442–1452. [CrossRef] [PubMed]
19. Lkhagvasuren, B.; Oka, T.; Nakamura, Y.; Hayashi, H.; Sudo, N.; Nakamura, K. Distribution of Fos-immunoreactive cells in rat forebrain and midbrain following social defeat stress and diazepam treatment. *Neuroscience* **2014**, *272*, 34–57. [CrossRef] [PubMed]
20. Mohammed, M.; Ootsuka, Y.; Blessing, W. Brown adipose tissue thermogenesis contributes to emotional hyperthermia in a resident rat suddenly confronted with an intruder rat. *Am. J. Physiol. Regul. Integr. Comp. Physiol.* **2014**, *306*, R394–R400. [CrossRef]
21. Yokoi, Y. Effect of ambient temperature upon emotional hyperthermia and hypothermia in rabbits. *J. Appl. Physiol.* **1966**, *21*, 1795–1798. [CrossRef] [PubMed]
22. Kohlhause, S.; Hoffmann, K.; Schlumbohm, C.; Fuchs, E.; Flügge, G. Nocturnal hyperthermia induced by social stress in male tree shrews: Relation to low testosterone and effects of age. *Physiol. Behav.* **2011**, *104*, 786–795. [CrossRef] [PubMed]

23. Schmelting, B.; Corbach-Söhle, S.; Kohlhause, S.; Schlumbohm, C.; Flügge, G.; Fuchs, E. Agomelatine in the tree shrew model of depression: Effects on stress-induced nocturnal hyperthermia and hormonal status. *Eur. Neuropsychopharmacol.* **2014**, *24*, 437–447. [CrossRef] [PubMed]
24. Pedernera-Romano, C.; Ruiz de la Torre, J.L.; Badiella, L.; Manteca, X. Effect of perphenazine enanthate on open-field test behaviour and stress-induced hyperthermia in domestic sheep. *Pharmacol. Biochem. Behav.* **2010**, *94*, 329–332. [CrossRef] [PubMed]
25. Muchlinski, A.E.; Baldwin, B.C.; Padick, D.A.; Lee, B.Y.; Salguero, H.S.; Gramajo, R. California ground squirrel body temperature regulation patterns measured in the laboratory and in the natural environment. *Comp. Biochem. Physiol. A Mol. Integr. Physiol.* **1998**, *120*, 365–372. [CrossRef] [PubMed]
26. Lee, B.Y.; Padick, D.A.; Muchlinski, A.E. Stress fever magnitude in laboratory-maintained California ground squirrels varies with season. *Comp. Biochem. Physiol. A Mol. Integr. Physiol.* **2000**, *125*, 325–330. [CrossRef]
27. Parr, L.A.; Hopkins, W.D. Brain temperature asymmetries and emotional perception in chimpanzees, Pan troglodytes. *Physiol. Behav.* **2000**, *71*, 363–371. [CrossRef]
28. Meyer, L.C.R.; Fick, L.; Matthee, A.; Mitchell, D.; Fuller, A. Hyperthermia in captured impala (*Aepyceros melampus*): A fright not flight response. *J. Wildl. Dis.* **2008**, *44*, 404–416. [CrossRef]
29. Gray, D.A.; Maloney, S.K.; Kamerman, P.R. Restraint increases afebrile body temperature but attenuates fever in Pekin ducks (*Anas platyrhynchos*). *Am. J. Physiol. Regul. Integr. Comp. Physiol.* **2008**, *294*, R1666–R1671. [CrossRef] [PubMed]
30. de Aguiar Bittencourt, M.; Melleu, F.F.; Marino-Neto, J. Stress-induced core temperature changes in pigeons (*Columba livia*). *Physiol. Behav.* **2015**, *139*, 449–458. [CrossRef] [PubMed]
31. Williams, J.W.; Rudy, T.A.; Yaksh, T.L.; Viswanathan, C.T. An extensive exploration of the rat brain for sites mediating prostaglandin-induced hyperthermia. *Brain Res.* **1977**, *120*, 251–262. [CrossRef]
32. Nakamura, K.; Matsumura, K.; Hübschle, T.; Nakamura, Y.; Hioki, H.; Fujiyama, F.; Boldogköi, Z.; König, M.; Thiel, H.-J.; Gerstberger, R.; et al. Identification of sympathetic premotor neurons in medullary raphe regions mediating fever and other thermoregulatory functions. *J. Neurosci.* **2004**, *24*, 5370–5380. [CrossRef] [PubMed]
33. Rathner, J.A.; Madden, C.J.; Morrison, S.F. Central pathway for spontaneous and prostaglandin E2 evoked cutaneous vasoconstriction. *Am. J. Physiol. Regul. Integr. Comp. Physiol.* **2008**, *295*, R343–R354. [CrossRef]
34. Lazarus, M.; Yoshida, K.; Coppari, R.; Bass, C.E.; Mochizuki, T.; Lowell, B.B.; Saper, C.B. EP3 prostaglandin receptors in the median preoptic nucleus are critical for fever responses. *Nat. Neurosci.* **2007**, *10*, 1131–1133. [CrossRef]
35. Morrison, S.F.; Nakamura, K. Central neural pathways for thermoregulation. *Front. Biosci.* **2011**, *16*, 74–104. [CrossRef] [PubMed]
36. Nakamura, K.; Matsumura, K.; Kaneko, T.; Kobayashi, S.; Katoh, H.; Negishi, M. The rostral raphe pallidus nucleus mediates pyrogenic transmission from the preoptic area. *J. Neurosci.* **2002**, *22*, 4600–4610. [CrossRef] [PubMed]
37. Kataoka, N.; Hioki, H.; Kaneko, T.; Nakamura, K. Psychological stress activates a dorsomedial hypothalamus-medullary raphe circuit driving brown adipose tissue thermogenesis and hyperthermia. *Cell Metab.* **2014**, *20*, 346–358. [CrossRef]
38. Kataoka, N.; Shima, Y.; Nakajima, K.; Nakamura, K. A central master driver of psychosocial stress responses in the rat. *Science* **2020**, *367*, 1105–1112. [CrossRef]
39. Kuroshima, A.; Habara, Y.; Uehara, A.; Murazumi, K.; Yahata, T.; Ohno, T. Cross adaption between stress and cold in rats. *Pflug. Arch.* **1984**, *402*, 402–408. [CrossRef]
40. Kuroshima, A.; Yahata, T. Changes in the colonic temperature and metabolism during immobilization stress in repetitively immobilized or cold-acclimated rats. *Jpn. J. Physiol.* **1985**, *35*, 591–597. [CrossRef]
41. Nozu, T.; Okano, S.; Kikuchi, K.; Yahata, T.; Kuroshima, A. Effect of immobilization stress on in vitro and in vivo thermogenesis of brown adipose tissue. *Jpn. J. Physiol.* **1992**, *42*, 299–308. [CrossRef]
42. Kaneda, Y.; Tsuji, S.; Oka, T. Age distribution and gender differences in psychogenic fever patients. *Biopsychosoc. Med.* **2009**, *3*, 6. [CrossRef]
43. Oka, T.; Oka, K. Age and gender differences of psychogenic fever: A review of the Japanese literature. *Biopsychosoc. Med.* **2007**, *1*, 11. [CrossRef]
44. Hiramoto, T.; Oka, T.; Yoshihara, K.; Kubo, C. Pyrogenic cytokines did not mediate a stress interview-induced hyperthermic response in a patient with psychogenic fever: A case report. *Psychosom. Med.* **2009**, *71*, 932–936. [CrossRef] [PubMed]
45. McNeil, G.N.; Leighton, L.H.; Elkins, A.M. Possible psychogenic fever of 103.5 degrees F in a patient with borderline personality disorder. *Am. J. Psychiatry* **1984**, *141*, 896–897. [PubMed]
46. Oka, T.; Hayashida, S.; Kaneda, Y.; Kodama, N.; Hashimoto, T.; Tsuji, S. Why do chronic stress-induced hyperthermia patients worry about slightly elevated body temperature? *Jpn. J. Psychosom. Intern. Med.* **2006**, *10*, 243–246.
47. Petersdorf, R.G.; Beeson, P.B. Fever of unexplained origin: Report on 100 cases. *Medicine* **1961**, *40*, 1–30. [CrossRef]
48. Naito, T.; Mizooka, M.; Mitsumoto, F.; Kanazawa, K.; Torikai, K.; Ohno, S.; Morita, H.; Ukimura, A.; Mishima, N.; Otsuka, F.; et al. Diagnostic workup for fever of unknown origin: A multicenter collaborative retrospective study. *BMJ Open* **2013**, *3*, e003971. [CrossRef]
49. Naito, T.; Tanei, M.; Ikeda, N.; Ishii, T.; Suzuki, T.; Morita, H.; Yamasaki, S.; Tamura, J.; Akazawa, K.; Yamamoto, K.; et al. Key diagnostic characteristics of fever of unknown origin in Japanese patients: A prospective multicentre study. *BMJ Open.* **2019**, *9*, e032059. [CrossRef]

50. Goto, M.; Koyama, H.; Takahashi, O.; Fukui, T. A retrospective review of 226 hospitalized patients with fever. *Intern. Med.* **2007**, *46*, 17–22. [CrossRef]
51. Ryuko, H.; Otsuka, F. A comprehensive analysis of 174 febrile patients admitted to Okayama University Hospital. *Acta Med. Okayama* **2013**, *67*, 227–237.
52. Araki, J.; Oka, K.; Yamamoto, K.; Hanayama, Y.; Tokumasu, K.; Hagiya, H.; Ogawa, H.; Itoshima, K.; Otsuka, F. Interrelationships Between Serum Levels of Procalcitonin and Inflammatory Markers in Patients Who Visited a General Medicine Department. *Acta Med. Okayama* **2021**, *75*, 299–306.
53. Oka, K.; Hanayama, Y.; Sato, A.; Omura, D.; Yasuda, M.; Hasegawa, K.; Obika, M.; Otsuka, F. Clinical Characteristics of Febrile Outpatients: Possible Involvement of Thyroid Dysfunction in Febrile Tachycardia. *Acta Med. Okayama* **2018**, *72*, 447–456.
54. Kanda, Y. Investigation of the freely available easy-to-use software "EZR" for medical statistics. *Bone Marrow Transpl.* **2013**, *48*, 452–458. [CrossRef]
55. Knockaert, D.C.; Dujardin, K.S.; Bobbaers, H.J. Long-term follow-up of patients with undiagnosed fever of unknown origin—PubMed. *Arch. Intern. Med.* **1996**, *156*, 618–620. [CrossRef]
56. Oka, T. Functional hyperthermia and comorbid psychiatric disorders. *Biopsychosoc. Med.* **2023**, *17*, 39. [CrossRef] [PubMed]
57. Hickie, I.; Davenport, T.; Wakefield, D.; Vollmer-Conna, U.; Cameron, B.; Vernon, S.D.; Reeves, W.C.; Lloyd, A. Post-infective and chronic fatigue syndromes precipitated by viral and non-viral pathogens: Prospective cohort study. *BMJ* **2006**, *333*, 575–578. [CrossRef] [PubMed]
58. Salit, I.E. Precipitating factors for the chronic fatigue syndrome. *J. Psychiatr. Res.* **1997**, *31*, 59–65. [CrossRef] [PubMed]
59. Oka, T.; Kanemitsu, Y.; Sudo, N.; Hayashi, H.; Oka, K. Psychological stress contributed to the development of low-grade fever in a patient with chronic fatigue syndrome: A case report. *Biopsychosoc. Med.* **2013**, *7*, 7. [CrossRef] [PubMed]
60. Ginier-Gillet, M. "Functional hyperthermia": A historical overview. *Biopsychosoc. Med.* **2023**, *17*, 38. [CrossRef] [PubMed]
61. Wee, C.C.; Mukamal, K.J.; Huang, A.; Davis, R.B.; McCarthy, E.P.; Mittleman, M.A. Obesity and C-reactive protein levels among white, black, and hispanic US adults. *Obesity* **2008**, *16*, 875–880. [CrossRef] [PubMed]
62. Choi, J.; Joseph, L.; Pilote, L. Obesity and C-reactive protein in various populations: A systematic review and meta-analysis. *Obes. Rev.* **2013**, *14*, 232–244. [CrossRef] [PubMed]
63. Visser, M.; Bouter, L.M.; McQuillan, G.M.; Wener, M.H.; Harris, T.B. Elevated C-reactive protein levels in overweight and obese adults. *JAMA* **1999**, *282*, 2131–2135. [CrossRef] [PubMed]
64. Kunimatsu, J. *Gairai de Miru Humeinetsu*, 1st ed.; Nakayama-Shoten: Tokyo, Japan, 2017; pp. 19–30, ISBN 978-4-521-74539-8.

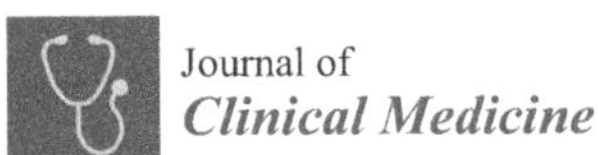

Journal of
Clinical Medicine

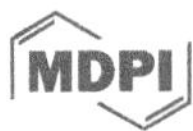

Article

Autoinflammatory Diseases and COVID-19 Vaccination: Analysis of SARS-CoV-2 Anti-S-RBD IgG Levels in a Cohort of Patients Receiving IL-1 Inhibitors

Sara Bindoli [1,†], Chiara Baggio [1,†], Paola Galozzi [2], Filippo Vesentini [1], Andrea Doria [1], Chiara Cosma [2], Andrea Padoan [2] and Paolo Sfriso [1,*]

[1] Rheumatology Unit, Department of Medicine, University of Padova, 35128 Padova, Italy; sara.bindoli@phd.unipd.it (S.B.); chiara.baggio@unipd.it (C.B.); filippo.vesentini@studenti.unipd.it (F.V.); adoria@unipd.it (A.D.)
[2] Laboratory Medicine Unit, Department of Medicine, University of Padova, 35128 Padova, Italy; paola.galozzi@unipd.it (P.G.); chiara.cosma@aopd.veneto.it (C.C.); andrea.padoan@unipd.it (A.P.)
* Correspondence: paolo.sfriso@unipd.it; Tel.: +49-8211206
† These authors contributed equally to this work.

Abstract: The purpose of the study was to evaluate the antibody response after COVID-19 vaccination in patients affected by systemic autoinflammatory diseases (SAID) undertaking IL-1 inhibitors (IL-1i) compared to healthy vaccinated controls (HC). The course of COVID-19 in vaccinated patients on IL-1i was also assessed. The serological response was evaluated in SAID patients using the CLIA MAGLUMI TM 2000 Plus test after the first vaccination cycle and the booster dose. Fifty-four fully vaccinated healthcare workers were enrolled as HCs. GraphPad Prism 8 software was used for statistical analysis. All patients developed an adequate antibody response. No differences were observed between the antibody titers of patients on IL-1i and those not on IL-1i, either after the first vaccination cycle or the booster dose ($p = 0.99$), and to HC ($p = 0.99$). With increasing age, a decrease in antibody production was assessed after the second vaccine in SAID ($r = 0.67$, $p = 0.0003$). In general, 11.6% of SAID patients had COVID-19 after receiving vaccination. None of them developed severe disease or experienced flares of their autoinflammatory disease. In conclusion, patients receiving IL-1i develop an antibody response comparable to HC. No side effects after vaccination were observed; IL-1i was continued before and after injections to avoid flare-ups.

Keywords: COVID-19; SARS-CoV-2 vaccination; anti-IL-1 drugs; anakinra; canakinumab; antibody response

Citation: Bindoli, S.; Baggio, C.; Galozzi, P.; Vesentini, F.; Doria, A.; Cosma, C.; Padoan, A.; Sfriso, P. Autoinflammatory Diseases and COVID-19 Vaccination: Analysis of SARS-CoV-2 Anti-S-RBD IgG Levels in a Cohort of Patients Receiving IL-1 Inhibitors. *J. Clin. Med.* **2023**, *12*, 4741. https://doi.org/10.3390/jcm12144741

Academic Editor: Erkan Demirkaya

Received: 27 April 2023
Revised: 7 July 2023
Accepted: 16 July 2023
Published: 18 July 2023

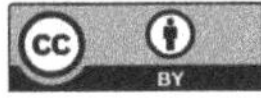

1. Introduction

The introduction of anti-SARS-CoV2 vaccination, which started in early 2021, has dramatically changed the severity course of COVID-19, not only in the general population but also in patients affected by different pathologies, such as cardiovascular diseases, diabetes, oncological disease, and rheumatological diseases (RD). In this field, a great deal of attention was directed toward those affected by autoimmune diseases, in particular those receiving conventional synthetic disease-modifying drugs (csDMARDs), biologics/target synthetic (b/ts) DMARDs, or anti-CD-20 drugs (rituximab). It is well known that patients affected by autoimmune and autoinflammatory syndromes [1] who undertake immunosuppressant and immunomodulatory therapies may have reduced immunogenicity after vaccination [2]. Indeed, those treated with mycophenolate mofetil, rituximab, abatacept, or glucocorticoids may present with reduced serological response [2]. A recent meta-analysis of 20 seroprevalence studies on SARS-CoV-2 vaccination reported the highest seroconversion rates with hydroxychloroquine and sulfasalazine. At the same time, methotrexate (either used in monotherapy or combination with other treatments) and rituximab were associated with the lowest response rates (81.9% and 36.3%, respectively); however anti-cytokine treatments were associated with a good seroconversion rate (>89%) either for TNF-alpha inhibitors, IL-6 inhibitors, IL-17 inhibitors, IL-1 receptor antagonist (anakinra) and Janus Kinases Inhibitors (JAK-I) [3]. In systemic autoinflammatory diseases (SAID), the effect of vaccination has hardly been reported. In a recent prospective study, it was observed that patients affected by severe COVID-19 and treated with anakinra alone or in combination with tocilizumab subsequently did not have an altered antibody response [4]; another study investigating the effect of vaccination on autoinflammatory diseases showed that the anti-SARS-CoV-2 vaccine was well tolerated in patients with pathologies mediated by IL-1, IL-18, and interferon (IFN)-γ, with no disease relapses requiring hospitalization, and presenting an adequate antibody production after the booster dose [5]. Regarding safety and adverse events (AEs), a recent study on Familial Mediterranean Fever (FMF) observed that 93 out of 161 patients reported adverse events/fever attacks after vaccination, with 54.7% of AEs occurring after mRNA vaccines [6]. A cross-sectional observational study in Turkey involving patients affected by FMF, Behçet Disease (BD), and rheumatic diseases (RD) other than FMF and BD observed a similar frequency of AEs in FMF/BD compared to RD. However, data on immunogenicity were not reported [7]. In general, anti-SARS-CoV-2 vaccination was well tolerated in patients with RD, with the vast majority obtaining a consistent serological response and reassuring patients treated with immunomodulatory therapies on the immunogenicity and short-term safety of the injections [8]. The present work aims to evaluate the levels of SARS-CoV-2 Spike protein Receptor Binding Domain (S-RBD) IgG antibody in a group of patients treated with IL-1 inhibitors (IL-1i), anakinra and canakinumab to observe whether IL-1i may be associated or not with a reduced serological response compared to a group of fully vaccinated healthy controls (HCs).

2. Materials and Methods

2.1. Clinical and Demographic Characteristics of the Patients Included in the Study

Forty-six SAID patients and fifty-four age- and sex-matched HCs were included in the study. The demographical and clinical data of SAID patients are depicted in Table 1 and graphically presented in Figure 1. SAID patients were included if they were injected with the anti-SARS-CoV-2 vaccine and if they were treated with IL-1i (anakinra or canakinumab) alone or in combination with colchicine or glucocorticoids (GCs) if they received colchicine, GCs, or if they were not on treatment for disease remission (but previously treated with colchicine or GCs). No relevant comorbidities (cardiovascular or oncological pathologies, pre-existing lung disease, or diabetes) were reported in the cohort, and disease activity remained stable throughout the study. Three patients were excluded from the study because they did not receive IL-1i or colchicine but were on therapy with rituximab (two patients) and adalimumab. Eight out of 43 (18.6%) patients had a previous diagnosis of COVID-19 infection (COVID+), based on the positivity to nasopharyngeal swab test, and therefore were excluded from the analysis. Concerning the type of vaccine, 40 patients received Comirnaty BNT162b2 mRNA (BioNTech-Pfizer, Mainz, Germany/New York, NY, USA), 2 received mRNA Spikevax 1273 (Moderna, Cambridge, MA, USA), and one patient received AZD1222 ChAdOx1 (University of Oxford/AstraZeneca, Oxford/Cambridge, UK) at the first two doses. HCs were chosen among healthcare workers of Padova University Hospital and were not affected by relevant comorbidities. The mean age was 40 (range, 25–67) years with a standard deviation (SD) of $\pm$11 years. All of them received the Comirnaty BNT162b2 mRNA vaccine. Among the HCs included in this study, 33 (61%) were women, and 21 (39%) were men. A total of 20/54 (37%) HCs had a previous diagnosis of COVID-19 infection (COVID+), based on the positivity to nasopharyngeal swab test and therefore excluded from the analysis. Patients and HCs underwent a primary vaccination cycle at the local vaccination hub; for SAID patients, the first dose was followed by a second after 21 days, between March and May 2021; the booster dose was between October and December 2021. For HCs: first dose, followed by a second after 21 days, between January and March 2021; booster dose between October and December 2021. Blood samples were prospectively collected in June 2021 (T3), October–November 2021 (T6), and February–April 2022 (T9). The biological samples obtained from patients and HCs were deidentified. Patients' sera were collected at Rheumatology Unit and sent to Laboratory Medicine Unit for analysis. The anti-SARS-CoV-2 Spike protein receptor binding domain (S-RBD) IgG levels were assessed in SAID and HCs at different time points (T3, T6, and T9). For this reason, we decided to conduct the subsequent analysis only in COVID-negative SAID and HCs. All the subjects gave their fully informed written consent to participate in the study, which was carried out per the Declaration of Helsinki. The protocol follows the guidelines of the Ethics Committee of Padova University Hospital. The flow diagram depicted in Figure 1 shows the study size and the number of participants included in the final analysis.

Table 1. Characteristics of SAID patients included in the study.

Demographic Characteristics	
Patients, *n*	43
Age, years (IQR)	49 (37–60)
Sex, *n* (%)	F, 26 (60.5); M, 17 (39.5)
Type of SAID	
AOSD, *n* (%)	20 (46.5)
FMF, *n* (%)	17 (39.5)
TRAPS, *n* (%)	3 (7.0)
CAPS, *n* (%)	2 (4.7)
Schnitzler, *n* (%)	1 (2.3)
Therapy	
IL-1i (alone), *n* (%)	18 (42.8)
IL-1i + colchicine, *n* (%)	6 (14)
IL-1i + GCs < 10 mg/day, *n* (%)	4 (9)
IL-1i + JAK inhibitors, *n* (%)	1 (2)
IL-1i + methotrexate, *n* (%)	2 (4)
Colchicine, *n* (%)	6 (14)
GCs < 10 mg/day, *n* (%)	1 (2)
None, *n* (%)	5 (11)
Type of Vaccine	
mRNA Comirnaty BNT162b2 (%)	40 (93.0)
mRNA Spikevax 1273 (%)	2 (4.7)
AZD1222 ChAdOx1 (%)	1 (2.3)

Data are expressed as the median and interquartile range (IQR) or number of patients (*n*) and percentage (%). IL-1i, IL-1 inhibitors; AOSD, Adult-Onset Still's Disease; FMF, Familial Mediterranean Fever; GCs = glucocorticoids; TRAPS, TNF receptor-associated periodic syndrome; CAPS, Cryopyrin-Associated Autoinflammatory Syndromes; IQR, interquartile range; *n*, number of patients.

2.2. Evaluation of Binding IgG Antibodies against the RBD Portion of the SARS-CoV-2 Spike Protein

SARS-CoV-2 S-RBD IgG were measured by chemiluminescent immunoassays (CLIA) on Maglumi 2000 plus (Snibe Diagnostics, Shenzhen, China), validated elsewhere [9], with results expressed in kilo Binding Antibody Unit (kBAU). The cutoff value is 33.0 kBAU/mL. Thus values $\geq$ 33.0 kBAU were accepted as positive and <33.0 kBAU as negative. IgG levels in SAID patients were measured 2–4 weeks after the second dose (T3), six months after the second dose (T6), and 90 days after the third dose (T9). Due to technical issues (limited reagent availability) and reduced compliance of some SAID patients, not all samples were assessed at each time point. Furthermore, not all SAID patients completed the analysis due to the limited ability to reach the Hospital during the pandemic. Therefore, the number of samples evaluated for SAID patients was: 43/43 (100%) in T3, 28/43 (65%) in T6, and 23/43 (54%) in T9. The numbers of samples evaluated for HCs were 48/54 (89%) in T3, 54/54 (100%) in T6, and 54/54 (100%) in T9.

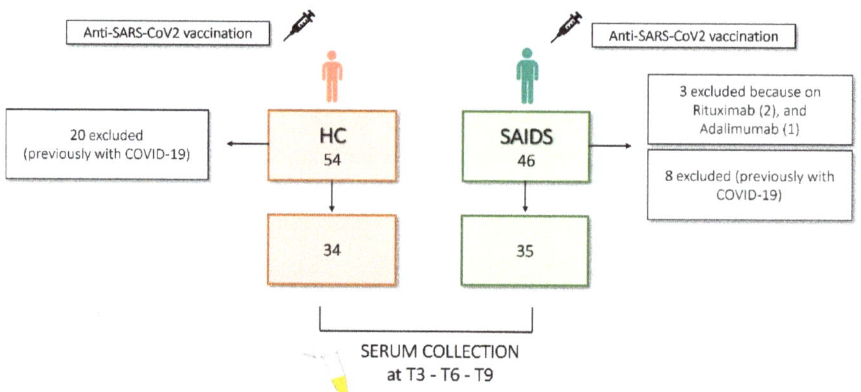

Figure 1. Flow diagram illustrating study size and participants.

2.3. Statistical Analysis

Data are reported as the median and interquartile range (IQR). The Shapiro-Wilk test was used to analyze the distribution of continuous variables. As data distribution was non-normal, Kruskal Wallis followed by Dunnet post hoc tests were used for multiple comparisons. Spearman correlation analysis was used to determine the correlations. Statistical analysis was performed with GraphPad Prism 8 (GraphPad Software Inc., La Jolla, CA, USA). A p-value < 0.05 was considered significant.

3. Results

We evaluated the anti-SARS-CoV-2 Spike protein receptor binding domain (S-RBD) IgG levels in SAID patients and HCs at different time points (T3, T6, and T9). As previously reported by Padoan et al. [10], S-RBD IgG levels were significantly higher in COVID+ HCs than in COVID− HCs ($p < 0.05$) (Figure 2A). For this reason, we decided to perform the subsequent analysis only in COVID-negative SAID and HCs. We evaluated S-RBD IgG levels in patients with SAID and HCs at different time points (Figure 2B). The number of samples evaluated for SAID patients was: 35/35 (100%) in T3, 24/35 (69%) in T6, and 19/35 (54%) in T9. In both analyzed groups (HC and SAID patients), the S-RBD IgG levels were significantly higher at T3 and T9 than at T6 ($p < 0.0001$). We found no differences between the patient group and the HCs at any of the time points considered. No significant associations were found between age and S-RBD IgG levels in T9 ($p = 0.61$) in SAID patients, while a negative correlation was found between age and S-RBD IgG in T6 ($p = 0.0003$, r = −0.67) (Figure 2C). Median levels of S-RBD IgG and interquartile range (IQR) of HCs and SAID patients are shown in Table 2.

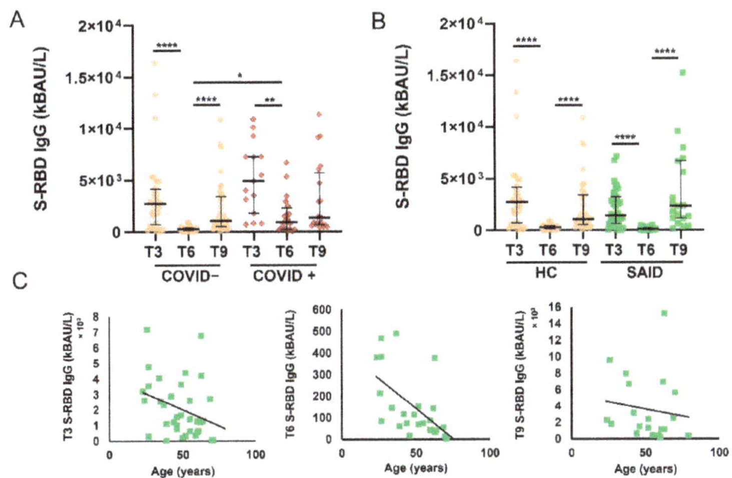

Figure 2. Levels of S-RBD IgG at different time points in patients with SAID and HC. (**A**). S-RBD IgG levels in COVID and COVID+ HC were measured at T3, T6, and T9. Data are reported as median and IQR. *p* was calculated according to the Kruskal-Wallis test. Dunn post hoc test, **** $p < 0.0001$, ** $p < 0.01$, * $p < 0.05$. (**B**). S-RBD IgG levels in COVID− SAID patients and COVID-HCs were measured at T3, T6, and T9. Data are reported as median and IQR. *p* was calculated according to the Kruskal-Wallis test. Dunn's post hoc test, **** $p < 0.0001$. (**C**). Correlation of S-RBD IgG levels in SAID patients measured at T3, T6, T9, and age. Spearman correlation analysis was used to determine the correlations. HC, healthy controls; SAID, Systemic autoinflammatory diseases; IQR, interquartile range.

Table 2. Anti-SARS-CoV-2 spike protein receptor binding domain (S-RBD) IgG levels at different time points in SAID patients and HC.

		T3	T6	T9
HC	S-RBD IgG, kBAU/L (IQR)	2719 (724–4154) *	275 (149–443)	1077 (529–3409) *
female		2934 (1690–4796) *	345 (137–514)	1150 (529–3755) °
male		1878 (413–3334) #	197 (147–296)	828 (497–2943) #
SAID, patients	S-RBD IgG, kBAU/L (IQR)	1400 (637–3206) *	86 (45–198)	2316 (1155–6681) *
female		1600 (852–3079) #	74 (43–378)	2316 (1155–6938) °
male		1261 (595–3548) #	87 (42–152)	1969 (594–5005) #

S-RBD IgG levels in COVID− SAID patients and COVID− HC were measured at T3, T6, and T9 using CLIA Maglumi 2000 plus as described in Materials and Methods. Data are reported as median and IQR. *p* was calculated according to the Kruskal-Wallis test. Dunn post hoc test, * $p < 0.0001$, ° $p < 0.001$, # $p < 0.01$ vs. T6. HC, healthy controls; SAID, Systemic autoinflammatory diseases; IQR, interquartile range.

Among the COVID- SAID patients included in this study, 57% were females, and 43% were males. The overall mean value for age, which did not differ significantly by sex (Mann-Whitney, $p = 0.67$), was 48 years with a standard deviation (SD) of ±14 years. The number of samples evaluated for female SAID patients was: 20/20 (100%) in T3, 13/20 (65%) in T6, and 11/35 (31%) in T9. The number of samples evaluated for male SAID patients was: 15/15 (100%) in T3, 11/15 (65%) in T6, and 8/15 (31%) in T9. Table 2 and Figure 3 show that S-RBD IgG levels did not differ between male and female patients with SAID.

Finally, we evaluated S-RBD IgG levels in COVID-negative patients treated with IL-1i. Figure 4A shows no significant differences between S-RBD IgG levels in T3, T6, and T9 in SAID patients treated with IL-1i and HCs. Furthermore, no significant differences were observed in S-RBD IgG levels in SAID patients treated with IL-1i and those who did not receive these treatments (Figure 4B). The number of samples evaluated for SAID treated with IL-1i was: 26/26 (100%) at T3, 16/26 (62%) at T6, and 15/26 (58%) at T9. The number of samples evaluated for patients with SAID not treated with IL-1i was: 9/9 (100%) in T3, 8/9 (89%) in T6, and 4/9 (44%) in T9.

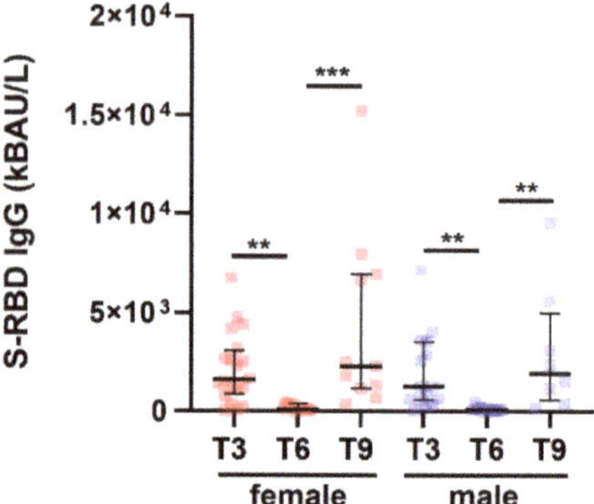

Figure 3. S-RBD IgG levels in patients with SAID and subdivided by sex. S-RBD IgG levels in SAID patients (COVID−) divided by gender measured at T3, T6, and T9. Data are reported as median and IQR. p was calculated according to the Kruskal-Wallis test. Dunn post hoc test, ** $p < 0.01$, *** $p < 0.0003$. SAID, Systemic autoinflammatory diseases. IQR, interquartile range.

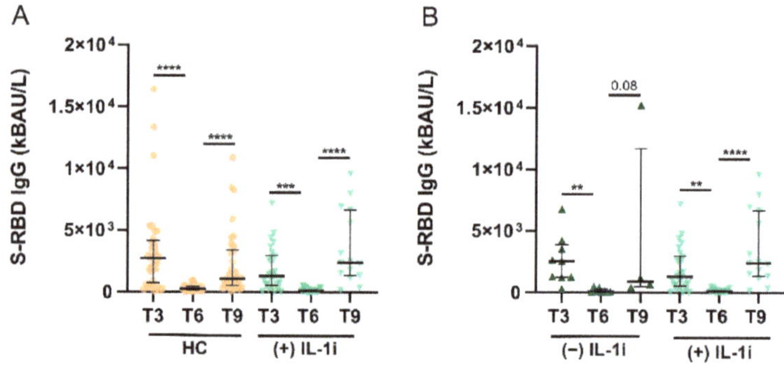

Figure 4. Levels of S-RBD IgG in SAID patients treated with IL-1i. (**A**). S-RBD IgG levels were measured in COVID− HC and COVID− SAID patients treated with IL-1i at T3, T6, and T9. Data are reported as median and IQR. p was calculated according to Kruskal-Wallis's test. Dunn post hoc test, **** $p < 0.0001$, *** $p < 0.001$. (**B**). S-RBD IgG levels in SAID patients treated or not with IL-1i were measured at T3, T6, and T9. Data are reported as mean ± SEM. p was calculated according to Kruskal-Wallis's test. Dunn post hoc test, ** $p < 0.005$, **** $p < 0.0001$. HC, healthy controls; SAID, Systemic autoinflammatory diseases; IL-1i, interleukin 1 inhibitors, IQR, interquartile range.

Through e-mail or telephone surveillance, patients were asked to report if they had disease relapses after anti-SARS-CoV-2 injection; none of them complained of hyperpyrexia, joint manifestations, skin rash, or serosis after vaccination, in addition to canonical injection site reactions as observed in the general population, or mild fever and arm pain for a few days after the injection. Regarding the five patients with a breakthrough infection, no disease relapses were observed during COVID-19, and none discontinued IL-1i. Table 3 illustrates the clinical features of COVID-19 in the five SAID infected and the ongoing therapies.

Table 3. The course of COVID-19 in 5 SAID patients after receiving three injections of anti-SARS-CoV-2 vaccine.

Patients	1	2	3	4	5
Disease	TRAPS	FMF	AOSD	FMF	AOSD
Date of the booster dose	21 November	21 November	21 December	21 November	21 December
Date of infection	22 January	22 May	22 January	22 March	22 June
COVID-19 symptoms	Sore throat, running nose	Fever < 38°, sore throat, cough, running nose	Fever < 38°, cough, running nose	Arthralgias, sore throat	Fever < 38°, sore throat
Therapy during COVID-19	CAM 300 mg/4 weeks	CAM 300 mg/4 weeks	Anakinra 200 mg/day	CAM 150 mg/4 weeks	Anakinra 100 mg/day
Therapy for COVID-19	Antipyretics	Antipyretics	Antipyretics	Monoclonal antibodies	Antipyretics

TRAPS, TNF-associated periodic syndrome; FMF, familial Mediterranean fever; AOSD, adult-onset Still's disease; CAM, canakinumab.

4. Discussion

The introduction of SARS-CoV-2 vaccination has profoundly changed the clinical outcome of those affected. It aims to prevent the more severe consequences of the infection itself, either in the general population or in patients affected by RD. Patients receiving immunomodulatory treatments are usually considered to have an increased risk of infections, and several factors such as older age, male sex, comorbidities, and the intake of a high dose of glucocorticoids (e.g., prednisone > 10 mg/day) or B-cell depleting therapies may increase the risk of hospitalization and death [11,12]. However, several biologics used in cohorts of patients with RD have been associated with a lower risk of hospitalization. Furthermore, different immunomodulatory therapies have been evaluated in the last two years as potential strategies for hyperinflammation, also called the 'cytokine storm', caused by SARS-CoV2, and have shown beneficial effects to date [13]. With the results obtained from our analysis, it is possible to observe that patients receiving anakinra and canakinumab did not show reduced antibody production after vaccination after both the complete cycle (I-II dose) and the booster dose, with titers that are compatible with those observed in HCs. A significant reduction in antibody levels was reported at T6 (6 months after the second injection) compared to T3, but this result is consistent with the normal decrease in serological response commonly observed in the general population and, in our case, in HCs. In T9, SAID patients presented with higher antibody titers. However, the difference was not significant compared to HCs. This data may be interpreted as a bias since SAID patients analysed in T9 were fewer than in T3, and the variability was elevated. Regarding the age differences between SAID patients and controls, we observed a reduction in T6 titer in both groups, in line with the increase in age. Overall, in this cohort, no patient was a no responder, and all 43 subjects developed antibody titers that exceeded the established cutoff, fixed at 33 kBAU/L, and were adequate to protect the patients from serious infection. Our data are consistent with other reports in which the serological response to vaccination was not impaired in those treated with IL-1i [14]. Similar results were also observed in adults treated with canakinumab who received influenza and meningococcal vaccines and had antibody titers comparable to controls [15]. Furthermore, comprehensive data on the safety and efficacy of inactivated vaccines were also reported in children taking IL-1i [16,17]. Therefore, patients on therapy with IL-1i should be encouraged not to discontinue the treatment during SARS-CoV-2 vaccination [18], given the risk of disease relapses and the possible additional increase of IL-1 if breakthrough infections by COVID-19 appear. Regarding safety and AEs, in a real-life observational study reported by Peet et al. and carried out in autoinflammatory patients treated with different biologics (IL-1i, IL-6 inhibitors, TNF-alpha inhibitors), side effects after vaccination against COVID-19 were reported after 71 of 138 (51.4%) administrations and were consistent with a flare of the underlying disease only in 26 of 138 (18.8%). Fatigue, myalgia, headache, and fever were the most frequent side effects observed after mRNA and adenovirus vaccines, but no serious AEs or death were reported [19]. Similarly, in the cohort reported by Shechtman et al., 273 FMF patients vaccinated with the BNT162b2 vaccine reported local reactions and mild systemic events; moreover, the Authors observed a recurrence of FMF-attacks (mostly abdominal serositis and joint involvement) after two doses in 12% of the subjects. However, the disease activity remained stable in most patients, with a rate of attacks higher the month before the vaccination than that after vaccination [20]. Moreover, they also observed that FMF patients treated with colchicine and canakinumab had a significantly higher rate of attacks following vaccination than those treated with colchicine alone. The explanation given is that patients under combination therapy usually have a high disease activity, thus, are more prone to develop attacks, but it is not an effect of IL-1 inhibition itself [20]. Güven and Colleagues observed a considerable number of FMF patients (54.7%) who suffered from vaccine-related adverse events and/or FMF attacks (mostly abdominal pain and fever), especially after receiving BNT162b2. They observed an increased rate of AEs after the booster dose. However, no serious events or increased mortality due to vaccination were detected [6]. Episodes of serositis (peritonitis, pleuritis), fever attacks and articular manifestations were observed in the Turkish cohort of 247 FMF patients reported by Ozdede et al.: an overall rate of 13.4% flares occurred after the BioNTech vaccine; however, in general, a similar AEs profile and frequency was observed in FMF/BD patients when compared to RD patients [7]. Concerning COVID-19 breakthrough infections, 5 out of 43 patients (11.6%) were infected with SARS-CoV-2 after the booster dose (third dose) but did not exhibit severe manifestations of COVID-19 nor disease flare-ups or symptoms related to long COVID-19 in the follow-up (Table 3). This could be explained by the fact that they received three vaccine shots. Therefore, the course of the disease resulted in mild; however, they all received IL-1i too, which could have down-regulated an eventual hyperinflammatory response caused by SARS-CoV-2. It is well-assessed that IL-1i, especially anakinra, may be beneficial in dampening the cytokine boost typical of the severe phases of COVID-19 infection. Therefore, the already in-place blockage of the inflammasome-IL-1β axis and the effect exerted by vaccination could have protected these patients more from developing a major infection and, in turn, from hyperinflammation. Our data are consistent with the clinical profile of SARS-CoV-2 breakthrough infections in double or triple-vaccinated, in which a lower rate of hospitalization and fatal outcome was reported compared to unvaccinated RD patients [21]. However, the sample size is too small to conclude the positive effect exerted by IL-1i, but the intake of certain drugs should be considered. Notably, in this cohort, two patients affected by IgG4-related diseases and receiving rituximab were not included in the analysis, as it is widely recognized that anti-CD-20 drugs can severely hamper the serological response [22]. No differences were observed between patients on IL-1i and those on colchicine or not treated. Almost all patients (42/43, 97.6%) received mRNA vaccines, and only one subject received the adenovirus vectored vaccine (AZD1222) in the first cycle but received a dose of mRNA vaccine at the booster dose (heterologous vaccination). Regarding safety, none of our patients treated with IL-1i or colchicine developed disease flares or serious AEs after receiving anti-SARS-CoV-2 vaccination, data consistent with the previously discussed literature. According to the EULAR recommendation for vaccination in subjects with RD, we suggested the administration of the vaccine to patients with 'quiet disease' (low disease activity or clinical remission), and we advise not discontinuing medications during the vaccination period to avoid possible disease flare-ups [23].

5. Conclusions

In conclusion, the present study supports that the anti-SARS-CoV-2 vaccines are equally immunogenic in SAID and HCs. Treatment with IL-1i is not associated with a delayed or hampered serological response, and no adverse events were observed after vaccination in those treated, providing evidence of excellent safety and tolerance in patients affected by autoinflammatory diseases. A limitation of the study is the small sample size of patients enrolled. However, considering that SAIDs are rare pathologies, the total number of patients is acceptable to present sufficient data on the vaccine's tolerability and efficacy during IL-1i. Further studies are necessary to understand if a fourth and a fifth dose or even annual vaccination against SARS-CoV-2 will be necessary for patients with RD or if guidelines for the general population should be followed.

Author Contributions: Conceptualization, S.B., C.B. and P.S.; methodology, S.B., C.B., P.G. and C.C.; formal analysis, S.B. and C.B.; investigation, S.B., C.B., F.V. and C.C.; resources, A.P. and P.S.; writing—orting—review and editing, S.B., C.B., P.G., A.D. and P.S.; visualization, S.B., C.B., P.G., F.V., A.D., C.C., A.P. and P.S.; supervision, P.G., A.D., A.P. and P.S.; S.B. and C.B. contributed equally to this work. All authors have read and agreed to the published version of the manuscript.

Funding: This research received no external funding.

Institutional Review Board Statement: The study was conducted according to the guidelines of the Declaration of Helsinki and approved by the Institutional Review Board of Padova University Hospital (Local Ethical Committee Number 27444).

Informed Consent Statement: Informed consent was obtained from all subjects involved in the study.

Data Availability Statement: Not applicable.

Conflicts of Interest: A.D. received consultancy fees from GSK, Eli Lilly, AstraZeneca, and Otsuka. P.S. received grants from Novartis and Sobi. The other authors declare no conflict of interest.

References

1. Galeazzi, M.; Gasbarrini, G.; Ghirardello, A.; Grandemange, S.; Hoffman, H.M.; Manna, R.; Podswiadek, M.; Punzi, L.; Sebastiani, G.D.; Touitou, I.; et al. Autoinflammatory syndromes. *Clin. Exp. Rheumatol.* **2006**, *24*, 79–85.
2. Furer, V.; Eviatar, T.; Zisman, D.; Peleg, H.; Paran, D.; Levartovsky, D.; Zisapel, M.; Elalouf, O.; Kaufman, I.; Meidan, R.; et al. Immunogenicity and safety of the BNT162b2 mRNA COVID-19 vaccine in adult patients with autoimmune inflammatory rheumatic diseases and the general population: A multicentre study. *Ann. Rheum. Dis.* **2021**, *80*, 1330–1338. [CrossRef] [PubMed]
3. Auroux, M.; Laurent, B.; Coste, B.; Massy, E.; Mercier, A.; Durieu, I.; Confavreux, C.B.; Lega, J.C.; Mainbourg, S.; Coury, F. Serological response to SARS-CoV-2 vaccination in patients with inflammatory rheumatic disease treated with disease-modifying anti-rheumatic drugs: A cohort study and a meta-analysis. *Joint Bone Spine* **2022**, *89*, 105380. [PubMed]
4. Başaran, S.; Şimşek-Yavuz, S.; Meşe, S.; Çağatay, A.; Medetalibeyoğlu, A.; Öncül, O.; Özsüt, H.; Ağaçfidan, A.; Gül, A.; Eraksoy, H. The effect of tocilizumab, anakinra and prednisolone on antibody response to SARS-CoV-2 in patients with COVID-19: A prospective cohort study with multivariate analysis of factors affecting the antibody response. *Int. J. Infect. Dis.* **2021**, *105*, 756–762. [CrossRef] [PubMed]
5. Alehashemi, S.; van Gelderen, E.; Rastegar, A.; de Jesus, A.A.; Goldbach-Mansky, R. Post-SARS-CoV-2 Vaccine Monitoring of Disease Flares in Autoinflammatory Diseases. *J. Clin. Immunol.* **2022**, *42*, 732–735. [CrossRef]
6. Güven, S.C.; Karakaş, Ö.; Atalar, E.; Konak, H.E.; Akyüz Dağlı, P.; Kayacan Erdoğan, E.; Armağan, B.; Gök, K.; Doğan, İ.; Maraş, Y.; et al. A single-center COVID-19 vaccine experience with CoronaVac and BNT162b2 in familial Mediterranean fever patients. *Int. J. Rheum. Dis.* **2022**, *25*, 787–794. [CrossRef]
7. Ozdede, A.; Guner, S.; Ozcifci, G.; Yurttas, B.; Toker Dincer, Z.; Atli, Z.; Uygunoğlu, U.; Durmaz, E.; Uçar, D.; Uğurlu, S.; et al. Safety of SARS-CoV-2 vaccination in patients with Behcet's syndrome and familial Mediterranean fever: A cross-sectional comparative study on the effects of M-RNA based and inactivated vaccine. *Rheumatol. Int.* **2022**, *42*, 973–987. [CrossRef]
8. Braun-Moscovici, Y.; Kaplan, M.; Braun, M.; Markovits, D.; Giryes, S.; Toledano, K.; Tavor, Y.; Dolnikov, K.; Balbir-Gurman, A. Disease activity and humoral response in patients with inflammatory rheumatic diseases after two doses of the Pfizer mRNA vaccine against SARS-CoV-2. *Ann. Rheum. Dis.* **2021**, *80*, 1317–1321. [CrossRef]
9. Padoan, A.; Bonfante, F.; Cosma, C.; Di Chiara, C.; Sciacovelli, L.; Pagliari, M.; Bortolami, A.; Costenaro, P.; Musso, G.; Basso, D.; et al. Analytical and clinical performances of a SARS-CoV-2 S-RBD IgG assay: Comparison with neutralization titers. *Clin. Chem. Lab Med.* **2021**, *59*, 1444–1452. [CrossRef]
10. Padoan, A.; Cosma, C.; Della Rocca, F.; Barbaro, F.; Santarossa, C.; Dall'Olmo, L.; Galla, L.; Cattelan, A.; Cianci, V.; Basso, D.; et al. A cohort analysis of SARS-CoV-2 anti-spike protein receptor binding domain (RBD) IgG levels and neutralizing antibodies in fully vaccinated healthcare workers. *Clin. Chem. Lab Med.* **2022**, *60*, 1110–1115. [CrossRef]
11. Strangfeld, A.; Schäfer, M.; Gianfrancesco, M.A.; Lawson-Tovey, S.; Liew, J.W.; Ljung, L.; Mateus, E.F.; Richez, C.; Santos, M.J.; Schmajuk, G.; et al. COVID-19 Global Rheumatology Alliance. Factors associated with COVID-19-related death in people with rheumatic diseases: Results from the COVID-19 Global Rheumatology Alliance physician-reported registry. *Ann. Rheum. Dis.* **2021**, *80*, 930–942. [CrossRef] [PubMed]

12. Gianfrancesco, M.; Hyrich, K.L.; Al-Adely, S.; Carmona, L.; Danila, M.I.; Gossec, L.; Izadi, Z.; Jacobsohn, L.; Katz, P.; Lawson-Tovey, S.; et al. COVID-19 Global Rheumatology Alliance. Characteristics associated with hospitalisation for COVID-19 in people with rheumatic disease: Data from the COVID-19 Global Rheumatology Alliance physician-reported registry. *Ann. Rheum. Dis.* **2020**, *79*, 859–866. [CrossRef] [PubMed]

13. Kyriazopoulou, E.; Poulakou, G.; Milionis, H.; Metallidis, S.; Adamis, G.; Tsiakos, K.; Fragkou, A.; Rapti, A.; Damoulari, C.; Fantoni, M.; et al. Early treatment of COVID-19 with anakinra guided by soluble urokinase plasminogen receptor plasma levels: A double-blind, randomized controlled phase 3 trial. *Nat. Med.* **2021**, *27*, 1752–1760. [CrossRef]

14. Ugurlu, S.; Akcin, R.; Ayla, A.Y.; Kocazeybek, B.; Oztas, M.; Can, G.; Mustafayeva, L.; Saltoglu, N.; Yilmaz, B.; Ozdogan, H. Antibody responses to inactivated and mRNA SARS-CoV-2 vaccines in familial Mediterranean fever patients treated with interleukin-1 inhibitors. *Rheumatology* **2022**, *61*, SI194–SI196. [CrossRef]

15. Chioato, A.; Noseda, E.; Felix, S.D.; Stevens, M.; Del Giudice, G.; Fitoussi, S.; Kleinschmidt, A. Influenza and meningococcal vaccinations are effective in healthy subjects treated with the interleukin-1 beta-blocking antibody canakinumab: Results of an open-label, parallel group, randomized, single-center study. *Clin. Vaccine Immunol.* **2010**, *17*, 1952–1957. [CrossRef] [PubMed]

16. Brogan, P.; Hofer, M.; Kuemmerle-Deschner, J.; Lauwerys, B.; Speziale, A.; Abrams, K.; Leon, K.; Wei, X.; Laxer, R. Efficacy, safety, and post-vaccination antibody titer data in children with CAPS treated with Canakinumab. *Pediatr. Rheumatol.* **2015**, *13*, P1. [CrossRef]

17. Heijstek, M.W.; Kamphuis, S.; Armbrust, W.; Swart, J.; Gorter, S.; de Vries, L.D.; Smits, G.P.; van Gageldonk, P.G.; Berbers, G.A.; Wulffraat, N.M. Effects of the live attenuated measles-mumps-rubella booster vaccination on disease activity in patients with juvenile idiopathic arthritis: A randomized trial. *JAMA* **2013**, *309*, 2449–2456. [CrossRef]

18. Atagündüz, P.; Keser, G.; Soy, M. Interleukin-1 Inhibitors and Vaccination Including COVID-19 in Inflammatory Rheumatic Diseases: A Nonsystematic Review. *Front. Immunol.* **2022**, *12*, 734279. [CrossRef]

19. Peet, C.J.; Papadopoulou, C.; Sombrito, B.R.M.; Wood, M.R.; Lachmann, H.J. COVID-19 and autoinflammatory diseases: Prevalence and outcomes of infection and early experience of vaccination in patients on biologics. *Rheumatol. Adv. Pract.* **2021**, *5*, rkab043. [CrossRef]

20. Shechtman, L.; Lahad, K.; Livneh, A.; Grossman, C.; Druyan, A.; Giat, E.; Lidar, M.; Freund, S.; Manor, U.; Pomerantz, A.; et al. Safety of the BNT162b2 mRNA COVID-19 vaccine in patients with familial Mediterranean fever. *Rheumatology* **2022**, *61*, SI129–SI135. [CrossRef]

21. Hasseli, R.; Richter, J.G.; Hoyer, B.F.; Lorenz, H.M.; Pfeil, A.; Regierer, A.C.; Schmeiser, T.; Strangfeld, A.; Voll, R.E.; Krause, A.; et al. COVID-19 task force of the German Society of Rheumatology collaborators; COVID-19-Rheuma.de collaborators. Characteristics and outcomes of SARS-CoV-2 breakthrough infections among double-vaccinated and triple-vaccinated patients with inflammatory rheumatic diseases. *RMD Open* **2023**, *9*, e002998. [PubMed]

22. Simon, D.; Tascilar, K.; Schmidt, K.; Manger, B.; Weckwerth, L.; Sokolova, M.; Bucci, L.; Fagni, F.; Manger, K.; Schuch, F.; et al. Humoral and Cellular Immune Responses to SARS-CoV-2 Infection and Vaccination in Autoimmune Disease Patients with B Cell Depletion. *Arthritis Rheumatol.* **2022**, *74*, 33–37. [CrossRef] [PubMed]

23. Bijlsma, J.W. EULAR COVID-19 Task Force. EULAR 2021 updated viewpoints on SARS-CoV-2 vaccination in patients with RMDs: A guidance to answer patients' questions. *Ann. Rheum. Dis.* **2022**, *81*, 786–788. [CrossRef] [PubMed]

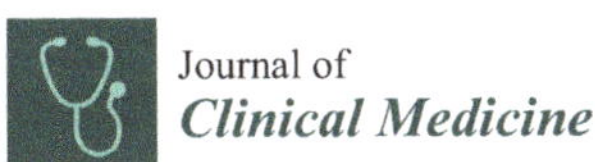

Journal of
Clinical Medicine

MDPI

Review

Targeting Interleukin-17 as a Novel Treatment Option for Fibrotic Diseases

Margherita Sisto * and Sabrina Lisi

Department of Translational Biomedicine and Neuroscience (DiBraiN), Section of Human Anatomy
and Histology, University of Bari "Aldo Moro", 70124 Bari, Italy; sabrina.lisi@uniba.it
* Correspondence: margherita.sisto@uniba.it; Tel.: +39-080-547-8315

Abstract: Fibrosis is the end result of persistent inflammatory responses induced by a variety of stimuli, including chronic infections, autoimmune reactions, and tissue injury. Fibrotic diseases affect all vital organs and are characterized by a high rate of morbidity and mortality in the developed world. Until recently, there were no approved antifibrotic therapies. In recent years, high levels of interleukin-17 (IL-17) have been associated with chronic inflammatory diseases with fibrotic complications that culminate in organ failure. In this review, we provide an update on the role of IL-17 in fibrotic diseases, with particular attention to the most recent lines of research in the therapeutic field represented by the epigenetic mechanisms that control IL-17 levels in fibrosis. A better knowledge of the IL-17 signaling pathway implications in fibrosis could design new strategies for therapeutic benefits.

Keywords: IL-17; fibrosis; autoimmune; epigenetics; biological drugs

Citation: Sisto, M.; Lisi, S. Targeting Interleukin-17 as a Novel Treatment Option for Fibrotic Diseases. *J. Clin. Med.* **2024**, *13*, 164. https://doi.org/10.3390/jcm13010164

Academic Editor: Eugen Feist

Received: 29 September 2023
Revised: 18 December 2023
Accepted: 21 December 2023
Published: 27 December 2023

1. Introduction

Fibrosis is a process that develops slowly and leads to tissue degeneration, with severe consequences for organs such as the heart, lung, liver, kidney, and skin [1]. In the last few years, fibrotic disorders have significantly increased and negatively impacted public health [2]. It is estimated that in the industrialized world, 45% of all deaths can be attributed to diseases where fibrosis plays a major etiological role [2,3]. Interestingly, in pathological disorders that are based on inflammatory processes, altered repair mechanisms can lead to the formation of fibrotic tissue upon wound healing [4], which may be responsible for aberrant tissue repair [1]. During the fibrotic process, an excessive accumulation of extracellular matrix (ECM) components occurs; collagen, fibronectin, and hyaluronic acid are released and synthesized to a greater level at the site of tissue injury, leading to organ failure and death [5].

In recent years, growing evidence has highlighted that aberrant fibrosis is also a major pathological feature of many chronic autoimmune diseases, including scleroderma, rheumatoid arthritis (RA), Crohn's disease, systemic lupus erythematosus (SLE), and Sjögren's syndrome (SS) [6,7]. These fibrotic diseases have, in common, a persistent inflammatory stimulus based on lymphocyte-monocyte interactions that produce growth factors and fibrogenic cytokines, inducing the deposition of connective tissue components that progressively destroy the healthy tissue structure [6,7]. These data confirmed that cytokines drive the acute and chronic inflammatory responses that culminate in fibrosis activation [8]. Recently, IL-17, a pro-inflammatory cytokine, has received growing attention derived from published results collected from the study of the correlation between inflammation and autoimmune diseases [9–11]. Based on this evidence, herein we review recent discoveries on the role of the members of the IL-17 family in the crucial events of organ fibrosis.

2. The IL-17 Cytokines Family and Its Receptors

The IL-17 family is a recently identified system of secretory regulatory peptides that show homology in amino acid sequences, including an extremely preserved cysteine-knot fold structure [12,13]. IL-17A was first identified in 1993 [14] and named human cytotoxic T lymphocyte-associated antigen 8 (CTLA8). It was subsequently termed IL-17 in 1995 [15] and, more recently, IL-17A. The IL-17A gene is inserted on the 6p12 chromosome, and human IL-17A is a homodimeric protein of 35 kDa that shares a different glycosylation [15,16]. Five other members of the IL-17 family were known: IL-17B, IL-17C, IL-17D, IL-17E (also named IL-25), and IL-17F [16–18]. IL-17A and F are the closest members, with 50% homology, followed by IL-17B (29%), IL-17D (25%), and IL-17C (23%); IL-17E displays the lowest degree of sequence conservation (16%), implicating that IL-17E is the most dissimilar protein [19,20]. The functions of these five proteins moderately overlap with those of IL-17A, whose precise role in health and disease remains elusive. IL-17, through its binding to the IL-17 receptors (IL-17Rs), is involved in chronic and persistent inflammation, autoimmunity, and the maintenance of epithelial layer integrity [21]. These receptors share a unique protein-protein interaction domain in their cytoplasmic tail called the SEF/IL-17R (SEFIR) domain [22]. Among the IL-17R family members, IL-17RA is the best-known receptor [23–25]. The IL-17R is a heterodimeric complex that is formed by the IL-17RA, IL-17RB, IL-17RC, IL-17RD, and IL-17RE, with the IL-17RA subunit in association with other subunits. IL-17A and IL-17F link to a dimeric IL17RA/RC system; IL-17B and IL-17E link to a dimeric 17RA/RB system; and IL-17C links to the IL17RA/RE complex [26]. In addition, IL-17D was recently reported to bind CD93 [27]. IL-17RA and IL-17RC, acting through the binding of the SEFIR domain with the ubiquitin ligase Act1, activate the TRAF6/TAK1/NF-κB pathway and the TRAF6/TAK1/MAPK/AP1 pathway [28]. Because IL-17RB, IL-17RD, and IL-17RE also contain a SEFIR domain, a similar mechanism of activation is probable. Moreover, a conserved intracellular subdomain homologous to Toll-IL-1R (TIR) domains was revealed which could be essential for signaling downstream of the IL-1 receptor and Toll-like receptors (TLRs) [24,29].

3. Production and Functions of the IL-17 Family Members

Functionally, IL-17 cytokines, critical for normal host immune responses, are potent drivers of inflammatory responses and cancer. Both in humans and in mice, IL-17 cytokines are produced by a broad spectrum of cell types that operate on multiple cellular targets [28,30,31], triggering the secretion of pro-inflammatory cytokines, chemokines, and prostaglandins [28,32]. In this context, IL-17A has been implicated in the pathogenesis of many disorders characterized by inflammatory complications, including cardiovascular and neurological diseases [33]. IL-17A is produced by CD4$^+$ and CD8$^+$ T cells and γδ T cells, and it acts on endothelial cells, macrophages, fibroblasts, osteoblasts, and chondrocytes [33]. This stimulation by IL-17A enhances the production of pro-inflammatory proteins from monocytes, such as TNF-α, IL-6, IL-1β, and IL-23. IL-17A also operates on mesenchymal cells derived from synovium and skin to stimulate the production of chemokines, thus involving neutrophil (IL-8/CXCL8), lymphocyte (CCL20), and macrophage recruitment [25]. However, if dysregulated, IL-17A responses can promote the development and chronicity of inflammatory disorders in a number of autoimmune diseases [34,35]. IL-17B was demonstrated to be highly expressed during the intestinal inflammatory state and is able to induce neutrophil migration upon intraperitoneal administration, suggesting a pro-inflammatory key role [18,36,37]. Interestingly, enhanced IL-17B levels are linked with poor prognosis in patients with various types of cancer, like breast, lung, and pancreatic, reinforcing the clinical relevance of this finding [38]. IL-17B expression was also detected in synovial tissues from patients with RA, where it is mainly produced by neutrophils and chondrocytes [39]. Likewise, IL-17A and IL-17C, produced by epithelial cells and immune cells, promote anti-microbial protective activity in the skin and in the intestine [28,40,41]. In addition, IL-17C is also secreted by keratinocytes and cutaneous neurons, but in a specific condition, represented by the reactivation of the herpes simplex virus [42]. IL-17D is the least understood of the IL-17 family of proteins. It is expressed in a broad variety of healthy tissues and has been found to be expressed at high levels in immunogenic cancer cells compared to poorly immunogenic tumor cells, leading to immune rejection mediated by NK cells. Therefore, it is well documented that IL-17D provokes exacerbated viral infections [43,44]. Some interesting studies have highlighted that IL-17D stimulating the endothelial cells promotes severe pro-inflammatory cytokine activity that leads to IL-6, IL-8, and GM-CSF secretion [43,45]. IL-17E, also known as IL-25, is involved in the pathogenesis of fungal infections, allergies, and autoimmune disorders. IL-17E is diverse from other proteins of the IL-17 family; in fact, it was considered a "mucosal barrier" molecule that confers immunity against parasitic infections. Indeed, large levels of IL-17E are secreted following infection with the parasitic helminth Nippostrongylus or Aspergillus [28]. Therefore, IL-17E induces expression of IL-4, IL-5, and IL-13, all of which are associated with type 2 immunity [46], and is able to promote epithelial-cell hyperplasia by increasing mucus secretion and hyperreactivity of the airway epithelium [47].

4. Role of IL-17 in Fibrotic Evolution

All fibrotic tissues exhibit characteristics of chronic immunologically-mediated inflammatory status during the initial periods of their development. IL-17 is expressed in an altered manner in several autoinflammatory diseases. Indeed, in inflammatory chronic conditions such as liver cirrhosis, idiopathic pulmonary fibrosis, and heart failure, IL-17 contributes to the severe fibrotic process through various mechanisms, including the induction of resident stromal cells and the progression of the inflammatory status. In liver fibrosis, IL-17, operating in synergy with IL-1β, IL-6, and IL-23, continues the inflammatory process by promoting transforming growth factor-β (TGFβ) expression in hepatic stellate cells [48,49]. IL-17 stimulates the hepatocytes, involved in fibroblast activation and collagen release, to secrete periostin [50]. Accordingly, inactivation of IL-17 signaling in hepatocytes diminished the fibrotic process in the liver of murine models affected by hepatitis-induced liver injury [51]. Therefore, IL-17 is markedly expressed in the bronchial mucosa of patients affected by severe asthma and drives the epithelial-to-mesenchymal transition (EMT) process when used to induce human small airway epithelial cells in in vitro cultures [52]. Supporting the involvement of IL-17 in EMT-dependent fibrosis, Sisto et al. recently demonstrated that IL-17, through the support of IL-22, contributes to triggering the EMT-dependent fibrotic process in healthy human salivary gland epithelial cells, clarifying the role of IL-17 in the fibrotic evolution observed in SS [53]. It is interesting to note that, in patients with idiopathic pulmonary fibrosis (IPF), Th17 cells secrete TGFβ and IL-17A at high levels; in addition, when lung fibrosis was induced in vitro through bleomycin (BLM) treatment of a murine model or when Th17 cells were cultured simultaneously in the presence of human lung fibroblasts, an increase in collagen deposition and other ECM factor production was revealed [54]. Indeed, blocking IL-17 improves the fibrotic condition in the lung of murine models affected by pulmonary disease following a post-bone marrow transplant [54]. Finally, IL-17 secreted by γδ T cells and Th17 cells plays a key role in several conditions of heart fibrosis, probably involving various inflammatory events in these organs. In fact, IL-17 induces cardiac myofibroblast transformation in murine models, in which ischemia causes heart injury, as well as in experimental models of hypertension [55]. Blockade of the IL-17 signaling pathway reduces cardiac fibrosis and improves myocardial contractile function [56]. A schematic representation of the role of IL-17 in autoimmune-related fibrosis is reported in Figure 1.

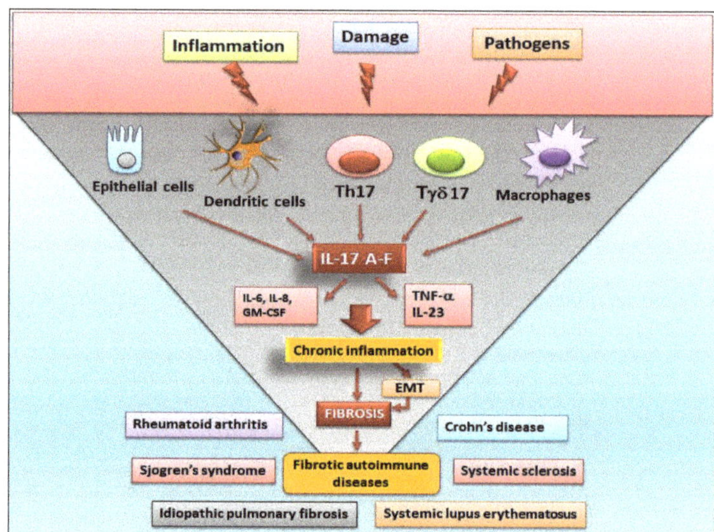

Figure 1. Role of IL-17 cytokines in fibrotic autoimmune diseases IL-17 is produced by epithelial cells, dendritic cells, macrophages, CD4 T helper 17 (Th17), and gamma/delta T cells (Tγδ17 cells). IL-17 signaling promotes the production of pro-inflammatory factors such as granulocyte-macrophage colony-stimulating factor (GM-CSF), tumor necrosis factor (TNFα), and the release of pro-inflammatory cytokines such as IL-6, IL-8, and IL-23. These pathogenic factors exacerbate chronic inflammation and, often through the epithelial-mesenchymal transition (EMT) process, cause the fibrotic evolution of autoimmune diseases.

5. Fibrosis Mediated by Several IL-17 Family Members

Dysregulated expression of IL-17 cytokines contributes to the triggering and exacerbation of fibrosis in a variable way, depending on the specific IL-17 family member. In this paragraph, we report the most recent knowledge regarding the role of IL-17 family members in the fibrotic evolution of inflammatory diseases.

5.1. IL-17A

Studies conducted using experimental animal models have demonstrated the role of IL-17A in regulating the complex interplay between lung inflammation and fibrosis. After BLM treatment to induce injury, IL-17A expression is upregulated, determining the release of pro-inflammatory cytokines and chemokines by endothelial cells and epithelial cells [54,57]. These factors recruit several types of inflammatory cells to the alveolar surface, and the resulting inflammation activates pulmonary fibrosis [58]. In addition, the same situations of inflammation, neutrophilia, and pulmonary fibrosis develop after IL-17A production following IL-1β treatment [54]. Confirming the pro-fibrotic role of IL-17A, blocking IL-17A through the intraperitoneal administration of an antibody against IL-17A reduces the acute inflammatory and fibrotic features in an experimental animal model [58]. Consequently, it is not surprising that the depletion of alveolar macrophages decreased the effects of IL-17 on the activation of lung fibrosis, supporting the hypothesis that these cells are involved first in the activation, producing pro-fibrotic factors such as IL-1β and IL-23 [59]. The IL-17A receptor is also ubiquitously expressed on the membrane surface of epithelial cells and fibroblasts; these cells are involved in the EMT-mediated pulmonary process correlated with pulmonary fibrosis; furthermore, these cells regulate fibroblast transformation into myofibroblasts, increasing extracellular matrix deposition [60]. Recently, it has been proposed that the IL-17A-mediated signaling and EMT of intrahepatic biliary epithelial cells are involved in the pathogenesis of primary biliary cirrhosis (PBC). This study demonstrated increased protein levels of the IL-17A receptor in intrahepatic biliary epithelial cells, and the IL-17A resulted in accumulation around those cells in the patients affected by PBC [48].

Additionally, IL-17A can act as a pro-fibrotic interleukin by suppressing autophagy in epithelial cells [59], although whether autophagy has a protective effect or not is yet to be determined. In addition, in some studies, after BLM treatment, an overexpression of IL-17R in fibroblasts was detected; furthermore, the addition of exogenous IL-17 can accelerate fibroblast proliferation, accompanied by an increased synthesis of specific proteins such as α-smooth muscle actin (α-SMA) and collagen [60]. The IL-17 stimulation of fibroblasts occurs, probably, via activation of NF-κB through the NF-κB activator 1 protein (Act1) [61], a critical mediator of IL-17 receptor family signaling, especially in autoimmune conditions [62].

5.2. IL-17B

Research on IL-17Bs role in fibrotic evolution has been limited, and in general, the function of IL-17B has not been thoroughly clarified. However, several studies support the possibility that the effects of IL-17A and IL-17B are very similar in the regulation of inflammation and fibrosis [63]. For example, IL-17B up-regulates the production of IL-6, IL-23, and IL-1α in the peritoneal neutrophils, macrophages, and lymphocytes [61]; in addition, it determines TNF-α and IL-1β release by the human monocyte/macrophage cell line [64]. IL-17B promotes the recruitment of cells that express the chemokine receptors CXCR4 or CXCR5, and the experimental intraperitoneal administration of recombinant human IL-17B determines the chemoattraction of neutrophils, which release chemoattractants for other cells [65]. Additionally, IL 17B can synergize with IL-33 to regulate T-helper (Th)-mediated immune responses [66]. These pro-inflammatory functions suggest that IL-17B may influence the progression of fibrosis, which follows the early stages of inflammation. This hypothesis was confirmed by the research group of Yang, who recently reported that the expression of IL-17B was affected by dysbiosis; this situation induces lung fibrosis by interacting with TNF-α to stimulate the secretion of Th17-cell-promoting genes and neutrophil-recruiting genes [67].

5.3. IL-17C

IL-17C has been shown to be expressed in CD4$^+$ T cells, dendritic cells (DCs), macrophages, and epithelial cells, which produce this interleukin during antimicrobial activity [68,69], determining an enhanced inflammatory response [68,69]. The activity of IL-17C occurs through binding to the IL-17 receptor complex, consisting of IL-17RA and IL-17RE subunits [70]. IL-17RE, in particular, was expressed mainly on epithelial cell surfaces and Th17 cells. Th17 cells react to stimulation with IL-17C, producing IL-17A and IL-17F, confirming that IL-17C might regulate the initial phase of the development of inflammation [68,69]. Once again, IL-17C production is dependent on NF-κB/Act1 activation, determined by IL-17C binding to the receptor complex IL-17RA/IL-17RE and, in turn, MAPK signaling molecules expression [70,71]. The function of the IL-17C isoform in the progression of fibrosis was mainly explored in IPF [72], using a lipopolysaccharide-induced lung injury as a model of IPF. Data collected on epithelial cell damage, the release of pro-inflammatory factors, and neutrophil recruitment mediated by the release of IL-17C confirmed the key role of IL-17C in lung inflammation. IL-17Cs role in Haemophilus influenzae and cigarette smoke-induced lung inflammation has been recently reported [73], mediating the expression of neutrophilic cytokines, the recruitment of neutrophils, and lung fibrotic damage [73].

5.4. IL-17D

IL-17D has a more limited expression and is detected in B lymphocytes and resting CD4$^+$ T cells; IL-17D acts, in particular, on endothelial cells, regulating their secretion of pro-inflammatory factors [74]. However, knowledge of the role of IL-17Ds in the exacerbation of pulmonary fibrosis remains poorly investigated and needs clarifying studies.

5.5. IL-17E

IL-17E, recently correlated with pulmonary fibrosis, was secreted by Th2 cells, epithelial cells, endothelial cells, T cells, alveolar macrophages, DCs, eosinophils, and basophils [75]. Xu and collaborators [76] not only demonstrated an increase in IL-17E secretion but also the activation of an EMT program in alveolar epithelial cells, determining EMT-dependent fibrosis activation in patients with IPF. These observations were confirmed by Hams [77] through the demonstration of increased levels of IL-17E in the lungs of IPF patients, which is correlated, interestingly, with IL-13 release that exacerbates collagen deposition during the IPF process. A schematic representation of the correlation between IL-17 subtypes A and E and EMT-dependent fibrosis is shown in Figure 2.

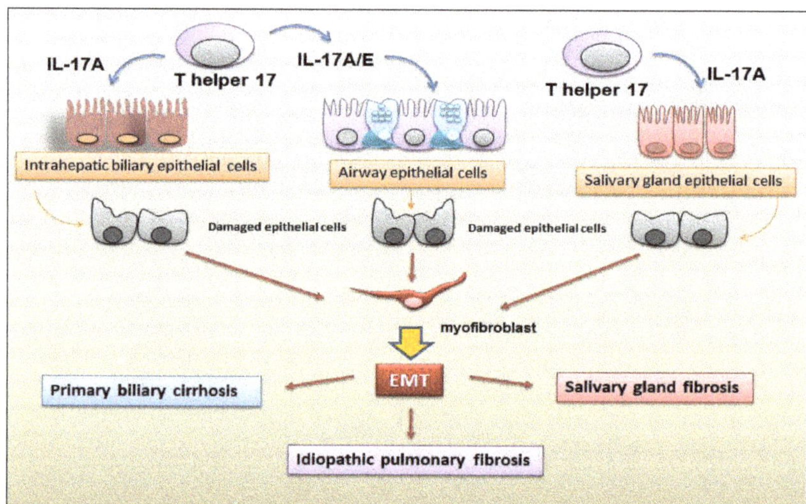

Figure 2. The main cellular sources and targets of IL-17A and IL-17E in the EMT-mediated fibrotic evolution of autoimmune diseases. IL-17A/E contributes to idiopathic pulmonary fibrosis, primary biliary cirrhosis, and salivary gland fibrosis through the activation of EMT, which leads to fibroblast proliferation and differentiation into myofibroblasts. EMT (epithelial-mesenchymal transition); T h17 cells (T helper 17 cells).

5.6. IL-17F

IL-17F shows a high homology of sequences and activities that mostly overlap with those of IL-17A [78]. The cells that produce IL-17F are the same as those releasing IL-17A. IL-17F is able to trigger the release of IL-6 and CXC chemokines from tracheal epithelial cells, inflammatory cells, endothelial cells, and fibroblasts, supporting the hypothesis that IL-17F could modulate autoimmune and inflammatory diseases [79,80]. However, the field of investigation into the pro-fibrotic activity of IL-17F is still pioneering.

The data related to IL-17 subtypes are reported in Table 1.

Table 1. Collective table reporting the mechanisms of action and related references for IL-17 subtypes.

Cytokines	Cellular Sources	Target Cells	Functions	References
IL-17A	Th17, γδT, macrophages, epithelial cells, dendritic cells	Epithelial cells, endothelial cells, inflammatory cells	Stimulation of inflammatory cells, release of profibrotic factors, pulmonary fibrosis, primary biliary cirrhosis, EMT, activation of NF-κB	[58–62]

Table 1. *Cont.*

Cytokines	Cellular Sources	Target Cells	Functions	References
IL-17B	Neutrophils, Th17, γδT, macrophages, epithelial cells, dendritic cells, B cells	Neutrophils, macrophages, lymphocytes	Release of IL-6, IL-23, IL-1α, TNF-α, IL-1β, regulation of the T helper (Th)-mediated immune responses, lung fibrosis, EMT	[63–65,67]
IL-17C	CD4$^+$ T cells, dendritic cells, macrophages, epithelial cells	Th17 cells, epithelial cells	Severe inflammatory response, NF-κB/Act1 activation, pro-inflammatory factors, pulmonary fibrosis	[68–73]
IL-17D	B lymphocytes, resting CD4$^+$ T cells	Endothelial cells	Secretion of inflammatory factors, exacerbation of pulmonary fibrosis	[73,74]
IL-17E	Th2 cells, epithelial cells, endothelial cells, T cells, alveolar macrophages, dendritic cells, eosinophils, basophils	Alveolar epithelial cells	EMT program, pulmonary fibrosis, increased levels of IL-17E in the lungs of IPF patients, IL-13 release	[75–77]
IL-17F	Th17, γδT, macrophages, epithelial cells, dendritic cells	Tracheal epithelial cells, inflammatory cells, endothelial cells, fibroblasts	IL-6 and CXC chemokines, autoimmune and inflammatory diseases, profibrotic activity	[78–80]

6. Epigenetic Regulation of IL-17 in Fibrotic Diseases

Dysregulated Th17 cell responses contribute to the immunopathogenesis of multiple inflammatory and autoimmune diseases [81]. Following aberrant activation stimuli, T helpers appear to be involved in triggering autoimmune responses against many organs, such as joints, brain, skin, gut, pancreas, salivary and lachrymal glands, and the eye. This abnormal and persistent activation leads to the onset of multiple autoimmune diseases, including multiple sclerosis (MS), psoriasis, Cröhn's disease, type I diabetes, SS, uveitis, systemic sclerosis (SSc), and SLE [82]. It is now accepted that the fibrotic evolution of autoimmune diseases presents an excessive release of pro-fibrotic factors as a result of the activation of molecular cascades depending on chronic inflammation, and the recent challenge consists of identifying anti-fibrotic therapies that can also have value in autoimmune diseases. Previous research has significantly increased our understanding of genetic susceptibility to fibrotic diseases based on the identification of sequence variants, polymorphisms, and mutations in several genes [83,84]. However, the concordance rate for some fibrotic diseases in monozygotic twins is low, indicating that genetic predisposition is insufficient to explain disease development and suggesting a potential role of epigenetics as the missing link that connects environmental exposure to disease development [85]. The following paragraphs explore findings related to the epigenetic regulation of IL-17 in fibrosis.

6.1. Histone Modification and IL-17 Production

As an epigenetically modulated mechanism, differentiation of T helper cells was acknowledged to imply total changes in histone modifications such as H3K4me3 and H3K27me3 [86]. Recently, it was reported that the histone deacetylase (HDAC) inhibitor, which has potential effects on epigenetic alterations, had been shown to mitigate renal fibrotic conditions. Findings have observed the conversion of CD4$^+$ forkhead box P3 (FOXP3)+ T regulatory (Treg) cells into T helper 17 cells (Th17), contributing to the progression of renal fibrosis. Worsening renal fibrosis was linked with the loss of CD4$^+$FOXP3+IL-17+ T cells in splenic single-cell suspensions. FOXP3+IL-17+ T cells expressed TGF-β1 both in vitro and in vivo, and, indeed, the loss of TGF-β1 expression was confirmed using IL-17 siRNA. It is now well established that these cells play a critical role in converting Tregs into IL-17- and TGF-β1-secreting cells [87]. Therefore, targeting the epigenetic process that induces the pathogenic activation of CD4$^+$ T helper cells may provide new therapeutic approaches to revolutionize the treatment of autoimmune conditions. Interestingly, removing acetyl groups by histone could occur through a series of HDACs that induce compact nucleosome structure and prevent active transcription; however, in some events, HDACs can directly activate transcription, although the exact processes by which they modulate transcription are currently poorly known [88]. In addition, HDACs seem to modulate the fibrotic process through fibroblast proliferation, senescence, and ECM production [89,90]. Based on this evidence, recent studies report that histone HDAC inhibitors can decrease the inflammatory status mediated by CD4$^+$ T cells and subsequent fibrotic evolution [91,92] (Figure 3).

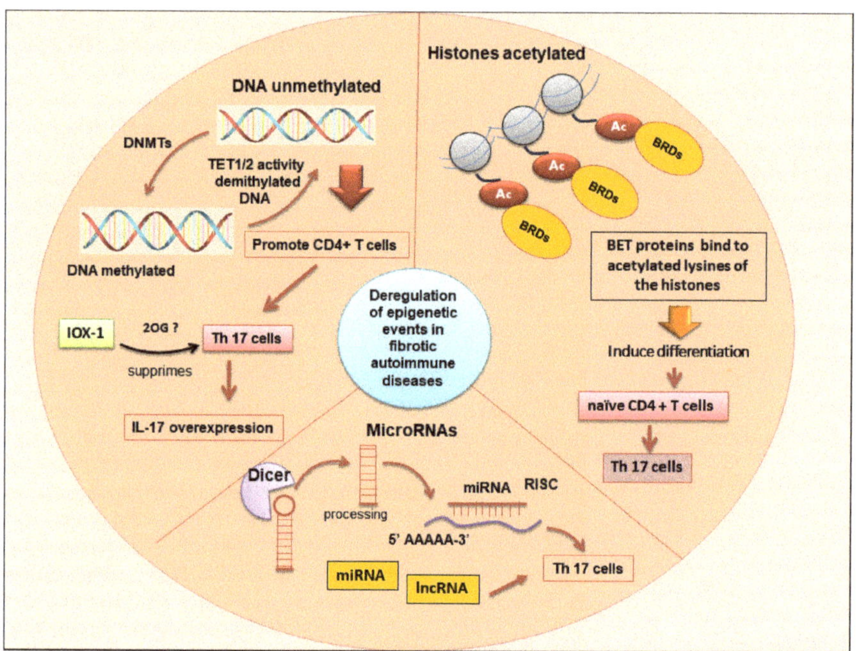

Figure 3. The main epigenetic changes associated with differentiation of T h17 cells and upregulation of IL-17 are DNA methylation, histone post-translational modifications, and ncRNA (lncRNA and miRNAs). Bet proteins (bromodomain and extra-terminal domain); BRDs (bromodomains); DNMTs (DNA methyltransferases); ncRNA (non-coding RNA); lncRNA (long non-coding RNA); miRNA (microRNA); Dicer (Endoribonuclease Dicer C-terminal complex); TET (ten-eleven translocation); 2OG (2Oxoglutarate Oxygenase); IOX-1 (Histone demethylase inhibitor); Risc (RNA-induced silencing complex); T h17 cells (T helper 17 cells); the symbol "?" indicates that the mechanism has not yet been clarified.

6.2. DNA Demethylation in the Control of IL-17 Pro-Fibrotic Activity

DNA demethylation, generally linked with gene silencing, has recently been identified as a strategy in the regulation of IL-17-dependent fibrosis. Ichiyama et al. demonstrated DNA methylation at T helper-specific IFNγ, IL17A, and Foxp3 [93]. Therefore, it was demonstrated that the H3K27me3 demethylase JMJD3 [94] and DNA demethylases Ten-Eleven-Translocation (TET)2/TET35 are key activators of IL-17 expression, and recent data have evidenced that H3K9me3 may also modulate the expression of IL-17 [95]. It is now accepted that bromodomain antagonists [96] and histone H3K27me3 demethylase inhibitors [97] are able to decrease the inflammatory status linked to CD4$^+$ T cell activation. Emerging evidence underscores the importance of bromodomain antagonists that interfere with epigenetic events on histones related to transcriptional processes. The bromodomain and extraterminal domain (BET) family proteins, consisting of BRD2, BRD3, BRD4, and

BRDT, are characterized by two bromodomains that recognize and bind to lysine-acetylated histones and other acetylated proteins with different degrees of affinity. Small-molecule BET inhibitors interact on the acetyl moiety inserted into the bromodomain acetyl-lysine-binding pocket, which is specific to the BET family proteins, and this allows BET inhibitors to be perfect candidates for blocking the constitutively active regions that have active histone marks. Indeed, BET inhibition has been shown to reduce the differentiation of naive T cells into Th17 cells [98]. Interestingly, studies in vitro have demonstrated that BET inhibition potently suppressed Th17 cell responses in explanted lung tissue from cystic fibrosis' patients with a history of chronic lung inflammation. Thus, these BET inhibitors are able to modulate T cell responses, specifically Th17-mediated inflammation, to inhibit IL-17-driven chemokine production in human bronchial epithelial cells through processes that include bromodomain-dependent inhibition of acetylated histones at the IL-17 gene locus [99]. In addition, in a murine model of acute pseudomonas aeruginosa lung infection, BET inhibition diminished inflammatory conditions without exacerbating infection, suggesting that BET inhibitors may be a potential therapeutic candidate in patients with cystic fibrosis [100].

Based on this evidence, targeting Th17 cells as well as those molecules mediating the differentiation and inflammatory functions of these cells can become a plausible therapeutic approach for many autoimmune diseases. While classical biologic agents (monoclonal antibodies or recombinant proteins) targeting IL-17 and IL-23, as well as inhibitors of RORγt, have shown potent efficacy only in some fibrotic diseases such as psoriasis and RA, unfortunately, this potential has not been observed in other diseases, such as uveitis and Cröhn's disease [101]. This has led to the identification of new potential therapeutic targets, and recently, IOX1 (a histone demethylase inhibitor) was identified as the potential candidate that suppresses Th17 function, targeting TET2 activity on the IL-17a promoter. The TET proteins TET1, TET2, and TET3 catalyze 5-methylcytosine (5 mC) conversion to 5-hydroxymethylcytosine (5 hmC) to regulate the DNA demethylation mechanism [102]. However, the potential therapeutic effect of the inhibitors of TET proteins has, until now, not been fully appreciated or developed. IOX1 is a general 2-Oxoglutarate Oxygenase (2OG) inhibitor that can also target other histone and DNA demethylases. Interestingly, IOX1 does not seem to have any direct interaction with demethylases, which could potentially activate IL-17A expression but, probably, suppress Th17 cells through targeting other 2OG enzymes [103]. From early studies conducted in the laboratory, IOX1 appears to have the advantage of similar efficacy with less cellular toxicity when compared to previously known inhibitors of IL-17-mediated inflammation, such as Tofacitinib [103] (Figure 3).

6.3. Correlations of Non-Coding RNA Expression and IL-17 Levels in Fibrosis

Different cascades and signaling pathways regulate fibrosis [6,104]. Recently, in addition to the large number of factors involved in fibrotic evolution, a number of non-coding RNAs (ncRNAs) have been found to affect fibrotic processes. The ncRNAs include a vast number of transcripts, within which long ncRNAs (lncRNAs) and microRNAs (miRNAs) have been extensively investigated in recent years, as they have demonstrated extensive regulatory activity on mRNA-coding genes. miRNAs are single-stranded transcripts with sizes of about 22 nucleotides, produced from precursors of 60–100 nucleotides by modifications conducted by an RNase III endonuclease, namely Dicer [105]. These small transcripts suppress the synthesis of proteins through base pairing to the 3′ untranslated region (3′UTR) of mRNA or, rarely, to the 5′UTR and coding regions [106]. When created, one or both strands of the miRNA duplex can be assimilated into the RNA-induced silencing complex regulating gene transcription [107]. On the other hand, lncRNAs have sizes greater than 200 nucleotides and represent a quantity higher than protein-coding genes [108]. With a total amount higher than that of protein-coding genes, their variability is correlated with the complexity of the organism and with the type of molecular pathway that they regulate. In fact, lncRNAs influence fundamental biological processes such as imprinting, chromosomal configuration, and enzymatic activation [109]. Many studies have revealed that miRNAs and lncRNAs are key regulators of the development of fibrotic processes, often correlated with autoimmune conditions. Probably they act on the most common fibrotic pathway, mediated by TGF-β, phosphatidylinositol 3-kinase/protein kinase B (PI3K/AKT), and Wnt/β-catenin. An example is represented by liver fibrosis, in which the activation and proliferation of hepatic stellate cells were regulated by miRNA or lncRNA that exerted their pro-fibrotic activity precisely by acting on the pathways just reported [110,111]. There is recent evidence that this pro- or anti-fibrotic activity may be mediated by a dysregulation of T helper cells with consequent variability in the release of IL-17. Positive correlations in miRNA expression and IL-17 levels have been observed in different studies related to fibrotic diseases or autoimmune diseases with a fibrotic evolution of the tissue or organs involved (Table 2). In experimental autoimmune uveoretinitis (EAU), an overexpression of miR-142-5p and miR-21 was detected to be correlated with increased IL-17 levels, but miR-182 was decreased [112]. In psoriasis, characterized by the fibrotic evolution of skin lesions, miR-1266 and miR-146, which are known to regulate IL-17A synthesis, were increased in the sera of these patients [113,114], also in association with RA [115,116]. A positive correlation was also observed in cardiac interstitial fibrosis, characterized by myocardial fibrosis, between IL-17 and lncRNA-AK081284 [117]. On the contrary, complicating the scenario, overexpression of ncRNA is accompanied by a reduction in IL-17 release in autoimmune conditions and other fibrotic diseases (Table 2), as observed, for example, in RA [116,118]. In an experimental model of autoimmune myasthenia gravis (EAMG), the administration of lentiviral miR-145 decreased EAMG disease, determining a concomitant decreased secretion of IL-17 [106]. In the prototypic fibrotic disease SSc, there is an increase in leucocytes in the skin, including primarily T cells. These T cells that are residing in the skin are in close proximity to the myofibroblasts, suggesting that they are governing their transdifferentiation [119] and may activate other immune cells in the inflammatory foci. It has been described in SSc fibroblasts that miRNA-129-5p is repressed compared with healthy control fibroblasts [120]. The authors also show that the T-cell cytokine IL-17 can increase miRNA-129-5p levels, and using siRNA to knock down IL-17 receptors in dermal fibroblasts reduced miRNA-129-5p levels. The actual target mRNA of miRNA-129-5p appears to be collagen alpha-1 [120]. This all suggests that the Th17 cells reduce collagen expression via the upregulation of the negative regulator miRNA-129-5p. Recently, Zhang and colleagues demonstrated that miR-125a-3p decreases levels of interlukin-17 and suppresses renal fibrosis via down-regulating TGF-β1 in Lupus nephritis (LN), an autoimmune disorder mediated by SLE. The condition of LN is accompanied by inflammation via a progressive suppression of kidney function, mediated by developing fibrosis [121]. In MS patients, the downregulation of miR-20b was revealed. In experimental autoimmune encephalomyelitis (EAE), primarily used as an animal model of human autoimmune inflammatory MS, miR-20b overexpression decreased disease severity by decreasing Th17 differentiation by targeting RORγt and STAT3 [122]. In the EAE model, miR-873 induced by IL-17 stimulation aggravated disease severity and increased inflammation by targeting Tumor Necrosis Factor Alpha-Induced Protein 3, or TNFAIP3 (A20)/NF-κ [123]. The same effect was obtained by the overexpression of miR-132 in the EAE [124]. Importantly, Du et al. reported that miR-326 expression correlated with MS disease severity in human patients, and in EAE mice, miR-326 regulates Th-17 cell differentiation through translational inhibition of Ets-1, a negative regulator of Th17 differentiation [125]. All these findings suggest that miRNA or lncRNA regulation and correlation with IL-17 are dependent on the fibrotic disease model (Table 2 and Figure 3).

Table 2. Positive or negative correlations in lncRNA/miRNA expression and IL-17 levels in fibrotic diseases or autoimmune fibrotic diseases.

lncRNA/miRNA	Effect on IL-17	Signalling Pathway	Fibrotic Diseases	References
miR-21	positive		liver fibrosis	[110,111]
lmiR-142-5p; miR-21	positive		autoimmune uveoretinitis	[112]
miR-182	negative		autoimmune uveoretinitis	[112]
lmiR-1266; lmiR-146	positive		psoriasis, also linked to RA	[113–115]
lmiR-21	negative	STAT3	RA	[116]
lmiR-145	negative		experimental autoimmune myasthenia gravis	[106]
lmiR-132	negative		EAE	[124]
lmiR-20b	negative	RORγt; STAT3	MS/EAE	[122]
lmiR-873; lmiR-326	positive	A20; NF-kB; ets-1	MS/EAE	[123]
miR-326	positive	Ets-1 inhibition	MS/EAE	[125]
lncRNA-AK081284	positive		cardiac fibrosis	[117]
miRNA-129-5p	negative	collagen alpha-1	SSc	[120]
miR-125a-3p	negative		Lupus nephritis	[121]

RA: rheumatoid arthritis; EAE: experimental autoimmune encephalomyelitis; MS: multiple sclerosis; SSc: systemic sclerosis.

7. IL-17 Inhibitors as a New Therapeutic Strategy

Given the strong pro-inflammatory role of IL-17, drugs that target IL-17 or the IL-17R are potential therapeutic candidates for inflammatory autoimmune diseases [126,127]. In 2016, anti-IL-17A monoclonal antibodies (mAbs), such as the IL-17 inhibitor secukinumab and the IL-17R inhibitor brodalumab, were both approved for the treatment of psoriasis [128]. More recently, the Food and Drug Administration has approved a novel drug, Ixekizumab, for the treatment of moderate-to-severe plaque psoriasis as well as active psoriatic arthritis. Ixekizumab is a humanized IgG4 mAb that selectively binds IL-17A and prevents interactions with IL-17R [128]. By targeting cells, it hampers the release of pro-inflammatory proteins, subsequently involving cellular components [127]. However, these drugs have unexpectedly demonstrated low efficacy in the diseases linked to IL-17, such as RA and MS [128]. Investigating in this context, Luo et al. discovered that a molecular complex containing the adaptor molecule Act1 and the tyrosine phosphatase SHP2 mediates autonomous IL-17R signaling, sustaining an intense inflammatory state. The resulting Act1–SHP2 complex is aberrantly increased in various autoimmune diseases, facilitating resistance to IL-17-directed therapy. The authors discovered that SHP2 inhibitors, as well as iguratimod, a small molecule that disrupts the Act1–SHP2 interaction, show promise in mouse models of MS and RA [129]. However, all monoclonal antibodies targeting the IL-17-IL-17R pathway and approved as treatments have several disadvantages, such as non-oral administration, poor tissue penetration, and various adverse effects as an escalation of the immune system's inflammatory response. Indeed, intensive research is being performed to discover potent small molecules targeting the IL-17A/IL-17 RA protein-protein interaction to modulate immune responses as an attractive approach for immunotherapy [130]. These new small-molecule drugs (SMDs), which are orally bioavailable, are beneficial in terms of production cost, convenience of delivery, and potentially higher efficacy. Actually, numerous clinical trials of anti-IL-17A and IL-17RA antibodies are currently in progress [130,131].

8. Conclusions

IL-17 is critical for host defense, but its role in the regulation of many chronic inflammatory, fibrotic, and/or autoimmune diseases becomes more and more evident. Although the pivotal roles of IL-17 in chronic inflammatory conditions are increasingly enumerated, these new concepts are not enough to clarify the function of IL-17 in fibrosis, which often represents the evolution of autoimmune diseases. Overall, the thin differences in IL-17 cytokines and their receptors seem to influence their role in fibrotic evolution. A thriving field of research concerns the inflammatory mechanisms mediated by the activation of EMT, which may have links to fibrotic evolution. In addition, in recent years, various experimental data have demonstrated the key role of epigenetics in the genetic regulation of fibrosis [107]. Several epigenetic modifications are involved in this process, such as histone modifications, DNA demethylation, or miRNAs and lncRNAs. Currently, however, there is no known clinical research on fibrotic diseases that is based on epigenetics. This would be essential to identify not only new therapies but also predictive biomarkers for the diagnosis of fibrotic diseases, such as many autoimmune diseases. In an attempt to optimize the general application and effectiveness of therapies targeted against IL-17 subtypes and to clarify the multiple molecular pathways in which they appear to carry out their regulatory activity, it will be necessary to elucidate the immunological and genetic circumstances under which IL-17 becomes pro-fibrotic.

Author Contributions: All authors were involved in drafting this article or revising it critically for important intellectual content, and all authors approved the final version for publication. M.S. and S.L. had full access to the data collected in this review, took responsibility for their integrity, and performed a critical reading. All authors have read and agreed to the published version of the manuscript.

Funding: This research received no external funding.

Institutional Review Board Statement: Not applicable.

Informed Consent Statement: Not applicable.

Data Availability Statement: Not applicable.

Conflicts of Interest: The authors declare no conflicts of interest.

References

1. Distler, J.H.W.; Gyorfi, A.H.; Ramanujam, M.; Whitfield, M.L.; Konigshoff, M.; Lafyatis, R. Shared and distinct mechanisms of fibrosis. *Nat. Rev. Rheumatol.* **2019**, *15*, 705–730. [CrossRef] [PubMed]
2. Mehal, W.Z.; Iredale, J.; Friedman, S.L. Scraping fibrosis: Expressway to the core of fibrosis. *Nat. Med.* **2011**, *17*, 552–553. [CrossRef] [PubMed]
3. Wick, G.; Grundtman, C.; Mayerl, C.; Wimpissinger, T.F.; Feichtinger, J.; Zelger, B.; Sgonc, R.; Wolfram, D. The immunology of fibrosis. *Annu. Rev. Immunol.* **2013**, *31*, 107–135. [CrossRef]
4. Enderson, N.C.; Rieder, F.; Wynn, T.A. Fibrosis: From mechanisms to medicines. *Nature* **2020**, *587*, 555–566. [CrossRef] [PubMed]
5. Miao, H.; Wu, X.Q.; Zhang, D.D.; Wang, Y.N.; Guo, Y.; Li, P.; Xiong, Q.; Zhao, Y.Y. Deciphering the cellular mechanisms underlying fibrosis-associated diseases and therapeutic avenues. *Pharmacol. Res.* **2021**, *163*, 105316. [CrossRef] [PubMed]
6. Sisto, M.; Ribatti, D.; Lisi, S. Organ Fibrosis and Autoimmunity: The Role of Inflammation in TGFβ-Dependent EMT. *Biomolecules* **2021**, *11*, 310. [CrossRef] [PubMed]
7. Sisto, M.; Lisi, S. Towards a Unified Approach in Autoimmune Fibrotic Signalling Pathways. *Int. J. Mol. Sci.* **2023**, *24*, 9060. [CrossRef] [PubMed]
8. Kany, S.; Vollrath, J.T.; Relja, B. Cytokines in Inflammatory Disease. *Int. J. Mol. Sci.* **2019**, *20*, 6008. [CrossRef]
9. Kuwabara, T.; Ishikawa, F.; Kondo, M.; Kakiuchi, T. The Role of IL-17 and Related Cytokines in Inflammatory Autoimmune Diseases. *Mediat. Inflamm.* **2017**, *2017*, 3908061. [CrossRef]
10. Ramani, K.; Biswas, P.S. Interleukin-17: Friend or foe in organ fibrosis. *Cytokine* **2019**, *120*, 282–288. [CrossRef]
11. Ruiz de Morales, J.M.G.; Puig, L.; Daudén, E.; Cañete, J.D.; Pablos, J.L.; Martín, A.O.; Juanatey, C.G.; Adán, A.; Montalbán, X.; Borruel, N.; et al. Critical role of interleukin (IL)-17 in inflammatory and immune disorders: An updated review of the evidence focusing in controversies. *Autoimmun. Rev.* **2020**, *19*, 102429. [CrossRef] [PubMed]
12. Kawaguchi, M.; Adachi, M.; Oda, N.; Kokubu, F.; Huang, S.K. IL-17 cytokine family. *J. Allergy Clin. Immunol.* **2004**, *114*, 1265–1273. [CrossRef] [PubMed]
13. Rouvier, E.; Luciani, M.F.; Mattéi, M.G.; Denizot, F.; Golstein, P. CTLA-8, cloned from an activated T cell, bearing AU-rich messenger RNA instability sequences, and homologous to a herpesvirus saimiri gene. *J. Immunol.* **1993**, *150*, 5445–5456. [CrossRef] [PubMed]
14. Yao, Z.; Painter, S.L.; Fanslow, W.C.; Ulrich, D.; Macduff, B.M.; Spriggs, M.K.; Armitage, R.J. Human IL-17: A novel cytokine derived from T cells. *J. Immunol.* **1995**, *155*, 5483–5486. [CrossRef] [PubMed]
15. Moseley, T.A.; Haudenschild, D.R.; Rose, L.; Reddi, A.H. Interleukin-17 family and IL-17 receptors. *Cytokine Growth Factor. Rev.* **2003**, *14*, 155–174. [CrossRef]

16. Hymowitz, S.G.; Filvaroff, E.H.; Yin, J.P.; Lee, J.; Cai, L.; Risser, P.; Maruoka, M.; Mao, W.; Foster, J.; Kelley, R.F.; et al. IL-17s adopt a cystine knot fold: Structure and activity of a novel cytokine, IL-17F, and implications for receptor binding. *EMBO J.* **2001**, *20*, 5332–5341. [CrossRef] [PubMed]
17. Lee, J.; Ho, W.-H.; Maruoka, M.; Corpuz, R.T.; Baldwin, D.T.; Foster, J.S.; Goddard, A.D.; Yansura, D.G.; Vandlen, R.L.; Wood, W.I.; et al. IL-17E, a novel proinflammatory ligand for the IL-17 receptor homolog IL-17Rh1. *J. Biol. Chem.* **2001**, *276*, 1660–1664. [CrossRef] [PubMed]
18. Bie, Q.; Jin, C.; Zhang, B.; Dong, H. IL-17B: A new area of study in the IL-17 family. *Mol. Immunol.* **2017**, *90*, 50–56. [CrossRef]
19. Kolls, J.K.; Lindén, A. Interleukin-17 family members and inflammation. *Immunity* **2004**, *21*, 467–476. [CrossRef]
20. Huang, X.D.; Zhang, H.; He, M.X. Comparative and evolutionary analysis of the interleukin 17 gene family in invertebrates. *PLoS ONE* **2015**, *10*, e0132802. [CrossRef]
21. Yang, X.O.; Chang, S.H.; Park, H.; Nurieva, R.; Shah, B.; Acero, L.; Wang, Y.H.; Schluns, K.S.; Broaddus, R.R.; Zhu, Z.; et al. Regulation of inflammatory responses by IL-17F. *J. Exp. Med.* **2008**, *205*, 1063–1075. [CrossRef] [PubMed]
22. Goepfert, A.; Lehmann, S.; Blank, J.; Kolbinger, F.; Rondeau, J.M. Structural Analysis Reveals that the Cytokine IL-17F Forms a Homodimeric Complex with Receptor IL-17RC to Drive IL-17RA-Independent Signaling. *Immunity* **2020**, *52*, 409–412. [CrossRef]
23. Yao, Z.; Fanslow, W.C.; Seldin, M.F.; Rousseau, A.M.; Painter, S.L.; Comeau, M.R. Herpesvirus Saimiri encodes a new cytokine, IL-17, which binds to a novel cytokine receptor. *Immunity* **1995**, *3*, 811–821. [CrossRef] [PubMed]
24. Monin, L.; Gaffen, S.L. Interleukin 17 family cytokines: Signaling mechanisms, biological activities, and therapeutic implications. *Cold Spring Harb. Perspect. Biol.* **2018**, *10*, a028522. [CrossRef] [PubMed]
25. Beringer, A.; Noack, M.; Miossec, P. IL-17 in chronic inflammation: From discovery to targeting. *Trends Mol. Med.* **2016**, *22*, 230–241. [CrossRef] [PubMed]
26. Gaffen, S.L. Structure and signalling in the IL-17 receptor family. *Nat. Rev. Immunol.* **2009**, *9*, 556–567. [CrossRef] [PubMed]
27. Huang, J.; Lee, H.Y.; Zhao, X.; Han, J.; Su, Y.; Sun, Q.; Shao, J.; Ge, J.; Zhao, Y.; Bai, X.; et al. Interleukin-17D regulates group 3 innate lymphoid cell function through its receptor CD93. *Immunity* **2021**, *54*, 673–686. [CrossRef] [PubMed]
28. McGeachy, M.J.; Cua, D.J.; Gaffen, S.L. The IL-17 family of cytokines in health and disease. *Immunity* **2019**, *50*, 892. [CrossRef]
29. Pande, S.; Yang, X.; Friesel, R. Interleukin-17 receptor D (Sef) is a multi functional regulator of cell signaling. *Cell Commun. Signal.* **2021**, *19*, 6. [CrossRef]
30. Amatya, N.; Garg, A.V.; Gaffen, S.L. IL-17 Signaling: The Yin and the Yang. *Trends Immunol.* **2017**, *38*, 310–322. [CrossRef]
31. Nies, J.F.; Panzer, U. IL-17C/IL-17RE: Emergence of a Unique Axis in TH17 Biology. *Front. Immunol.* **2020**, *11*, 341. [CrossRef] [PubMed]
32. Patel, D.D.; Kuchroo, V.K. Th17 Cell Pathway in Human Immunity: Lessons from Genetics and Therapeutic Interventions. *Immunity* **2015**, *43*, 1040–1051. [CrossRef] [PubMed]
33. Tang, M.; Lu, L.; Yu, X. Interleukin-17A Interweaves the Skeletal and Immune Systems. *Front. Immunol.* **2021**, *11*, 625034. [CrossRef] [PubMed]
34. Rosine, N.; Miceli-Richard, C. Innate Cells: The Alternative Source of IL-17 in Axial and Peripheral Spondyloarthritis? *Front. Immunol.* **2021**, *11*, 553742. [CrossRef]
35. Mills, K.H.G. IL-17 and IL-17-producing cells in protection versus pathology. *Nat. Rev. Immunol.* **2023**, *23*, 38–44. [CrossRef] [PubMed]
36. Lee, Y.K.; Landuyt, A.E.; Lobionda, S.; Sittipo, P.; Zhao, Q.; Maynard, C.L. TCR-independent functions of Th17 cells mediated by the synergistic actions of cytokines of the IL-12 and IL-1 families. *PLoS ONE* **2017**, *12*, e0186351. [CrossRef]
37. Zhang, X.; Zhang, X.; Song, X.; Xiang, C.; He, C.; Xie, Y.; Zhou, Y.; Wang, N.; Guo, G.; Zhang, W.; et al. Interleukin 17 B regulates colonic myeloid cell infiltration in a mouse model of DSS-induced colitis. *Front. Immunol.* **2023**, *14*, 1055256. [CrossRef]
38. Bie, Q.; Song, H.; Chen, X.; Yang, X.; Shi, S.; Zhang, L.; Zhao, R.; Wei, L.; Zhang, B.; Xiong, H.; et al. IL-17B/IL-17RB signaling cascade contributes to self-renewal and tumorigenesis of cancer stem cells by regulating Beclin-1 ubiquitination. *Oncogene* **2021**, *40*, 220–2216. [CrossRef]
39. Bastid, J.; Dejou, C.; Docquier, A.; Bonnefoy, N. The Emerging Role of the IL-17B/IL-17RB Pathway in Cancer. *Front. Immunol.* **2020**, *11*, 718. [CrossRef]
40. Chung, S.H.; Ye, X.Q.; Iwakura, Y. Interleukin-17 family members in health and disease. *Int. Immunol.* **2021**, *33*, 723–729. [CrossRef]
41. Ramirez-Carrozzi, V.; Sambandam, A.; Luis, E.; Lin, Z.; Jeet, S.; Lesch, J.; Hackney, J.; Kim, J.; Zhou, M.; Lai, J.; et al. IL-17C regulates the innate immune function of epithelial cells in an autocrine manner. *Nat. Immunol.* **2011**, *12*, 1159–1166. [CrossRef] [PubMed]
42. Peng, T.; Chanthaphavong, R.S.; Sun, S.; Trigilio, J.A.; Phasouk, K.; Jin, L.; Layton, E.D.; Li, A.Z.; Correnti, C.E.; De van der Schueren, W.; et al. Keratinocytes produce IL-17c to protect peripheral nervous systems during human HSV-2 reactivation. *J. Exp. Med.* **2017**, *214*, 2315–2329. [CrossRef] [PubMed]
43. Saddawi-Konefka, R.; Seelige, R.; Gross, E.T.; Levy, E.; Searles, S.C.; Washington, A., Jr. Nrf2 Induces IL-17D to Mediate Tumor and Virus Surveillance. *Cell Rep.* **2016**, *16*, 2348–2358. [CrossRef] [PubMed]
44. Seelige, R.; Washington, A., Jr.; Bui, J.D. The ancient cytokine IL-17D is regulated by Nrf2 and mediates tumor and virus surveillance. *Cytokine* **2017**, *91*, 10–12. [CrossRef] [PubMed]

45. Starnes, T.; Broxmeyer, H.E.; Robertson, M.J.; Hromas, R. Cutting edge: IL-17D, a novel member of the IL-17 family, stimulates cytokine production and inhibits hemopoiesis. *J. Immunol.* **2002**, *169*, 642–646. [CrossRef] [PubMed]

46. Kleinschek, M.A.; Owyang, A.M.; Joyce-Shaikh, B.; Langrish, C.L.; Chen, Y.; Gorman, D.M.; Blumenschein, W.M.; McClanahan, T.; Brombacher, F.; Hurst, S.D.; et al. IL-25 regulates Th17 function in autoimmune inflammation. *J. Exp. Med.* **2007**, *204*, 161–170. [CrossRef] [PubMed]

47. Owyang, A.M.; Zaph, C.; Wilson, E.H.; Guild, K.J.; McClanahan, T.; Miller, H.R. Interleukin 25 regulates type 2 cytokine-dependent immunity and limits chronic inflammation in the gastrointestinal tract. *J. Exp. Med.* **2006**, *203*, 843–849. [CrossRef] [PubMed]

48. Huang, Q.; Chu, S.; Yin, X.; Yu, X.; Kang, C.; Li, X.; Qiu, Y. Interleukin-17A-Induced Epithelial-Mesenchymal Transition of Human Intrahepatic Biliary Epithelial Cells: Implications for Primary Biliary Cirrhosis. *Tohoku J. Exp. Med.* **2016**, *240*, 269–275. [CrossRef]

49. Gaffen, S.L.; Jain, R.; Garg, A.V.; Cua, D.J. The IL-23-IL-17 immune axis: From mechanisms to therapeutic testing. *Nat. Rev. Immunol.* **2014**, *14*, 585–600. [CrossRef]

50. Amara, S.; Lopez, K.; Banan, B.; Brown, S.K.; Whalen, M.; Myles, E.; Ivy, M.T.; Johnson, T.; Schey, K.L.; Tiriveedhi, V. Synergistic effect of pro-inflammatory TNFα and IL-17 in periostin mediated collagen deposition: Potential role in liver fibrosis. *Mol. Immunol.* **2015**, *64*, 26–35. [CrossRef]

51. Tan, Z.; Qian, X.; Jiang, R.; Liu, Q.; Wang, Y.; Chen, C.; Wang, X.; Ryffel, B.; Sun, B. IL-17A plays a critical role in the pathogenesis of liver fibrosis through hepatic stellate cell activation. *J. Immunol.* **2013**, *191*, 1835–1844. [CrossRef]

52. Jiang, G.; Liu, C.T.; Zhang, W.D. IL-17A and GDF15 are able to induce epithelial-mesenchymal transition of lung epithelial cells in response to cigarette smoke. *Exp. Ther. Med.* **2018**, *16*, 12–20. [CrossRef]

53. Sisto, M.; Lorusso, L.; Tamma, R.; Ingravallo, G.; Ribatti, D.; Lisi, S. Interleukin-17 and -22 synergy linking inflammation and EMT-dependent fibrosis in Sjögren's syndrome. *Clin. Exp. Immunol.* **2019**, *198*, 261–272. [CrossRef]

54. Wilson, M.S.; Madala, S.K.; Ramalingam, T.R.; Gochuico, B.R.; Rosas, I.O.; Cheever, A.W.; Wynn, T.A. Bleomycin and IL-1β-mediated pulmonary fibrosis is IL-17A dependent. *J. Exp. Med.* **2010**, *207*, 535–552. [CrossRef]

55. Liu, Y.; Zhu, H.; Su, Z.; Sun, C.; Yin, J.; Yuan, H.; Sandoghchian, S.; Jiao, Z.; Wang, S.; Xu, H. IL-17 contributes to cardiac fibrosis following experimental autoimmune myocarditis by a PKCβ/Erk1/2/NF-κB-dependent signaling pathway. *Int. Immunol.* **2012**, *24*, 605–612. [CrossRef]

56. Zhou, S.F.; Yuan, J.; Liao, M.Y.; Xia, N.; Tang, T.T.; Li, J.J.; Jiao, J.; Dong, W.Y.; Nie, S.F.; Zhu, Z.F.; et al. IL-17A promotes ventricular remodeling after myocardial infarction. *J. Mol. Med.* **2014**, *92*, 1105–1116. [CrossRef]

57. Gasse, P.; Riteau, N.; Vacher, R.; Michel, M.L.; Fautrel, A.; di Padova, F.; Fick, L.; Charron, S.; Lagente, V.; Eberl, G.; et al. IL-1 and IL-23 mediate early IL-17A production in pulmonary inflammation leading to late fibrosis. *PLoS ONE* **2011**, *6*, e23185. [CrossRef]

58. Todd, N.W.; Luzina, I.G.; Atamas, S.P. Molecular and cellular mechanisms of pulmonary fibrosis. *Fibrogenes. Tissue Repair.* **2012**, *5*, 11. [CrossRef]

59. Gurczynski, S.J.; Moore, B.B. IL-17 in the lung: The good, the bad, and the ugly. *Am. J. Physiol. Lung Cell Mol. Physiol.* **2018**, *314*, L6–L16. [CrossRef]

60. Nie, Y.J.; Wu, S.H.; Xuan, Y.H.; Yan, G. Role of IL-17 family cytokines in the progression of IPF from inflammation to fibrosis. *Mil. Med. Res.* **2022**, *9*, 21. [CrossRef]

61. Sønder, S.U.; Saret, S.; Tang, W.; Sturdevant, D.E.; Porcella, S.F.; Siebenlist, U. IL-17-induced NF-kappaB activation via CIKS/Act1: Physiologic significance and signaling mechanisms. *J. Biol. Chem.* **2011**, *286*, 12881–12890. [CrossRef] [PubMed]

62. Wu, L.; Zepp, J.; Li, X. Function of Act1 in IL-17 family signaling and autoimmunity. *Adv. Exp. Med. Biol.* **2012**, *946*, 223–235. [PubMed]

63. Reynolds, J.M.; Lee, Y.H.; Shi, Y.; Wang, X.; Angkasekwinai, P.; Nallaparaju, K.C. Interleukin-17B Antagonizes Interleukin-25-Mediated Mucosal Inflammation. *Immunity* **2015**, *42*, 692–703. [CrossRef] [PubMed]

64. Li, H.; Chen, J.; Huang, A.; Stinson, J.; Heldens, S.; Foster, J.; Dowd, P.; Gurney, A.L.; Wood, W.I. Cloning and characterization of IL-17B and IL-17C, two new members of the IL-17 cytokine family. *Proc. Natl. Acad. Sci. USA* **2000**, *97*, 773–778. [CrossRef] [PubMed]

65. Shi, Y.; Ullrich, S.J.; Zhang, J.; Connolly, K.; Grzegorzewski, K.J.; Barber, M.C.; Wang, W.; Wathen, K.; Hodge, V.; Fisher, C.L.; et al. A novel cytokine receptor-ligand pair. Identification, molecular characterization, and in vivo immunomodulatory activity. *J. Biol. Chem.* **2000**, *275*, 19167–19176. [CrossRef] [PubMed]

66. Morrow, K.N.; Coopersmith, C.M.; Ford, M.L. IL-17, IL-27, and IL-33: A Novel Axis Linked to Immunological Dysfunction During Sepsis. *Front. Immunol.* **2019**, *10*, 1982. [CrossRef] [PubMed]

67. Yang, D.; Chen, X.; Wang, J.; Lou, Q.; Lou, Y.; Li, L.; Wang, H.; Chen, J.; Wu, M.; Song, X.; et al. Dysregulated Lung Commensal Bacteria Drive Interleukin-17B Production to Promote Pulmonary Fibrosis through Their Outer Membrane Vesicles. *Immunity* **2019**, *50*, 692–706. [CrossRef]

68. Krohn, S.; Nies, J.F.; Kapffer, S.; Schmidt, T.; Riedel, J.H.; Kaffke, A.; Peters, A.; Borchers, A.; Steinmetz, O.M.; Krebs, C.F.; et al. IL-17C/IL-17 Receptor E Signaling in CD4+ T Cells Promotes TH17 Cell-Driven Glomerular Inflammation. *J. Am. Soc. Nephrol.* **2018**, *29*, 1210–1222. [CrossRef]

69. Vandeghinste, N.; Klattig, J.; Jagerschmidt, C.; Lavazais, S.; Marsais, F.; Haas, J.D.; Auberval, M.; Lauffer, F.; Moran, T.; Ongenaert, M.; et al. Neutralization of IL-17C Reduces Skin Inflammation in Mouse Models of Psoriasis and Atopic Dermatitis. *J. Investig. Dermatol.* **2018**, *138*, 1555–1563. [CrossRef]

70. Chang, S.H.; Reynolds, J.M.; Pappu, B.P.; Chen, G.; Martinez, G.J.; Dong, C. Interleukin-17C promotes Th17 cell responses and autoimmune disease via interleukin-17 receptor E. *Immunity* **2011**, *35*, 611–621. [CrossRef]

71. Conti, H.R.; Whibley, N.; Coleman, B.M.; Garg, A.V.; Jaycox, J.R.; Gaffen, S.L. Signaling through IL-17C/IL-17RE is dispensable for immunity to systemic, oral and cutaneous candidiasis. *PLoS ONE* **2015**, *10*, e0122807. [CrossRef] [PubMed]

72. Chen, S.; Zhang, X.; Yang, C.; Wang, S.; Shen, H. Essential role of IL-17 in acute exacerbation of pulmonary fibrosis induced by non-typeable *Haemophilus influenzae*. *Theranostics* **2022**, *12*, 5125–5137. [CrossRef] [PubMed]

73. Vella, G.; Ritzmann, F.; Wolf, L.; Kamyschnikov, A.; Stodden, H.; Herr, C.; Slevogt, H.; Bals, R.; Beisswenger, C. IL-17C contributes to NTHi-induced inflammation and lung damage in experimental COPD and is present in sputum during acute exacerbations. *PLoS ONE* **2021**, *16*, e0243484. [CrossRef] [PubMed]

74. Liu, X.; Sun, S.; Liu, D. IL-17D: A Less Studied Cytokine of IL-17 Family. *Int. Arch. Allergy Immunol.* **2020**, *181*, 618–623. [CrossRef] [PubMed]

75. Xu, M.; Dong, C. IL-25 in allergic inflammation. *Immunol. Rev.* **2017**, *278*, 185–191. [CrossRef] [PubMed]

76. Xu, X.; Luo, S.; Li, B.; Dai, H.; Zhang, J. IL-25 contributes to lung fibrosis by directly acting on alveolar epithelial cells and fibroblasts. *Exp. Biol. Med.* **2019**, *244*, 770–780. [CrossRef]

77. Hams, E.; Armstrong, M.E.; Barlow, J.L.; Saunders, S.P.; Schwartz, C.; Cooke, G.; Fahy, R.J.; Crotty, T.B.; Hirani, N.; Flynn, R.J.; et al. IL-25 and type 2 innate lymphoid cells induce pulmonary fibrosis. *Proc. Natl. Acad. Sci. USA* **2014**, *111*, 367–372. [CrossRef]

78. Chang, S.H.; Dong, C. IL-17F: Regulation, signaling and function in inflammation. *Cytokine* **2009**, *46*, 7–11. [CrossRef]

79. Hot, A.; Miossec, P. Effects of interleukin (IL)-17A and IL-17F in human rheumatoid arthritis synoviocytes. *Ann. Rheum. Dis.* **2011**, *70*, 727–732. [CrossRef]

80. Ritzmann, F.; Lunding, L.P.; Bals, R.; Wegmann, M.; Beisswenger, C. IL-17 Cytokines and Chronic Lung Diseases. *Cells* **2022**, *11*, 2132. [CrossRef]

81. Bettelli, E.; Carrier, Y.; Gao, W.; Korn, T.; Strom, T.B.; Oukka, M.; Weiner, H.L.; Kuchroo, V.K. Reciprocal developmental pathways for the generation of pathogenic effector Th17 cells and regulatory T cells. *Nature* **2006**, *441*, 235–238. [CrossRef] [PubMed]

82. Raphael, I.; Joern, R.R.; Forsthuber, T.G. Memory CD4+ T Cells in Immunity and Autoimmune Diseases. *Cells* **2020**, *9*, 531. [CrossRef] [PubMed]

83. Allen, R.J.; Porte, J.; Braybrooke, R.; Flores, C.; Fingerlin, T.E.; Oldham, J.M.; Guillen-Guio, B.; Ma, S.F.; Okamoto, T.; John, A.E.; et al. Genetic variants associated with susceptibility to idiopathic pulmonary fibrosis in people of European ancestry: A genome-wide association study. *Lancet Respir. Med.* **2017**, *5*, 869–880. [CrossRef] [PubMed]

84. Dagneaux, L.; Owen, A.R.; Bettencourt, J.W.; Barlow, J.D.; Amadio, P.C.; Kocher, J.P.; Morrey, M.E.; Sanchez-Sotelo, J.; Berry, D.J.; van Wijnen, A.J.; et al. Human Fibrosis: Is There Evidence for a Genetic Predisposition in Musculoskeletal Tissues? *J. Arthroplast.* **2020**, *35*, 3343–3352. [CrossRef] [PubMed]

85. Liu, Y.; Wen, D.; Ho, C.; Yu, L.; Zheng, D.; O'reilly, S.; Gao, Y.; Li, Q.; Zhang, Y. Epigenetics as a versatile regulator of fibrosis. *J. Transl. Med.* **2023**, *21*, 164. [CrossRef]

86. Wei, G.; Wei, L.; Zhu, J.; Zang, C.; Hu-Li, J.; Yao, Z.; Cui, K.; Kanno, Y.; Roh, T.Y.; Watford, W.T.; et al. Global mapping of H3K4me3 and H3K27me3 reveals specificity and plasticity in lineage fate determination of differentiating CD4+ T cells. *Immunity* **2009**, *30*, 155–167. [CrossRef]

87. Wu, W.P.; Tsai, Y.G.; Lin, T.Y.; Wu, M.J.; Lin, C.Y. The attenuation of renal fibrosis by histone deacetylase inhibitors is associated with the plasticity of FOXP3+IL-17+ T cells. *BMC Nephrol.* **2017**, *18*, 225. [CrossRef]

88. Seto, E.; Yoshida, M. Erasers of histone acetylation: The histone deacetylase enzymes. *Cold Spring Harb. Perspect. Biol.* **2014**, *6*, a018713. [CrossRef]

89. Felisbino, M.B.; McKinsey, T.A. Epigenetics in cardiac fibrosis. *JACC Basic. Transl. Sci.* **2018**, *3*, 704–715. [CrossRef]

90. Barcena-Varela, M.; Colyn, L.; Fernandez-Barrena, M.G. Epigenetic mechanisms in hepatic stellate cell activation during liver fibrosis and carcinogenesis. *Int. J. Mol. Sci.* **2019**, *20*, 2507. [CrossRef]

91. Göschl, L.; Preglej, T.; Boucheron, N.; Saferding, V.; Müller, L.; Platzer, A.; Hirahara, K.; Shih, H.-Y.; Backlund, J.; Matthias, P.; et al. Histone deacetylase 1 (HDAC1): A key player of T cell-mediated arthritis. *J. Autoimmun.* **2020**, *108*, 102379. [CrossRef] [PubMed]

92. Regna, N.L.; Chafin, C.B.; Hammond, S.E.; Puthiyaveetil, A.G.; Caudell, D.L.; Reilly, C.M. Class I and II histone deacetylase inhibition by ITF2357 reduces SLE pathogenesis in vivo. *Clin. Immunol.* **2014**, *151*, 29–42. [CrossRef] [PubMed]

93. Ichiyama, K.; Chen, T.; Wang, X.; Yan, X.; Kim, B.-S.; Tanaka, S.; Ndiaye-Lobry, D.; Deng, Y.; Zou, Y.; Zheng, P.; et al. The methylcytosine dioxygenase Tet2 promotes DNA demethylation and activation of cytokine gene expression in T cells. *Immunity* **2015**, *42*, 613–626. [CrossRef] [PubMed]

94. Li, Q.; Zou, J.; Wang, M.; Ding, X.; Chepelev, I.; Zhou, X.; Zhao, W.; Wei, G.; Cui, J.; Zhao, K.; et al. Critical role of histone demethylase Jmjd3 in the regulation of CD4+ T-cell differentiation. *Nat. Commun.* **2014**, *5*, 5780. [CrossRef] [PubMed]

95. Takada, I. DGCR14 induces Il17a gene expression through the RORgamma/BAZ1B/RSKS2 complex. *Mol. Cell Biol.* **2015**, *35*, 344–355. [CrossRef] [PubMed]

96. Bandukwala, H.S.; Gagnon, J.; Togher, S.; Greenbaum, J.A.; Lamperti, E.D.; Parr, N.J.; Molesworth, A.M.H.; Smithers, N.; Lee, K.; Witherington, J.; et al. Selective inhibition of CD4+ T-cell cytokine production and autoimmunity by BET protein and c-Myc inhibitors. *Proc. Natl. Acad. Sci. USA* **2012**, *109*, 14532–14537. [CrossRef]

97. Cribbs, A.P.; Terlecki-Zaniewicz, S.; Philpott, M.; Baardman, J.; Ahern, D.; Lindow, M.; Obad, S.; Oerum, H.; Sampey, B.; Mander, P.K.; et al. Histone H3K27me3 demethylases regulate human Th17 cell development and effector functions by impacting on metabolism. *Proc. Natl. Acad. Sci. USA* **2020**, *117*, 6056–6066. [CrossRef]

98. Mele, D.A.; Salmeron, A.; Ghosh, S.; Huang, H.R.; Bryant, B.M.; Lora, J.M. BET bromodomain inhibition suppresses TH17-mediated pathology. *J. Exp. Med.* **2013**, *210*, 2181–2190. [CrossRef]

99. Klein, K. Bromodomain protein inhibition: A novel therapeutic strategy in rheumatic diseases. *RMD Open* **2018**, *4*, e000744. [CrossRef]

100. Chen, K.; Campfield, B.T.; Wenzel, S.E.; McAleer, J.P.; Kreindler, J.L.; Kurland, G.; Gopal, R.; Wang, T.; Chen, W.; Eddens, T.; et al. Antiinflammatory effects of bromodomain and extraterminal domain inhibition in cystic fibrosis lung inflammation. *JCI Insight* **2016**, *1*, e87168. [CrossRef]

101. Fragoulis, G.E.; Siebert, S.; McInnes, I.B. Therapeutic targeting of IL-17 and IL-23 cytokines in immune-mediated diseases. *Ann. Rev. Med.* **2016**, *67*, 337–353. [CrossRef] [PubMed]

102. Pastor, W.A.; Aravind, L.; Rao, A. TETonic shift: Biological roles of TET proteins in DNA demethylation and transcription. *Nat. Rev. Mol. Cell Biol.* **2013**, *14*, 341–356. [CrossRef] [PubMed]

103. Hu, X.; Zou, Y.; Copland, D.A.; Schewitz-Bowers, L.P.; Li, Y.; Lait, P.J.P.; Stimpson, M.; Zhang, Z.; Guo, S.; Liang, J.; et al. Epigenetic drug screen identified IOX1 as an inhibitor of Th17-mediated inflammation through targeting TET2. *Ebiomedicine* **2022**, *86*, 104333. [CrossRef] [PubMed]

104. Antar, S.A.; Ashour, N.A.; Marawan, M.E.; Al-Karmalawy, A.A. Fibrosis: Types, Effects, Markers, Mechanisms for Disease Progression, and Its Relation with Oxidative Stress, Immunity, and Inflammation. *Int. J. Mol. Sci.* **2023**, *24*, 4004. [CrossRef] [PubMed]

105. Zapletal, D.; Kubicek, K.; Svoboda, P.; Stefl, R. Dicer structure and function: Conserved and evolving features. *EMBO Rep.* **2023**, *24*, e57215. [CrossRef] [PubMed]

106. Wang, B. Base Composition Characteristics of Mammalian miRNAs. *J. Nucleic Acids.* **2013**, *2013*, 951570. [CrossRef]

107. Ghafouri-Fard, S.; Abak, A.; Talebi, S.F.; Shoorei, H.; Branicki, W.; Taheri, M.; Akbari Dilmaghani, N. Role of miRNA and lncRNAs in organ fibrosis and aging. *Biomed. Pharmacother.* **2021**, *143*, 112132.

108. Quinn, J.J.; Chang, H.Y. Unique features of long non-coding RNA biogenesis and function. *Nat. Rev. Genet.* **2016**, *17*, 47–62. [CrossRef]

109. Mattick, J.S.; Amaral, P.P.; Carninci, P.; Carpenter, S.; Chang, H.Y.; Chen, L.-L.; Chen, R.; Dean, C.; Dinger, M.E.; Fitzgerald, K.A.; et al. Long non-coding RNAs: Definitions, functions, challenges and recommendations. *Nat. Rev. Mol. Cell Biol.* **2023**, *24*, 430–447. [CrossRef]

110. Li, Q.Y.; Gong, T.; Huang, Y.K.; Kang, L.; Warner, C.A.; Xie, H.; Chen, L.M.; Duan, X.Q. Role of noncoding RNAs in liver fibrosis. *World J. Gastroenterol.* **2023**, *29*, 1446–1459. [CrossRef]

111. Yao, S.X.; Zhang, G.S.; Cao, H.X.; Song, G.; Li, Z.T.; Zhang, W.T. Correlation between microRNA-21 and expression of Th17 and Treg cells in microenvironment of rats with hepatocellular carcinoma. *Asian Pac. J. Trop. Med.* **2015**, *8*, 762–765. [CrossRef] [PubMed]

112. Ishida, W.; Fukuda, K.; Sakamoto, S.; Koyama, N.; Koyanagi, A.; Yagita, H.; Fukushima, A. Regulation of experimental autoimmune uveoretinitis by anti-delta-like ligand 4 monoclonal antibody. *Investig. Ophthalmol. Vis. Sci.* **2011**, *52*, 8224–8230. [CrossRef] [PubMed]

113. Ichihara, A.; Jinnin, M.; Oyama, R.; Yamane, K.; Fujisawa, A.; Sakai, K.; Masuguchi, S.; Fukushima, S.; Maruo, K.; Ihn, H. Increased serum levels of miR-1266 in patients with psoriasis vulgaris. *Eur. J. Dermatol.* **2012**, *22*, 68–71. [CrossRef] [PubMed]

114. Xia, P.; Fang, X.; Zhang, Z.H.; Huang, Q.; Yan, K.X.; Kang, K.F.; Han, L.; Zheng, Z.Z. Dysregulation of miRNA146a versus IRAK1 induces IL-17 persistence in the psoriatic skin lesions. *Immunol. Lett.* **2012**, *148*, 151–162. [CrossRef]

115. Niimoto, T.; Nakasa, T.; Ishikawa, M.; Okuhara, A.; Izumi, B.; Deie, M.; Suzuki, O.; Adachi, N.; Ochi, M. MicroRNA-146a expresses in interleukin-17 producing T cells in rheumatoid arthritis patients. *BMC Musculoskelet. Disord.* **2010**, *11*, 209. [CrossRef]

116. Dong, L.; Wang, X.; Tan, J.; Li, H.; Qian, W.; Chen, J.; Chen, Q.; Wang, J.; Xu, W.; Tao, C.; et al. Decreased expression of microRNA-21 correlates with the imbalance of Th17 and Treg cells in patients with rheumatoid arthritis. *J. Cell Mol. Med.* **2014**, *18*, 2213–2224. [CrossRef]

117. Zhang, Y.; Zhang, Y.Y.; Li, T.T.; Wang, J.; Jiang, Y.; Zhao, Y.; Jin, X.X.; Xue, G.L.; Yang, Y.; Zhang, X.F.; et al. Ablation of interleukin-17 alleviated cardiac interstitial fibrosis and improved cardiac function via inhibiting long non-coding RNA-AK081284 in diabetic mice. *J. Mol. Cell Cardiol.* **2018**, *115*, 64–72. [CrossRef]

118. Castro-Villegas, C.; Pérez-Sánchez, C.; Escudero, A.; Filipescu, I.; Verdu, M.; Ruiz-Limón, P.; Aguirre, M.A.; Jiménez-Gomez, Y.; Font, P.; Rodriguez-Ariza, A.; et al. Circulating miRNAs as potential biomarkers of therapy effectiveness in rheumatoid arthritis patients treated with anti-TNFα. *Arthritis Res. Ther.* **2015**, *17*, 49. [CrossRef]

119. O'Reilly, S.; Hügle, T.; van Laar, J.M. T cells in systemic sclerosis: A reappraisal. *Rheumatology* **2012**, *51*, 1540–1549. [CrossRef]

120. Nakashima, T.; Jinnin, M.; Yamane, K.; Honda, N.; Kajihara, I.; Makino, T.; Masuguchi, S.; Fukushima, S.; Okamoto, Y.; Hasegawa, M.; et al. Impaired IL-17 signaling pathway contributes to the increased collagen expression in scleroderma fibroblasts. *J. Immunol.* **2012**, *188*, 3573–3583. [CrossRef]

121. Zhang, Y.; Chen, X.; Deng, Y. miR-125a-3p decreases levels of interlukin-17 and suppresses renal fibrosis via down-regulating TGF-β1 in systemic lupus erythematosus mediated Lupus nephritic mice. *Am. J. Transl. Res.* **2019**, *11*, 1843–1853. [PubMed]

122. Zhu, E.; Wang, X.; Zheng, B.; Wang, Q.; Hao, J.; Chen, S.; Zhao, Q.; Zhao, L.; Wu, Z.; Yin, Z. miR-20b suppresses Th17 differentiation and the pathogenesis of experimental autoimmune encephalomyelitis by targeting RORγt and STAT3. *J. Immunol.* **2014**, *192*, 5599–5609. [CrossRef] [PubMed]
123. Liu, X.; He, F.; Pang, R.; Zhao, D.; Qiu, W.; Shan, K.; Zhang, J.; Lu, Y.; Li, Y.; Wang, Y. Interleukin-17 (IL-17)-induced microRNA 873 (miR-873) contributes to the pathogenesis of experimental autoimmune encephalomyelitis by targeting A20 ubiquitin-editing enzyme. *J. Biol. Chem.* **2014**, *289*, 28971–28986. [CrossRef] [PubMed]
124. Hanieh, H.; Alzahrani, A. MicroRNA-132 suppresses autoimmune encephalomyelitis by inducing cholinergic anti-inflammation: A new Ahr-based exploration. *Eur. J. Immunol.* **2013**, *43*, 2771–2782. [PubMed]
125. Du, C.; Liu, C.; Kang, J.; Zhao, G.; Ye, Z.; Huang, S.; Li, Z.; Wu, Z.; Pei, G. MicroRNA miR-326 regulates TH-17 differentiation and is associated with the pathogenesis of multiple sclerosis. *Nat. Immunol.* **2009**, *10*, 1252–1259. [CrossRef] [PubMed]
126. Flemming, A. Why do IL-17-targeted therapies have limited efficacy? *Nat. Rev. Immunol.* **2023**, *23*, 543. [CrossRef]
127. Rafael-Vidal, C.; Pérez, N.; Altabás, I.; Garcia, S.; Pego-Reigosa, J.M. Blocking IL-17: A Promising Strategy in the Treatment of Systemic Rheumatic Diseases. *Int. J. Mol. Sci.* **2020**, *27*, 7100. [CrossRef]
128. Wang, J.; Wang, C.; Liu, L.; Hong, S.; Ru, Y.; Sun, X.; Chen, J.; Zhang, M.; Lin, N.; Li, B.; et al. Adverse events associated with anti-IL-17 agents for psoriasis and psoriatic arthritis: A systematic scoping review. *Front. Immunol.* **2023**, *14*, 993057. [CrossRef]
129. Luo, Q.; Liu, Y.; Shi, K.; Shen, X.; Yang, Y.; Liang, X.; Lu, L.; Qiao, W.; Chen, A.; Hong, D.; et al. An autonomous activation of interleukin-17 receptor signaling sustains inflammation and promotes disease progression. *Immunity* **2023**, *56*, 2006–2020. [CrossRef]
130. Zhang, B.; Dömling, A. Small molecule modulators of IL-17A/IL-17RA: A patent review (2013–2021). *Expert Opin. Ther. Pat.* **2022**, *32*, 1161–1173. [CrossRef]
131. Huangfu, L.; Li, R.; Huang, Y.; Wang, S. The IL-17 family in diseases: From bench to bedside. *Signal Transduct. Target. Ther.* **2023**, *8*, 402. [CrossRef] [PubMed]

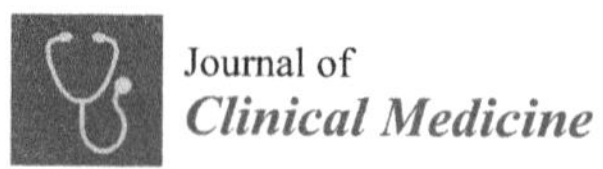
Journal of
Clinical Medicine

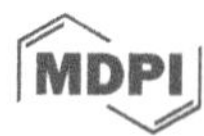

Review

The Role of Sclerostin in Rheumatic Diseases: A Review

Łukasz Jaśkiewicz [1,*], Grzegorz Chmielewski [2], Jakub Kuna [2], Tomasz Stompór [3] and Magdalena Krajewska-Włodarczyk [2,*]

[1] Department of Human Physiology and Pathophysiology, School of Medicine, Collegium Medicum, University of Warmia and Mazury in Olsztyn, 10-082 Olsztyn, Poland
[2] Department of Rheumatology, School of Medicine, Collegium Medicum, University of Warmia and Mazury in Olsztyn, 10-900 Olsztyn, Poland
[3] Department of Nephrology, Hypertension and Internal Medicine, University of Warmia and Mazury in Olsztyn, 10-516 Olsztyn, Poland
*   Correspondence: lukasz.jaskiewicz@uwm.edu.pl (Ł.J.); magdalenakw@op.pl (M.K.-W.)

Abstract: Systemic connective tissue disorders constitute a heterogenous group of autoimmune diseases with the potential to affect a range of organs. Rheumatoid arthritis (RA) is a chronic, progressive, autoimmune inflammatory disease affecting the joints. Systemic lupus erythematosus (SLE) may manifest with multiple system involvement as a result of inflammatory response to autoantibodies. Spondyloarthropathies (SpAs) such as ankylosing spondylitis (AS) or psoriatic arthritis (PsA) are diseases characterised by the inflammation of spinal joints, paraspinal tissues, peripheral joints and enthesitis as well as inflammatory changes in many other systems and organs. Physiologically, sclerostin helps to maintain balance in bone tissue metabolism through the Wnt/β-catenin pathway, which represents a major intracellular signalling pathway. This review article aims to present the current knowledge on the role of sclerostin in the Wnt/β-catenin pathway and its correlation with clinical data from RA, SLE, AS and PsA patients.

Keywords: rheumatoid arthritis; systemic lupus erythematosus; ankylosing spondylitis; psoriatic arthritis; sclerostin; Wnt/β-catenin pathway

Citation: Jaśkiewicz, Ł.; Chmielewski, G.; Kuna, J.; Stompór, T.; Krajewska-Włodarczyk, M. The Role of Sclerostin in Rheumatic Diseases: A Review. *J. Clin. Med.* **2023**, *12*, 6248. https://doi.org/10.3390/jcm12196248

Academic Editor: Eugen Feist

Received: 18 August 2023
Revised: 21 September 2023
Accepted: 26 September 2023
Published: 28 September 2023

1. Introduction

Systemic connective tissue disorders constitute a heterogenous group of autoimmune diseases with the potential to affect a range of organs. The presence of autoantibodies can be recognised as their characteristic feature. They are usually disease-specific, and so they have been included into the classification criteria [1,2].

Rheumatoid arthritis (RA) is a chronic autoimmune disease involving the joints, but may also be associated with serious systemic symptoms, e.g., interstitial lung disease or hematologic disorders [3–5]. It is a progressive disease and the persistent inflammatory process leads to cartilage damage and the formation of erosions, gradually causing disability [6].

Systemic lupus erythematosus (SLE) is a systemic autoimmune disorder, which may involve multiple systems. Its exact aetiology is still unclear [7]. The disease may have different clinical presentations, which complicates prognostic assessment in this patient group [8,9]. It has been demonstrated that environmental and genetic factors, through their mutual interaction, may be implicated in triggering the immune response, resulting in excessive autoantibody production, which leads to inflammation-mediated tissue and organ injury. SLE is characterised by the presence of antibodies targeted at nuclear and cytoplasmic antigens [10,11].

Spondyloarthropathies (SpAs) are inflammatory diseases involving spinal joints, peripheral joints and tendons. These include the following: ankylosing spondylitis (AS), psoriatic arthritis (PsA), reactive arthritis and non-specific inflammatory bowel disease-associated arthritis [12–15].

Sclerostin, a glycoprotein produced and released primarily by mature osteocytes, is an inhibitor of Wnt/β-catenin pathway-dependent osteoblast proliferation and differentiation from mesenchymal stem cells [16]. Physiologically, sclerostin is a regulator of bone tissue metabolism. As a result of mechanical loading and microtraumas, and with oestrogen deficiency, the release of sclerostin is inhibited, which stimulates the processes of bone formation and repair [17–20]. With age, there is an increase in plasma sclerostin concentration in both sexes, and this may be associated with age-related osteoporosis [21]. Apart from inhibiting the Wnt/β-catenin pathway, sclerostin can stimulate RANKL secretion in osteocytes, osteoclastogenesis and bone resorption [22,23]. Sclerostin was originally discovered as a result of studies on inactivating mutations in the coding and enhancer regions of the *SOST* gene [24]. The function of sclerostin as an inhibitor of osteogenesis has been confirmed in a study involving transgenic mice. Sclerostin knock-out (SOST KO) mice showed high bone mass and increased bone formation and bone strength [25,26], whereas animals with sclerostin overexpression presented with low bone mass and bone fragility [27].

To date, only a few publications have investigated the role of sclerostin as a potential biomarker in rheumatic diseases.

2. Wnt/β-Catenin Pathway

The Wnt pathway is recognised as a major intracellular signalling pathway that is also in osteocytes [28,29]. It may involve the activation of the best-studied, β-catenin-dependent, canonical pathway, or a few non-canonical pathways [30]. The canonical pathway regulates the activity of T-cell factor (TCF), impacting the embryogenesis, differentiation and proliferation of cells [31]. Wnt proteins are implicated in initiating intracellular signalling pathways by binding to specific Frizzled transmembrane receptors, showing a high degree of affinity to Wnt proteins [32]. Apart from the interaction of a Wnt protein with a Frizzled receptor, the activation of the signalling pathway requires the binding of a co-receptor from the family of low-density lipoprotein receptor (LDLR)-related proteins, particularly LRP5 and LRP6. This leads to the formation of a trimeric complex capable of signal transduction [33]. Additionally, Dishevelled (Dvl) protein [34] and axin [35] bind to the cytoplasmic parts of the Frizzled receptor and LRP co-receptor, respectively. The activation of the complex is associated with the heterodimerisation of Dvl proteins and axin, which results in the re-configuration of the complex and the activation and detachment of β-catenin [36]. Free, active β-catenin accumulates in the cytoplasm and is then transported to the cell nucleus, where it binds to the TCF protein, constituting one of the major transcription factors. The interaction of β-catenin with CF leads to chromatin remodelling, adjacent to the TCF binding site, and is a key stimulator in commencing gene transcription [37]. With no signal stimulating the Wnt pathway, the amount and activity of β-catenin are limited by the operation of the so-called destruction complex, formed by axin (here, unbound to the LRP co-receptor), protein APC (adenomatous polyposis coli) and two serine-threonine kinases: CKIα (casein kinase 1α) and GSK3 (glycogen synthase kinase 3). The activity of kinases in the axin/APC/CKIα/GSK3 complex leads to β-catenin phosphorylation, its identification via β-TrCP ligase (β-transducing repeat-containing protein ligase) and ubiquitination, with its ultimate degradation in proteasomes [38]. The inhibition of the Wnt signalling pathway may involve extracellular inhibitors of Wnt activators such as sFRP (secreted Frizzled-related protein) [39] and WIF (Wnt inhibitory factor) [40], as well as inhibitors of the LRP co-receptor including Wise proteins [41], Dkk-1 (Dickkopf-related protein-1) [42] and sclerostin [43]. See Figure 1.

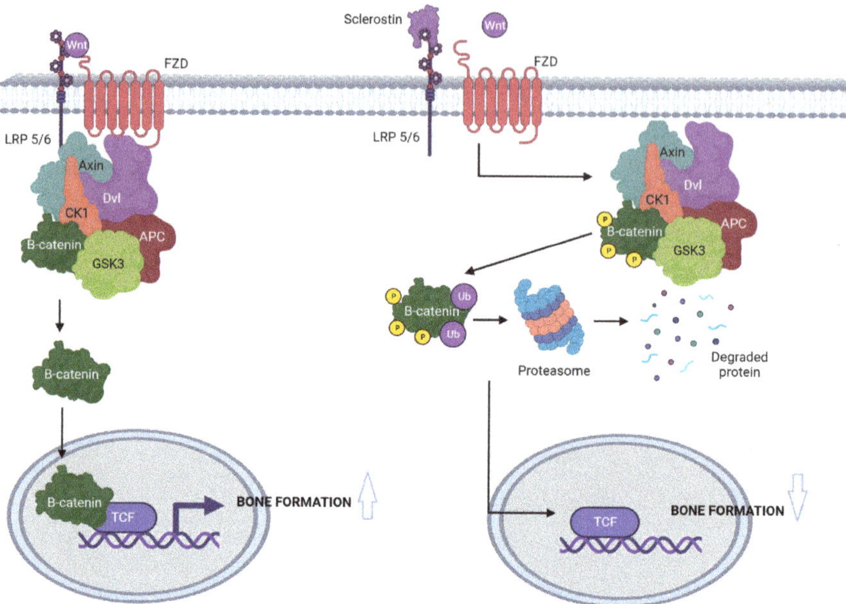

Figure 1. The effect of sclerostin on the Wnt/β-catenin pathway. When the Wnt signalling pathway is not inhibited by sclerostin, it leads to increased bone formation. Sclerostin inhibits the canonical Wnt-signalling pathway through its binding to the Wnt LRP 5/6 co-receptors and leads to decreased bone formation. APC: adenomatous polyposis coli; CK1α: casein kinase 1 α; Dvl: Dishevelled protein; FZD: Frizzled receptor; GSK3: glycogen synthase kinase 3; LRP 5/6: low-density lipoprotein receptor-related protein 5/6; P: phosphorus; Ub: ubiquitin; TCF: transcription factor. Created using BioRender.com (accessed on 16 August 2023).

3. The Role of Sclerostin in Rheumatoid Arthritis

Rheumatoid arthritis (RA) involves, as its integral component, disorders of bone tissue metabolism manifested by erosions, periarticular osteoporosis and generalised osteoporosis [4,44,45]. The stage of the disease and the rate of bone involvement progression depend on the intensity of bone resorption and inadequate bone formation, which may be conditioned by a range of factors connected with inflammatory joint disease, such as pro-inflammatory cytokine overproduction, limited physical activity or medications used. They may also include well-recognised risk factors for osteoporosis, i.e., old age, endocrine disorders, genetic susceptibility, low peak bone mass, nutrient-deficient diet and smoking [46,47]. The ethology of RA is still not entirely clear. Many factors, such as genetic background, smoking or infections, play a role in the process of converting arginine into citrulline by the Peptidyl Arginine Deiminase 4 (PADI4) enzyme [48,49]. A genetic predisposition was identified, which was located in a common epitope in the HLA-DRB1 locus of major histocompatibility complex (MHC) class II antigens [50]. The key factor in the development of RA is the occurrence of anti-citrullinated protein antibody (ACPA) and/or rheumatoid factor (RF) produced by plasma cells of the synovial membrane [51], which results in the stimulation of monocytes, mast cells and dendritic cells, but also Th1, Th17, B lymphocytes and plasma cells, to produce mediators of the inflammatory reaction [52]. RF interacts directly with the Fc region of IgG and forms immune complexes that increase vascular permeability and have a chemotactic effect [53]. ACPA is directed against, among others, the following: citrullinated filaggrin, fibrinogen, vimentin and α-enolase, which activates the complement system and induces the secretion of TNF-α by macrophages [54]. T lymphocytes recognise the antigen through antigen-presenting cells (APCs) and trigger a specific response. The pathogenesis of RA involves Th1 lymphocytes producing IFN-γ and

Th17 lymphocytes, which are often found in the synovium of RA patients and rarely in the synovium of the joints of healthy people. Th17 lymphocytes, through the secretion of IL-17 and IL-22, strongly stimulate macrophages to secrete pro-inflammatory cytokines such as TNF-α, IL-1 and IL-6 [55–57]. B lymphocytes differentiate into antibody-producing plasma cells, and also produce pro-inflammatory cytokines and play the role of antigen-presenting cells and cells regulating the humoral response [58]. Fibroblast-like synoviocytes (FSCs) are activated and, together with other inflammatory cells, produce RANKL [59]. Ultimately, this leads to increased production of osteoclasts and the formation of erosions. In RA, in particular, macrophages produce large amounts of pro-inflammatory cytokines, i.e., TNF-alpha, IL-6, IL-1, IL-15, IL-18, IL-32 and chemotactic factors [57]. TNF-α increases the expression of sclerostin in primary osteocytes and also enhances the formation of osteoclasts induced by RANKL, which promotes the formation of erosions [60,61].

The risk for cardiovascular diseases observed in RA patients is significantly higher than in the general population [5,6] and exceeds the risk assessed according to traditional factors contributing to arteriosclerosis [7–9]. Chronic inflammation in RA is associated with endothelial dysfunction and the formation of arteriosclerotic lesions. Advanced arteriosclerosis is marked by particularly severe arterial calcification [10–12], mainly involving the intimal layer [13]; calcification of the medial layer (Mönckeberg's calcification) may develop independently of changes observed in arteriosclerosis [14]. While intimal calcifications occupy focal areas and are mainly found in arteriosclerotic plaque, calcifications in the medial layer display a linear pattern [15].

In the few studies conducted to date investigating the association between sclerostin and the course of RA, serum sclerostin concentrations were higher [62–64], the same [65,66] or lower [67] when compared to the results obtained in control groups of healthy individuals. The discrepancies may have been due to differences between patient groups participating in the study. They could have also been due to the effect of using different assays to determine sclerostin concentrations. Somewhat unexpectedly, the sclerostin concentration was observed to rise during successful therapy with etanercept [68] and tocilizumab [69], while it decreased with greater disease activity, as measured via DAS28 [62–64,68], the number of tender joints [65] and an increase in the C-reactive protein (CRP) level [64,66]. There seems to be no association between sclerostin concentration and advanced stage of the disease radiologically [63,65,70], although there was a significant correlation reported between its level and local occurrence of severe osteoarticular lesions, as assessed using the Larsen scoring system [64]. Moreover, there was no correlation found between sclerostin concentration and bone mineral density in the forearm or femoral neck bone in RA patients [64,71]. In a study by Paccou et al., there was an association identified between increased BMD of the lumbar region and rise in sclerostin concentration, similarly to the control group, where a high sclerostin level was consistent with high BMD values in the femoral neck bone [71]. These results may suggest the involvement of total mass of active osteocytes and potential engagement of other excited cells, including synoviocytes, in the process of sclerostin production and release [72].

In a study by Wehmeyer et al. in an arthritis model in hTNFtg mice, SOST expression was not only present in osteocytes but was TNF-α-induced in FLS cells, which were the main source of sclerostin. Interestingly, also in this study, sclerostin seemed to exert a protective effect, as the administration of sclerostin inhibitor led to greater joint swelling, weaker grip and progression of bone lesions in the joints. In a mouse model of antigen (G6PI)-induced, partially TNF-α-dependent arthritis, sclerostin was found to have no effect on bone loss; however, it diminished the disease activity in a TNF-α-independent, serum-derived model in K/BxN mice. Additionally, the administration of recombinant sclerostin inhibited, through LRP6, the activity of TNF-α-induced (but not IL-1-induced) MAP: p38 and ERK kinases, and as a result, the activity of NFκB in synoviocytes from mice and in those obtained from RA patients as well. Moreover, it was associated with decreased expression of the RANK ligand on human FLS [72]. In a study using a collagen-induced arthritis model, using sclerostin inhibitor prevented the loss of total bone mass, having no effect on the formation of local bone erosions [73]. In another study, although blocking sclerostin in hTNFtg mice inhibited bone destruction, this was only after the additional administration of TNF-α inhibitor [74]. Of note, animal models of arthritis used in the studies do not truly represent human rheumatoid arthritis, and so the reported discrepancies in the results may be due to the dominant activity of particular cytokines in these models.

4. The Role of Sclerostin in Systemic Lupus Erythematosus

Systemic lupus erythematosus (SLE) may cause disorders of the locomotor system which usually include painful conditions of joints and muscles, tendonitis or tenosynovitis. However, periarticular structures usually remain unaffected [75]. Tendonitis, tenosynovitis or capsulitis may lead to Jaccoud arthropathy, which is characterised by joint deformity, but, unlike in RA, no erosions are observed [76]. In the pathophysiology of SLE, we observed increased formation of autoantigen–antibody complexes by autoreactive B lymphocytes, which were then recognised by plasmacytoid dendritic cells. This leads to the stimulation of Toll-like receptor [TLR]-7 and TLR-9-dependent pathways, as well as the secretion of endogenous IFN-α [77]. This causes the additional stimulation of both groups of lymphocytes: B and T. Hyperactivity of T lymphocytes, in particular the CD4+ subpopulation [78], may affect the Wnt/β-catenin pathway, which has also been described in animal models of lupus nephritis [79].

In the few studies conducted to date, aiming to assess the association between sclerostin and the course of SLE, the serum sclerostin concentration was found to be elevated. Fayed et al. compared a group of 100 patients with a control group of 50 and demonstrated increased sclerostin concentration in patients with SLE and its statistically significant correlation with proteinuria in these patients. This confirms a key role of Wnt/β-catenin signalling in SLE pathogenesis, which means that sclerostin may become a potential biomarker of lupus nephritis in the future [80]. The research to date has shown that the Wnt/β-catenin signalling pathway plays a role in cell protection against stress factors and apoptosis [81]. However, excessive and long-lasting activation of Wnt/β-catenin signalling may enhance the expression of matrix metalloproteinases (MMPs), particularly MMP-2 and MMP-9, in glomeruli. Metalloproteinases, through the degradation of the matrix, lead to the loss of membrane and extracellular matrix integrity, and, moreover, may lead to renal fibrosis and progressive renal dysfunction [82]. Garcia-de los Ríos et al. reported on the association of sclerostin with the presence of atherosclerotic plaque in the carotid arteries of women with SLE [83]. To date, there have been reports on a correlation between sclerostin concentration and arterial calcification in RA [71].

5. The Role of Sclerostin in Psoriatic Arthritis

Psoriatic arthritis (PsA) is a chronic disease manifesting with synovitis, enthesitis and dermatitis, with no rheumatoid factor present. The disease has a heterogenous clinical presentation regarding the number of joints affected and the degree of their damage, as well as the severity of skin lesions, if seen, as these may be absent [84,85]. IL-17 plays an important role in the pathogenesis of PsA, affecting bone formation in inflammatory places as a result of mechanical injury, as is the case with entheses in animal models of SpA [86]. In addition, TNF-α, IL22 and IL23 play an important role. IL23, which is secreted mainly by macrophages and dendritic cells, but also by keratinocytes, is primarily responsible for the induction of Th17 cells [87]. Th17 cells produce IL-17, which enhances the production of pro-inflammatory cytokines such as IL1-β, IL-6 and TNF-alpha by synovial fibroblasts and macrophages [88]. Ultimately, this leads to the destruction of bone tissue as a result of the inflammatory process. Moreover, IL-23 promotes the expression of RANK, which leads to the differentiation of precursor cells toward osteoclasts, which intensifies bone tissue damage [89]. In turn, IL-22 has a bone-forming effect by inducing the formation of osteoblasts [90].

Fassio et al. assessed the sclerostin concentration in 33 women with PsA comparing the obtained results with a group of 28 women with RA and 35 healthy women of the control group. No statistically significant differences were found between the groups for sclerostin [91]. Fassio et al. assessed the efficacy of treatment with secukinumab (anti-IL-17) in a group of 28 patients, as compared to a control group (n = 43), at a follow-up after 1, 3 and 6 months, and demonstrated that it may have an effect on the activity of osteocytes, including Wnt/β-catenin pathway inhibitors, which may suggest the potential of the drug to inhibit local excessive bone proliferation, being a typical component of PsA. The treatment used did not cause a statistically significant increase in sclerostin concentration in the study groups in comparison to the control group [92]. In 2019, Diani et al. compared a group of 50 patients with psoriasis with a group of 50 patients with PsA and a group of 20 healthy individuals in order to identify potential differences in the concentrations of predictive osteoimmunological biomarkers. The study mentioned above showed that both the patients with psoriasis and the patients with PsA had higher sclerostin concentrations than the individuals from the control group. Moreover, the study provided evidence for a positive correlation between sclerostin concentration and the duration of psoriasis [93]. Tasende et al. conducted a study on a group of 45 patients, including 15 individuals with a diagnosis of PsA, 8 individuals with RA, 15 patients with chronic arthritis and 4 patients diagnosed with AS. In the above-mentioned study, there was no statistically significant increase in mRNA expression in synovium, or in sclerostin concentration in patients with PsA in comparison to patients with RA, chronic arthritis or ankylosing spondylitis [94].

6. The Role of Sclerostin in Ankylosing Spondylitis

Ankylosing spondylitis (AS) is an inflammatory disease affecting sacroiliac joints, spinal joints, fibrous rings and spinal ligaments. The underlying inflammatory process results in gradual spinal damage. The aetiology of this condition has not been fully elucidated [15,95,96]. AS is characterised by chronic inflammation and bone remodelling as a result of osteogenesis, mainly in the axial skeleton [97]. The link between inflammation and bone remodelling has not been fully explained. TNF-α as a pro-inflammatory cytokine in AS is responsible for the induction of Dkk-1 and sclerostin [98], which in turn downregulate bone formation via the inhibition of Wnt and bone morphogenic proteins (BMPs) [28]. However, bone formation is also responsible for mechanical load, which stimulates osteocytes to produce BMP, and thus activates the Wnt pathway and inhibits the production of Dkk-1 and sclerostin [99]. In vivo studies in a mouse model of SpA demonstrated that mechanical stress causes enthesitis and bone remodelling [100].

The first publication discussing the role of sclerostin in the course of AS appeared in 2009. Appel et al. reported a lower sclerostin concentration in patients diagnosed with AS in comparison to a control group of healthy volunteers. Additionally, they found that a low sclerostin level was correlated with syndesmophyte formation [101]. In the years to follow, some publications reported decreased [102–112] or increased [113–115] sclerostin levels in the course of AS, while according to other reports its values did not differ from those found in the control group [116–118]. Consequently, the role of sclerostin remains unclear. A low sclerostin concentration is correlated with an increased Dkk1 concentration, which confirms its inhibitory effect on the Wnt/β-catenin pathway [101,102]. The association of sclerostin and syndesmophyte formation was also confirmed by Heiland et al. [102,119]. However, this correlation remains unclear [103,120]. Korkosz et al. demonstrated that sclerostin levels in patients treated with TNF inhibitor remained unchanged [121]. Similar observations were made by Ustun et al., who found that sclerostin by itself did not induce inflammation or damage which could be visualised via radiological examination [122,123]. In a study assessing sclerostin concentration during 12-week therapy with apremilast, a PDE4 inhibitor, a significant reduction in sclerostin levels was seen. However, the clinical relevance of this report remains uncertain [120].

In Table 1, detailed data are presented comparing patients and healthy controls, as well as the type of assay used.

Table 1. Summary of study results comparing a group of patients to healthy controls.

Authors (Ref)	Number of Patients	Number of Healthy Controls	Patient Group		Age (Mean ± SD)	Level of Sclerostin	Assay Name	Producer	Tissue
			Number of Females	Number of Males					
			RA						
Dhakad U et al. [62]	47	28	47	0	32.7 ± 6.8	Elevated	ELISA	No data	Serum
El-Bakry S et al. [63]	31	10	28	3	40 (without SD)	Elevated	ELISA	Biomedica	Serum
Singh A et al. [64]	50	50	41	9	41.30 ± 12.971	Elevated	ELISA	RayBio	Serum
Mehaney DA et al. [65]	40	40	33	7	46.7 ± 13.6	No difference	ELISA	TECO Medical	Serum
Świerkot J et al. [66]	27	12	27	0	54.7 (without SD)	No difference	ELISA	TECO Medical	Serum
Seror R et al. [67]	694	453	694	0	48.5 (without SD)	Decreased	ELISA	Biomedica	Serum
			SLE						
Fayed A et al. [80]	100	50	100	0	25.9 ± 5.8	Elevated	ELISA	Quantikine	Serum
Garcia-de los Ríos C et al. [83]	68	No control group	68	0	43.8 ± 11.0	Elevated	ELISA	BI-20472	Serum
			PsA						
Fassio A et al. [91]	33	35	33	0	58.8 ± 8.8	No difference	ELISA	Biomedica	Serum
Fassio A et al. [92]	28	43	18	10	57 ± 10	No difference	ELISA	Biomedica	Serum
Diani M et al. [93]	50	20	11	39	48 (without SD)	No difference	ELISA	Quantikine	Serum
Pinto Tasende JA et al. [94]	15	No control group	5	10	48.0 (without SD)	No difference	ELISA Quantitative real-time PCR	DAS Superscript® VILO (Thermo Fisher Scientific, Waltham, MA, USA)	Serum Synovial tissue
			AS						
Appel H et al. [101]	46	50	16	30	No data	Decreased	ELISA	R&D Systems	Serum
Heiland GR et al. [102]	65	No control group	19	46	35.2 ± 10.4	Decreased	ELISA	No data	Serum
Saad CG et al. [103]	30	36	6	24	35.7 ± 11.0	Decreased	ELISA	Biomedica	Serum
Klingberg E et al. [104]	204	80	87	117	49 (without SD)	Decreased	ELISA	Biomedica	Serum
Sakellariou GT et al. [105]	65	36	4	61	41.3 (without SD)	Decreased	ELISA	Aviscera Bioscience	Serum
Rossini M. et al. [106]	71	70	12	59	Men 43 ± 12 Women 49 ± 12	Decreased	ELISA	Biomedica	Serum
Solmaz D et al. [107]	97	48	21	76	38 ± 14.0	Decreased	ELISA	PeloBiotech, Planegg	Serum
Genre F et al. [108]	119	63	46	73	44.9 ± 11.9	Decreased	ELISA	TECO Medical	Serum
Luchetti MM et al. [109]	45 *	20	20	25	43 (without SD)	Decreased	ELISA ELISA	ICL Lab Inc	Serum Serum
Perrotta FM et al. [110]	40	20	10	30	50 (without SD)	Decreased	ELISA	AUROGENE srl	Serum
Gercik O et al. [111]	55	57	21	34	41 (without SD)	No difference	ELISA	Elabscience	Serum
Iaremenko O et al. [112]	102	15	35	67	38.1 ± 11.2	Decreased	ELISA	Biomedica	Serum
Korkosz M et al. [113]	50—high activity 28—low activity	23	8 No data	42 No data	37.8 ± 11.6 32.0 ± 6.6	Increased No difference	ELISA	Biomedica	Serum
Sun W et al. [115]	88	26	22	66	36.5 ± 13.5	Increased	ELISA	Biomedica	Serum
Sakellariou GT et al. [116]	57	34	4	53	39.1 ± 1.4	No difference	ELISA	Aviscera Bioscience Inc.	Serum
Taylan A et al. [117]	55	33	7	48	36 (without SD)	No difference	ELISA	Biomedica	Serum
Tuylu T et al. [118]	45—syndesmophyte (+) 49—syndesmophyte (−)	68	13 16	32 33	43.9 ± 9.9 40.7 ± 8.7	No difference	ELISA	Biomedica	Serum

* Inflammatory bowel disease (IBD)-associated spondyloarthritis (SpA/IBD).

Differences in the results obtained between individual studies may result from the use of tests from different manufacturers, despite the use of the same testing technique in most cases, as well as the accompanying additional diseases. The concentration of sclerostin largely depends on the test used for measurement. Delanaye P. et al. showed that the concentrations obtained using the R&D Systems and MesoScaleDiscovery tests were lower than those obtained using Biomedica or TECO Medical, which means that the results must be interpreted with great caution [124]. Moreover, the results were influenced by the heterogeneity of the study groups, as well as the use of various exclusion criteria from the studies, which are presented in Table S1 of the Supplementary Materials. So far, higher sclerostin concentrations have been observed in older patients and patients with chronic kidney disease or type 2 diabetes mellitus [125,126].

7. Conclusions

Among numerous clinical aspects connected with the course of rheumatoid arthritis, disorders of bone metabolism and resultant complications significantly contribute to a worse prognosis as negative regulators of bone growth. It may influence the development of osteoporosis and erosions. In both RA and AS, TNF-α appears to play a key role in sclerostin levels and increased osteoclast activity, but this is only reflected in studies in RA. In AS, it appears that mechanical stress has a greater effect on inhibiting sclerostin formation than TNF-α has on its increased production. It seems that in patients with PsA, the concentration of IL-17 and IL-23 should be of key importance for the concentration of sclerostin and the Wnt/β-catenin pathway itself; however, previous studies comparing groups of patients with PsA with a control group of healthy people do not confirm this, which may also mean that other factors may play a role. For patients with SLE, the sclerostin concentration appears to be a promising biomarker associated with lupus nephropathy or increased cardiovascular risk, which is related to an increased production of IFN-α and effects on T lymphocytes. In spondyloarthropathy, the significance of sclerostin remains unclear and requires further investigation. The Wnt/β-catenin pathway is a key regulator in bone remodelling, but its role requires further research to gain a better understanding of this issue.

Supplementary Materials: The following supporting information can be downloaded at: https://www.mdpi.com/article/10.3390/jcm12196248/s1, Table S1: Summary of exclusion criteria.

Author Contributions: Conceptualisation, Ł.J., T.S. and M.K.-W.; methodology, Ł.J. and M.K.-W.; software, Ł.J.; formal analysis, Ł.J.; investigation, Ł.J., T.S., G.C., J.K. and M.K.-W.; data curation, Ł.J.; writing—original draft preparation, Ł.J., T.S., G.C., J.K. and M.K.-W.; writing—review and editing, Ł.J., T.S. and M.K.-W.; visualisation, Ł.J.; supervision, M.K.-W.; project administration, M.K.-W.; funding acquisition, M.K.-W. All authors have read and agreed to the published version of the manuscript.

Funding: This study was supported by the School of Medicine (61.610.001-110), University of Warmia and Mazury, in Olsztyn, Poland.

Institutional Review Board Statement: Not applicable.

Informed Consent Statement: Not applicable.

Data Availability Statement: No new data were created in this work.

Conflicts of Interest: The authors declare no conflict of interest.

References

1. Mulhearn, B.; Tansley, S.L.; McHugh, N.J. Autoantibodies in connective tissue disease. *Best Pract. Res. Clin. Rheumatol.* **2019**, *34*, 101462. [CrossRef] [PubMed]
2. Fernandez, A.P. Connective Tissue Disease. *Dermatol. Clin.* **2019**, *37*, 37–48. [CrossRef] [PubMed]
3. O'Dwyer, D.N.; Armstrong, M.E.; Cooke, G.; Dodd, J.D.; Veale, D.J.; Donnelly, S.C. Rheumatoid Arthritis (RA) associated interstitial lung disease (ILD). *Eur. J. Intern. Med.* **2013**, *24*, 597–603. [CrossRef] [PubMed]
4. Scott, D.L.; Wolfe, F.; Huizinga, T.W.J. Rheumatoid arthritis. *Lancet* **2010**, *376*, 1094–1108. [CrossRef] [PubMed]
5. Smolen, J.S.; Aletaha, D.; McInnes, I.B. Rheumatoid arthritis. *Lancet* **2016**, *388*, 2023–2038. [CrossRef] [PubMed]

6. Lin, Y.-J.; Anzaghe, M.; Schülke, S. Update on the Pathomechanism, Diagnosis, and Treatment Options for Rheumatoid Arthritis. *Cells* **2020**, *9*, 880. [CrossRef]

7. Rekvig, O.P.; Van der Vlag, J. The pathogenesis and diagnosis of systemic lupus erythematosus: Still not resolved. *Semin. Immunopathol.* **2014**, *36*, 301–311. [CrossRef]

8. Dörner, T.; Furie, R. Novel paradigms in systemic lupus erythematosus. *Lancet* **2019**, *393*, 2344–2358. [CrossRef]

9. Trentin, F.; Zucchi, D.; Signorini, V.; Elefante, E.; Bortoluzzi, A.; Tani, C. One year in review 2021: Systemic lupus erythematosus. *Clin. Exp. Rheumatol.* **2021**, *39*, 231–241. [CrossRef]

10. Pan, L.; Lu, M.-P.; Wang, J.-H.; Xu, M.; Yang, S.-R. Immunological pathogenesis and treatment of systemic lupus erythematosus. *World J. Pediatr.* **2020**, *16*, 19–30. [CrossRef]

11. Moulton, V.R.; Suarez-Fueyo, A.; Meidan, E.; Li, H.; Mizui, M.; Tsokos, G.C. Pathogenesis of Human Systemic Lupus Erythematosus: A Cellular Perspective. *Trends Mol. Med.* **2017**, *23*, 615–635. [CrossRef] [PubMed]

12. Denison, H.J.; Curtis, E.M.; A Clynes, M.; Bromhead, C.; Dennison, E.M.; Grainger, R. The incidence of sexually acquired reactive arthritis: A systematic literature review. *Clin. Rheumatol.* **2016**, *35*, 2639–2648. [CrossRef]

13. Gutiérrez-Sánchez, J.; Parra-Izquierdo, V.; Flórez-Sarmiento, C.; Jaimes, D.A.; De Ávila, J.; Bello-Gualtero, J.M.; Ramos-Casallas, A.; Chila-Moreno, L.; Pacheco-Tena, C.; Beltrán-Ostos, A.; et al. Implementation of screening criteria for inflammatory bowel disease in patients with spondyloarthritis and its association with disease and endoscopic activity. *Clin. Rheumatol.* **2023**, *42*, 415–422. [CrossRef] [PubMed]

14. Rudwaleit, M.; Taylor, W.J. Classification criteria for psoriatic arthritis and ankylosing spondylitis/axial spondyloarthritis. *Best Pract. Res. Clin. Rheumatol.* **2010**, *24*, 589–604. [CrossRef] [PubMed]

15. Braun, J.; van den Berg, R.; Baraliakos, X.; Boehm, H.; Burgos-Vargas, R.; Estévez, E.C.; Dagfinrud, H.; Dijkmans, B.; Dougados, M.; Emery, P.; et al. 2010 update of the ASAS/EULAR recommendations for the management of ankylosing spondylitis. *Ann. Rheum. Dis.* **2011**, *70*, 896–904. [CrossRef]

16. Wang, J.S.; Mazur, C.M.; Wein, M.N. Sclerostin and Osteocalcin: Candidate Bone-Produced Hormones. *Front. Endocrinol.* **2021**, *12*, 584147. [CrossRef]

17. Khosla, S.; Westendorf, J.J.; Oursler, M.J. Building bone to reverse osteoporosis and repair fractures. *J. Clin. Investig.* **2008**, *118*, 421–428. [CrossRef]

18. Gaudio, A.; Pennisi, P.; Bratengeier, C.; Torrisi, V.; Lindner, B.; Mangiafico, R.A.; Pulvirenti, I.; Hawa, G.; Tringali, G.; Fiore, C.E. Increased Sclerostin Serum Levels Associated with Bone Formation and Resorption Markers in Patients with Immobilization-Induced Bone Loss. *J. Clin. Endocrinol. Metab.* **2010**, *95*, 2248–2253. [CrossRef]

19. Tu, X.; Rhee, Y.; Condon, K.W.; Bivi, N.; Allen, M.R.; Dwyer, D.; Stolina, M.; Turner, C.H.; Robling, A.G.; Plotkin, L.I.; et al. Sost downregulation and local Wnt signaling are required for the osteogenic response to mechanical loading. *Bone* **2012**, *50*, 209–217. [CrossRef]

20. Kim, B.-J.; Bae, S.J.; Lee, S.-Y.; Lee, Y.-S.; Baek, J.-E.; Park, S.-Y.; Lee, S.H.; Koh, J.-M.; Kim, G.S. TNF-α mediates the stimulation of sclerostin expression in an estrogen-deficient condition. *Biochem. Biophys. Res. Commun.* **2012**, *424*, 170–175. [CrossRef]

21. I Mödder, U.; A Hoey, K.; Amin, S.; McCready, L.K.; Achenbach, S.J.; Riggs, B.L.; Melton, L.J.; Khosla, S. Relation of age, gender, and bone mass to circulating sclerostin levels in women and men. *J. Bone Miner. Res.* **2011**, *26*, 373–379. [CrossRef] [PubMed]

22. Wijenayaka, A.R.; Kogawa, M.; Lim, H.P.; Bonewald, L.F.; Findlay, D.M.; Atkins, G.J. Sclerostin Stimulates Osteocyte Support of Osteoclast Activity by a RANKL-Dependent Pathway. *PLoS ONE* **2011**, *6*, e25900. [CrossRef] [PubMed]

23. Tu, X.; Delgado-Calle, J.; Condon, K.W.; Maycas, M.; Zhang, H.; Carlesso, N.; Taketo, M.M.; Burr, D.B.; Plotkin, L.I.; Bellido, T. Osteocytes mediate the anabolic actions of canonical Wnt/β-catenin signaling in bone. *Proc. Natl. Acad. Sci. USA* **2015**, *112*, E478–E486. [CrossRef] [PubMed]

24. Li, X.; Zhang, Y.; Kang, H.; Liu, W.; Liu, P.; Zhang, J.; Harris, S.E.; Wu, D. Sclerostin Binds to LRP5/6 and Antagonizes Canonical Wnt Signaling. *J. Biol. Chem.* **2005**, *280*, 19883–19887. [CrossRef]

25. Li, X.; Ominsky, M.S.; Niu, Q.-T.; Sun, N.; Daugherty, B.; D'Agostin, D.; Kurahara, C.; Gao, Y.; Cao, J.; Gong, J.; et al. Targeted Deletion of the Sclerostin Gene in Mice Results in Increased Bone Formation and Bone Strength. *J. Bone Miner. Res.* **2008**, *23*, 860–869. [CrossRef]

26. Lin, C.; Jiang, X.; Dai, Z.; Guo, X.; Weng, T.; Wang, J.; Li, Y.; Feng, G.; Gao, X.; He, L. Sclerostin Mediates Bone Response to Mechanical Unloading Through Antagonizing Wnt/β-Catenin Signaling. *J. Bone Miner. Res.* **2009**, *24*, 1651–1661. [CrossRef]

27. Kramer, I.; Loots, G.G.; Studer, A.; Keller, H.; Kneissel, M. Parathyroid hormone (PTH)–induced bone gain is blunted in SOST overexpressing and deficient mice. *J. Bone Miner. Res.* **2009**, *25*, 178–189. [CrossRef]

28. Maeda, K.; Kobayashi, Y.; Koide, M.; Uehara, S.; Okamoto, M.; Ishihara, A.; Kayama, T.; Saito, M.; Marumo, K. The Regulation of Bone Metabolism and Disorders by Wnt Signaling. *Int. J. Mol. Sci.* **2019**, *20*, 5525. [CrossRef]

29. Manolagas, S.C. Wnt signaling and osteoporosis. *Maturitas* **2014**, *78*, 233–237. [CrossRef]

30. Komiya, Y.; Habas, R. Wnt signal transduction pathways. *Organogenesis* **2008**, *4*, 68–75. [CrossRef]

31. Logan, C.Y.; Nusse, R. The wnt signaling pathway in development and disease. *Annu. Rev. Cell Dev. Biol.* **2004**, *20*, 781–810. [CrossRef] [PubMed]

32. Hsieh, J.-C.; Kodjabachian, L.; Rebbert, M.L.; Rattner, A.; Smallwood, P.M.; Samos, C.H.; Nusse, R.; Dawid, I.B.; Nathans, J. A new secreted protein that binds to Wnt proteins and inhibits their activites. *Nature* **1999**, *398*, 431–436. [CrossRef] [PubMed]

33. Tamai, K.; Semenov, M.; Kato, Y.; Spokony, R.; Liu, C.; Katsuyama, Y.; Hess, F.; Saint-Jeannet, J.-P.; He, X. LDL-receptor-related proteins in Wnt signal transduction. *Nature* **2000**, *407*, 530–535. [CrossRef]
34. Umbhauer, M.; Djiane, A.; Goisset, C.; Penzo-Méndez, A.; Riou, J.; Boucaut, J.; Shi, D. The C-terminal cytoplasmic Lys-Thr-X-X-X-Trp motif in frizzled receptors mediates Wnt/beta-catenin signalling. *EMBO J.* **2000**, *19*, 4944–4954. [CrossRef] [PubMed]
35. Mao, J.; Wang, J.; Liu, B.; Pan, W.; Farr, G.H.; Flynn, C.; Yuan, H.; Takada, S.; Kimelman, D.; Li, L.; et al. Low-Density Lipoprotein Receptor-Related Protein-5 Binds to Axin and Regulates the Canonical Wnt Signaling Pathway. *Mol. Cell* **2001**, *7*, 801–809. [CrossRef] [PubMed]
36. Itoh, K.; Antipova, A.; Ratcliffe, M.J.; Sokol, S. Interaction of Dishevelled and *Xenopus* Axin-Related Protein Is Required for Wnt Signal Transduction. *Mol. Cell. Biol.* **2000**, *20*, 2228–2238. [CrossRef]
37. Hecht, A.; Vleminckx, K.; Stemmler, M.P.; van Roy, F.; Kemler, R. The p300/CBP acetyltransferases function as transcriptional coactivators of beta-catenin in vertebrates. *EMBO J.* **2000**, *19*, 1839–1850. [CrossRef]
38. Aberle, H.; Bauer, A.; Stappert, J.; Kispert, A.; Kemler, R. β-catenin is a target for the ubiquitin–proteasome pathway. *EMBO J.* **1997**, *16*, 3797–3804. [CrossRef]
39. Hoang, B.; Moos, M.; Vukicevic, S.; Luyten, F.P. Primary Structure and Tissue Distribution of FRZB, a Novel Protein Related to Drosophila Frizzled, Suggest a Role in Skeletal Morphogenesis. *J. Biol. Chem.* **1996**, *271*, 26131–26137. [CrossRef]
40. Liepinsh, E.; Bányai, L.; Patthy, L.; Otting, G. NMR Structure of the WIF Domain of the Human Wnt-Inhibitory Factor-1. *J. Mol. Biol.* **2006**, *357*, 942–950. [CrossRef]
41. Itasaki, N.; Jones, C.M.; Mercurio, S.; Rowe, A.; Domingos, P.M.; Smith, J.C.; Krumlauf, R. Wise, a context-dependent activator and inhibitor of Wnt signalling. *Development* **2003**, *130*, 4295–4305. [CrossRef] [PubMed]
42. Glinka, A.; Wu, W.; Delius, H.; Monaghan, A.P.; Blumenstock, C.; Niehrs, C. Dickkopf-1 is a member of a new family of secreted proteins and functions in head induction. *Nature* **1998**, *391*, 357–362. [CrossRef] [PubMed]
43. Choi, H.Y.; Dieckmann, M.; Herz, J.; Niemeier, A. Lrp4, a Novel Receptor for Dickkopf 1 and Sclerostin, Is Expressed by Osteoblasts and Regulates Bone Growth and Turnover In Vivo. *PLoS ONE* **2009**, *4*, e7930. [CrossRef] [PubMed]
44. Kay, J.; Upchurch, K.S. ACR/EULAR 2010 rheumatoid arthritis classification criteria. *Rheumatology* **2012**, *51*, vi5–vi9. [CrossRef] [PubMed]
45. Roux, C. Osteoporosis in inflammatory joint diseases. *Osteoporos. Int.* **2011**, *22*, 421–433. [CrossRef]
46. Wysham, K.D.; Baker, J.F.; Shoback, D.M. Osteoporosis and fractures in rheumatoid arthritis. *Curr. Opin. Rheumatol.* **2021**, *33*, 270–276. [CrossRef]
47. Aspray, T.J.; Hill, T.R. Osteoporosis and the Ageing Skeleton. In *Biochemistry and Cell Biology of Ageing: Part II Clinical Science*; Springer: Singapore, 2019; Volume 91, pp. 453–476. [CrossRef]
48. Rahman, P. Pharmacogenetics of rheumatoid arthritis: Potential targets from susceptibility genes and present therapies. *Pharmacogenom. Pers. Med.* **2010**, *3*, 15–31. [CrossRef]
49. Bagheri-Hosseinabadi, Z.; Mirzaei, M.R.; Esmaeili, O.; Asadi, F.; Ahmadinia, H.; Shamsoddini, B.; Abbasifard, M. Implications of Peptidyl Arginine Deiminase 4 gene transcription and polymorphisms in susceptibility to rheumatoid arthritis in an Iranian population. *BMC Med. Genom.* **2023**, *16*, 104. [CrossRef]
50. Matzaraki, V.; Kumar, V.; Wijmenga, C.; Zhernakova, A. The MHC locus and genetic susceptibility to autoimmune and infectious diseases. *Genome Biol.* **2017**, *18*, 76. [CrossRef]
51. McInnes, I.B.; Schett, G. The Pathogenesis of Rheumatoid Arthritis. *N. Engl. J. Med.* **2011**, *365*, 2205–2219. [CrossRef]
52. Yap, H.-Y.; Tee, S.Z.-Y.; Wong, M.M.-T.; Chow, S.-K.; Peh, S.-C.; Teow, S.-Y. Pathogenic Role of Immune Cells in Rheumatoid Arthritis: Implications in Clinical Treatment and Biomarker Development. *Cells* **2018**, *7*, 161. [CrossRef]
53. Chang, M.H.; Nigrovic, P.A. Antibody-dependent and -independent mechanisms of inflammatory arthritis. *J. Clin. Investig.* **2019**, *4*, 125278. [CrossRef] [PubMed]
54. Wu, C.-Y.; Yang, H.-Y.; Lai, J.-H. Anti-Citrullinated Protein Antibodies in Patients with Rheumatoid Arthritis: Biological Effects and Mechanisms of Immunopathogenesis. *Int. J. Mol. Sci.* **2020**, *21*, 4015. [CrossRef] [PubMed]
55. Maggi, L.; Mazzoni, A.; Cimaz, R.; Liotta, F.; Annunziato, F.; Cosmi, L. Th17 and Th1 Lymphocytes in Oligoarticular Juvenile Idiopathic Arthritis. *Front. Immunol.* **2019**, *10*, 450. [CrossRef] [PubMed]
56. Yang, P.; Qian, F.-Y.; Zhang, M.-F.; Xu, A.-L.; Wang, X.; Jiang, B.-P.; Zhou, L.-L. Th17 cell pathogenicity and plasticity in rheumatoid arthritis. *J. Leukoc. Biol.* **2019**, *106*, 1233–1240. [CrossRef]
57. Kondo, N.; Kuroda, T.; Kobayashi, D. Cytokine Networks in the Pathogenesis of Rheumatoid Arthritis. *Int. J. Mol. Sci.* **2021**, *22*, 10922. [CrossRef]
58. Wu, F.; Gao, J.; Kang, J.; Wang, X.; Niu, Q.; Liu, J.; Zhang, L. B Cells in Rheumatoid Arthritis: Pathogenic Mechanisms and Treatment Prospects. *Front. Immunol.* **2021**, *12*, 750753. [CrossRef]
59. Bartok, B.; Firestein, G.S. Fibroblast-like synoviocytes: Key effector cells in rheumatoid arthritis. *Immunol. Rev.* **2010**, *233*, 233–255. [CrossRef]
60. Marahleh, A.; Kitaura, H.; Ohori, F.; Kishikawa, A.; Ogawa, S.; Shen, W.-R.; Qi, J.; Noguchi, T.; Nara, Y.; Mizoguchi, I. TNF-α Directly Enhances Osteocyte RANKL Expression and Promotes Osteoclast Formation. *Front. Immunol.* **2019**, *10*, 2925. [CrossRef]
61. Kitaura, H.; Marahleh, A.; Ohori, F.; Noguchi, T.; Shen, W.-R.; Qi, J.; Nara, Y.; Pramusita, A.; Kinjo, R.; Mizoguchi, I. Osteocyte-Related Cytokines Regulate Osteoclast Formation and Bone Resorption. *Int. J. Mol. Sci.* **2020**, *21*, 5169. [CrossRef]

62. Sahoo, R.; Dhakad, U.; Goel, A.; Pradhan, S.; Srivastava, R.; Das, S. Serum sclerostin levels in rheumatoid arthritis and correlation with disease activity and bone mineral density. *Indian J. Rheumatol.* **2019**, *14*, 28. [CrossRef]
63. El-Bakry, S.; Saber, N.; Zidan, H.; Samaha, D. Sclerostin as an innovative insight towards understanding Rheumatoid Arthritis. *Egypt. Rheumatol.* **2016**, *38*, 71–75. [CrossRef]
64. Singh, A.; Gupta, M.K.; Mishra, S.P. Study of correlation of level of expression of Wnt signaling pathway inhibitors sclerostin and dickkopf-1 with disease activity and severity in rheumatoid arthritis patients. *Drug Discov. Ther.* **2019**, *13*, 22–27. [CrossRef] [PubMed]
65. Mehaney, D.A.; Eissa, M.; Anwar, S.; El-Din, S.F. Serum Sclerostin Level Among Egyptian Rheumatoid Arthritis Patients: Relation to Disease Activity, Bone Mineral Density and Radiological Grading. *Acta Reum. Port* **2015**, *40*, 268–274.
66. Świerkot, J.; Gruszecka, K.; Matuszewska, A.; Wiland, P. Assessment of the Effect of Methotrexate Therapy on Bone Metabolism in Patients with Rheumatoid Arthritis. *Arch. Immunol. Ther. Exp.* **2015**, *63*, 397–404. [CrossRef]
67. Seror, R.; Boudaoud, S.; Pavy, S.; Nocturne, G.; Schaeverbeke, T.; Saraux, A.; Chanson, P.; Gottenberg, J.-E.; Devauchelle-Pensec, V.; Tobón, G.J.; et al. Increased Dickkopf-1 in Recent-onset Rheumatoid Arthritis is a New Biomarker of Structural Severity. Data from the ESPOIR Cohort. *Sci. Rep.* **2016**, *6*, 18421. [CrossRef]
68. Lim, M.J.; Kwon, S.R.; Joo, K.; Son, M.J.; Park, S.-G.; Park, W. Early effects of tumor necrosis factor inhibition on bone homeostasis after soluble tumor necrosis factor receptor use. *Korean J. Intern. Med.* **2014**, *29*, 807–813. [CrossRef]
69. Terpos, E.; Fragiadaki, K.; Konsta, M.; Bratengeier, C.; Papatheodorou, A.; Sfikakis, P.P. Early effects of IL-6 receptor inhibition on bone homeostasis: A pilot study in women with rheumatoid arthritis. *Clin. Exp. Rheumatol.* **2011**, *29*, 921–925.
70. Register, T.C.; Hruska, K.A.; Divers, J.; Bowden, D.W.; Palmer, N.D.; Carr, J.J.; Wagenknecht, L.E.; Hightower, R.C.; Xu, J.; Smith, S.C.; et al. Plasma Dickkopf1 (DKK1) Concentrations Negatively Associate with Atherosclerotic Calcified Plaque in African-Americans with Type 2 Diabetes. *J. Clin. Endocrinol. Metab.* **2013**, *98*, E60–E65. [CrossRef]
71. Paccou, J.; Mentaverri, R.; Renard, C.; Liabeuf, S.; Fardellone, P.; Massy, Z.A.; Brazier, M.; Kamel, S. The Relationships Between Serum Sclerostin, Bone Mineral Density, and Vascular Calcification in Rheumatoid Arthritis. *J. Clin. Endocrinol. Metab.* **2014**, *99*, 4740–4748. [CrossRef]
72. Wehmeyer, C.; Frank, S.; Beckmann, D.; Böttcher, M.; Cromme, C.; König, U.; Fennen, M.; Held, A.; Paruzel, P.; Hartmann, C.; et al. Sclerostin inhibition promotes TNF-dependent inflammatory joint destruction. *Sci. Transl. Med.* **2016**, *8*, 330ra35. [CrossRef]
73. Marenzana, M.; Vugler, A.; Moore, A.; Robinson, M. Effect of sclerostin-neutralising antibody on periarticular and systemic bone in a murine model of rheumatoid arthritis: A microCT study. *Thromb. Haemost.* **2013**, *15*, R125. [CrossRef] [PubMed]
74. Chen, X.-X.; Baum, W.; Dwyer, D.; Stock, M.; Schwabe, K.; Ke, H.-Z.; Stolina, M.; Schett, G.; Bozec, A. Sclerostin inhibition reverses systemic, periarticular and local bone loss in arthritis. *Ann. Rheum. Dis.* **2013**, *72*, 1732–1736. [CrossRef] [PubMed]
75. Aringer, M.; Costenbader, K.; Daikh, D.; Brinks, R.; Mosca, M.; Ramsey-Goldman, R.; Smolen, J.S.; Wofsy, D.; Boumpas, D.T.; Kamen, D.L.; et al. 2019 European League Against Rheumatism/American College of Rheumatology classification criteria for systemic lupus erythematosus. *Rheumatology* **2019**, *78*, 1151–1159. [CrossRef]
76. Santiago, M.B. Jaccoud-type lupus arthropathy. *Lupus* **2022**, *31*, 398–406. [CrossRef] [PubMed]
77. Sutanto, H.; Yuliasih, Y. Disentangling the Pathogenesis of Systemic Lupus Erythematosus: Close Ties between Immunological, Genetic and Environmental Factors. *Medicina* **2023**, *59*, 1033. [CrossRef]
78. Niewold, T.B.; Clark, D.N.; Salloum, R.; Poole, B.D. Interferon Alpha in Systemic Lupus Erythematosus. *J. Biomed. Biotechnol.* **2010**, *2010*, 948364. [CrossRef]
79. Tveita, A.A.; Rekvig, O.P. Alterations in Wnt pathway activity in mouse serum and kidneys during lupus development. *Arthritis Rheum.* **2011**, *63*, 513–522. [CrossRef]
80. Fayed, A.; Soliman, A.; Elgohary, R. Measuring Serum Sclerostin in Egyptian Patients With Systemic Lupus Erythematosus and Evaluating Its Effect on Disease Activity. *Am. J. Clin. Oncol.* **2019**, *27*, 161–167. [CrossRef]
81. Chen, S.; Guttridge, D.C.; You, Z.; Zhang, Z.; Fribley, A.; Mayo, M.W.; Kitajewski, J.; Wang, C.-Y. WNT-1 Signaling Inhibits Apoptosis by Activating β-Catenin/T Cell Factor–Mediated Transcription. *J. Cell Biol.* **2001**, *152*, 87–96. [CrossRef]
82. A Cabral-Pacheco, G.; Garza-Veloz, I.; La Rosa, C.C.-D.; Ramirez-Acuña, J.M.; A Perez-Romero, B.; Guerrero-Rodriguez, J.F.; Martinez-Avila, N.; Martinez-Fierro, M.L. The Roles of Matrix Metalloproteinases and Their Inhibitors in Human Diseases. *Int. J. Mol. Sci.* **2020**, *21*, 9739. [CrossRef] [PubMed]
83. Ríos, C.G.-D.L.; Medina-Casado, M.; Díaz-Chamorro, A.; Sierras-Jiménez, M.; Lardelli-Claret, P.; Cáliz-Cáliz, R.; Sabio, J.M. Sclerostin as a biomarker of cardiovascular risk in women with systemic lupus erythematosus. *Sci. Rep.* **2022**, *12*, 21621. [CrossRef] [PubMed]
84. Geng, Y.; Song, Z.; Zhang, X.; Deng, X.; Wang, Y.; Zhang, Z. Improved diagnostic performance of CASPAR criteria with integration of ultrasound. *Front. Immunol.* **2022**, *13*, 935132. [CrossRef] [PubMed]
85. Eder, L.; Gladman, D.D. Psoriatic Arthritis: Phenotypic Variance and Nosology. *Curr. Rheumatol. Rep.* **2013**, *15*, 316. [CrossRef]
86. van Tok, M.N.; van Duivenvoorde, L.M.; Kramer, I.; Ingold, P.; Pfister, S.; Roth, L.; Bs, I.C.B.; van de Sande, M.G.H.; Taurog, J.D.; Kolbinger, F.; et al. Interleukin-17A Inhibition Diminishes Inflammation and New Bone Formation in Experimental Spondyloarthritis. *Arthritis Rheumatol.* **2019**, *71*, 612–625. [CrossRef]
87. Tsukazaki, H.; Kaito, T. The Role of the IL-23/IL-17 Pathway in the Pathogenesis of Spondyloarthritis. *Int. J. Mol. Sci.* **2020**, *21*, 6401. [CrossRef]

88. Sarkar, S.; A Cooney, L.; A Fox, D. The role of T helper type 17 cells in inflammatory arthritis. *Clin. Exp. Immunol.* **2010**, *159*, 225–237. [CrossRef]

89. Chen, L.; Wei, X.-Q.; Evans, B.; Jiang, W.; Aeschlimann, D. IL-23 promotes osteoclast formation by up-regulation of receptor activator of NF-κB (RANK) expression in myeloid precursor cells. *Eur. J. Immunol.* **2008**, *38*, 2845–2854. [CrossRef]

90. Mitra, A.; Raychaudhuri, S.K.; Raychaudhuri, S.P. Functional role of IL-22 in psoriatic arthritis. *Arthritis Res. Ther.* **2012**, *14*, R65. [CrossRef]

91. Fassio, A.; Idolazzi, L.; Viapiana, O.; Benini, C.; Vantaggiato, E.; Bertoldo, F.; Rossini, M.; Gatti, D. In psoriatic arthritis Dkk-1 and PTH are lower than in rheumatoid arthritis and healthy controls. *Clin. Rheumatol.* **2017**, *36*, 2377–2381. [CrossRef]

92. Fassio, A.; Gatti, D.; Rossini, M.; Idolazzi, L.; Giollo, A.; Adami, G.; Gisondi, P.; Girolomoni, G.; Viapiana, O. Secukinumab produces a quick increase in WNT signalling antagonists in patients with psoriatic arthritis. *Clin. Exp. Rheumatol.* **2019**, *37*, 133–136. [PubMed]

93. Diani, M.; Perego, S.; Sansoni, V.; Bertino, L.; Gomarasca, M.; Faraldi, M.; Pigatto, P.D.M.; Damiani, G.; Banfi, G.; Altomare, G.; et al. Differences in Osteoimmunological Biomarkers Predictive of Psoriatic Arthritis among a Large Italian Cohort of Psoriatic Patients. *Int. J. Mol. Sci.* **2019**, *20*, 5617. [CrossRef]

94. Tasende, J.A.P.; Fernandez-Moreno, M.; Vazquez-Mosquera, M.E.; Fernandez-Lopez, J.C.; Oreiro-Villar, N.; Santos, F.J.D.T.; Blanco-García, F.J. Increased synovial immunohistochemistry reactivity of TGF-β1 in erosive peripheral psoriatic arthritis. *BMC Musculoskelet. Disord.* **2023**, *24*, 246. [CrossRef]

95. Van Der Linden, S.; Valkenburg, H.A.; Cats, A. Evaluation of Diagnostic Criteria for Ankylosing Spondylitis. *Arthritis Rheum.* **1984**, *27*, 361–368. [CrossRef] [PubMed]

96. Ghasemi-Rad, M.; Attaya, H.; Lesha, E.; Vegh, A.; Maleki-Miandoab, T.; Nosair, E.; Sepehrvand, N.; Davarian, A.; Rajebi, H.; Pakniat, A.; et al. Ankylosing spondylitis: A state of the art factual backbone. *World J. Radiol.* **2015**, *7*, 236–252. [CrossRef]

97. Carter, S.; Braem, K.; Lories, R.J. The role of bone morphogenetic proteins in ankylosing spondylitis. *Ther. Adv. Musculoskelet. Dis.* **2012**, *4*, 293–299. [CrossRef]

98. Osta, B.; Benedetti, G.; Miossec, P. Classical and Paradoxical Effects of TNF-α on Bone Homeostasis. *Front. Immunol.* **2014**, *5*, 48. [CrossRef]

99. Santos, A.; Bakker, A.D.; Willems, H.M.E.; Bravenboer, N.; Bronckers, A.L.J.J.; Klein-Nulend, J. Mechanical Loading Stimulates BMP7, But Not BMP2, Production by Osteocytes. *Calcif. Tissue Int.* **2011**, *89*, 318–326. [CrossRef]

100. Jacques, P.; Lambrecht, S.; Verheugen, E.; Pauwels, E.; Kollias, G.; Armaka, M.; Verhoye, M.; Van der Linden, A.; Achten, R.; Lories, R.J.; et al. Proof of concept: Enthesitis and new bone formation in spondyloarthritis are driven by mechanical strain and stromal cells. *Ann. Rheum. Dis.* **2014**, *73*, 437–445. [CrossRef]

101. Appel, H.; Ruiz-Heiland, G.; Listing, J.; Zwerina, J.; Herrmann, M.; Mueller, R.; Haibel, H.; Baraliakos, X.; Hempfing, A.; Rudwaleit, M.; et al. Altered skeletal expression of sclerostin and its link to radiographic progression in ankylosing spondylitis. *Arthritis Rheum.* **2009**, *60*, 3257–3262. [CrossRef]

102. Heiland, G.R.; Appel, H.; Poddubnyy, D.; Zwerina, J.; Hueber, A.; Haibel, H.; Baraliakos, X.; Listing, J.; Rudwaleit, M.; Schett, G.; et al. High level of functional dickkopf-1 predicts protection from syndesmophyte formation in patients with ankylosing spondylitis. *Ann. Rheum. Dis.* **2012**, *71*, 572–574. [CrossRef] [PubMed]

103. Saad, C.G.; Ribeiro, A.C.; Moraes, J.C.; Takayama, L.; Goncalves, C.R.; Rodrigues, M.B.; de Oliveira, R.M.; A Silva, C.; Bonfa, E.; Pereira, R.M. Low sclerostin levels: A predictive marker of persistent inflammation in ankylosing spondylitis during anti-tumor necrosis factor therapy? *Thromb. Haemost.* **2012**, *14*, R216. [CrossRef] [PubMed]

104. Klingberg, E.; Nurkkala, M.; Carlsten, H.; Forsblad-D'elia, H. Biomarkers of Bone Metabolism in Ankylosing Spondylitis in Relation to Osteoproliferation and Osteoporosis. *J. Rheumatol.* **2014**, *41*, 1349–1356. [CrossRef] [PubMed]

105. Sakellariou, G.T.; Anastasilakis, A.D.; Bisbinas, I.; Oikonomou, D.; Gerou, S.; Polyzos, S.A.; Sayegh, F.E. Circulating periostin levels in patients with AS: Association with clinical and radiographic variables, inflammatory markers and molecules involved in bone formation. *Rheumatology* **2015**, *54*, 908–914. [CrossRef]

106. Rossini, M.; Viapiana, O.; Idolazzi, L.; Ghellere, F.; Fracassi, E.; Troplini, S.; Povino, M.R.; Kunnathully, V.; Adami, S.; Gatti, D. Higher Level of Dickkopf-1 is Associated with Low Bone Mineral Density and Higher Prevalence of Vertebral Fractures in Patients with Ankylosing Spondylitis. *Calcif. Tissue Int.* **2016**, *98*, 438–445. [CrossRef]

107. Solmaz, D.; Uslu, S.; Kozacı, D.; Karaca, N.; Bulbul, H.; Tarhan, E.F.; Ozmen, M.; Can, G.; Akar, S. Evaluation of periostin and factors associated with new bone formation in ankylosing spondylitis: Periostin may be associated with the Wnt pathway. *Int. J. Rheum. Dis.* **2018**, *21*, 502–509. [CrossRef]

108. Genre, F.; Rueda-Gotor, J.; Remuzgo-Martínez, S.; Corrales, A.; Ubilla, B.; Mijares, V.; Fernández-Díaz, C.; Portilla, V.; Blanco, R.; Hernandez, J.L.; et al. Implication of osteoprotegerin and sclerostin in axial spondyloarthritis cardiovascular disease: Study of 163 Spanish patients. *Clin. Exp. Rheumatol.* **2018**, *36*, 302–309.

109. Luchetti, M.M.; Ciccia, F.; Avellini, C.; Benfaremo, D.; Guggino, G.; Farinelli, A.; Ciferri, M.; Rossini, M.; Svegliati, S.; Spadoni, T.; et al. Sclerostin and Antisclerostin Antibody Serum Levels Predict the Presence of Axial Spondyloarthritis in Patients with Inflammatory Bowel Disease. *J. Rheumatol.* **2018**, *45*, 630–637. [CrossRef]

110. Perrotta, F.M.; Ceccarelli, F.; Barbati, C.; Colasanti, T.; De Socio, A.; Scriffignano, S.; Alessandri, C.; Lubrano, E. Serum Sclerostin as a Possible Biomarker in Ankylosing Spondylitis: A Case-Control Study. *J. Immunol. Res.* **2018**, *2018*, 9101964. [CrossRef]

111. Gercik, O.; Solmaz, D.; Coban, E.; Iptec, B.O.; Avcioglu, G.; Bayindir, O.; Kabadayi, G.; Topal, F.E.; Kozaci, D.; Akar, S. Evaluation of serum fibroblast growth factor-23 in patients with axial spondyloarthritis and its association with sclerostin, inflammation, and spinal damage. *Rheumatol. Int.* **2019**, *39*, 835–840. [CrossRef]
112. Iaremenko, O.; Shynkaruk, I.; Fedkov, D.; Iaremenko, K.; Petelytska, L. Bone turnover biomarkers, disease activity, and MRI changes of sacroiliac joints in patients with spondyloarthritis. *Rheumatol. Int.* **2020**, *40*, 2057–2063. [CrossRef] [PubMed]
113. Korkosz, M.; Gąsowski, J.; Leszczyński, P.; Pawlak-Buś, K.; Jeka, S.; Kucharska, E.; Grodzicki, T. High disease activity in ankylosing spondylitis is associated with increased serum sclerostin level and decreased wingless protein-3a signaling but is not linked with greater structural damage. *BMC Musculoskelet. Disord.* **2013**, *14*, 99. [CrossRef] [PubMed]
114. Muntean, L.; Lungu, A.; Gheorghe, S.; Valeanu, M.; Craciun, A.; Felea, I.; Petcu, A.; Filipescu, I.; Simon, S.-P.; Rednic, S. ORIGINAL ARTICLEElevated Serum Levels of Sclerostin are Associated with High Disease Activity and Functional Impairment in Patients with Axial Spondyloarthritis. *Clin. Lab.* **2016**, *59*, 150801. [CrossRef]
115. Sun, W.; Tian, L.; Jiang, L.; Zhang, S.; Zhou, M.; Zhu, J.; Xue, J. Sclerostin rather than Dickkopf-1 is associated with mSASSS but not with disease activity score in patients with ankylosing spondylitis. *Clin. Rheumatol.* **2019**, *38*, 989–995. [CrossRef] [PubMed]
116. Sakellariou, G.T.; Iliopoulos, A.; Konsta, M.; Kenanidis, E.; Potoupnis, M.; Tsiridis, E.; Gavana, E.; Sayegh, F.E. Serum levels of Dkk-1, sclerostin and VEGF in patients with ankylosing spondylitis and their association with smoking, and clinical, inflammatory and radiographic parameters. *Jt. Bone Spine* **2017**, *84*, 309–315. [CrossRef]
117. Taylan, A.; Sari, I.; Akinci, B.; Bilge, S.; Kozaci, D.; Akar, S.; Colak, A.; Yalcin, H.; Gunay, N.; Akkoc, N. Biomarkers and cytokines of bone turnover: Extensive evaluation in a cohort of patients with ankylosing spondylitis. *BMC Musculoskelet. Disord.* **2012**, *13*, 191. [CrossRef]
118. Tuylu, T.; Sari, I.; Solmaz, D.; Kozaci, D.L.; Akar, S.; Gunay, N.; Onen, F.; Akkoc, N. Fetuin-A is related to syndesmophytes in patients with ankylosing spondylitis: A case control study. *Clinics* **2014**, *69*, 688–693. [CrossRef]
119. Descamps, E.; Molto, A.; Borderie, D.; Lories, R.; Richard, C.M.; Pons, M.; Roux, C.; Briot, K. Changes in bone formation regulator biomarkers in early axial spondyloarthritis. *Rheumatology* **2021**, *60*, 1185–1194. [CrossRef]
120. Pathan, E.; Abraham, S.; Van Rossen, E.; Withrington, R.; Keat, A.; Charles, P.J.; Paterson, E.; Chowdhury, M.; McClinton, C.; Taylor, P.C. Efficacy and safety of apremilast, an oral phosphodiesterase 4 inhibitor, in ankylosing spondylitis. *Ann. Rheum. Dis.* **2013**, *72*, 1475–1480. [CrossRef]
121. Korkosz, M.; Gąsowski, J.; Leszczyński, P.; Pawlak-Buś, K.; Jeka, S.; Siedlar, M.; Grodzicki, T. Effect of tumour necrosis factor-α inhibitor on serum level of dickkopf-1 protein and bone morphogenetic protein-7 in ankylosing spondylitis patients with high disease activity. *Scand. J. Rheumatol.* **2014**, *43*, 43–48. [CrossRef]
122. Ustun, N.; Tok, F.; Kalyoncu, U.; Motor, S.; Yuksel, R.; E Yagiz, A.; Guler, H.; Turhanoglu, A.D. Sclerostin and Dkk-1 in patients with ankylosing spondylitis. *Acta Reum. Port.* **2014**, *39*, 146–151.
123. Özdemirel, A.E.; Güven, S.C.; Doğancı, A.; Sürmeli, Z.S.; Özyuvalı, A.; Kurt, M.; Rüstemova, D.; Hassan, S.; Sayın, A.P.Y.; Tutkak, H.; et al. Anti-tumor necrosis factor alpha treatment does not influence serum levels of the markers associated with radiographic progression in ankylosing spondylitis. *Arch. Rheumatol.* **2023**, *38*, 148–155. [CrossRef]
124. Delanaye, P.; Paquot, F.; Bouquegneau, A.; Blocki, F.; Krzesinski, J.-M.; Evenepoel, P.; Pottel, H.; Cavalier, E. Sclerostin and chronic kidney disease: The assay impacts what we (thought to) know. *Nephrol. Dial. Transplant.* **2018**, *33*, 1404–1410. [CrossRef] [PubMed]
125. De Maré, A.; Verhulst, A.; Cavalier, E.; Delanaye, P.; Behets, G.J.; Meijers, B.; Kuypers, D.; D'haese, P.C.; Evenepoel, P. Clinical Inference of Serum and Bone Sclerostin Levels in Patients with End-Stage Kidney Disease. *J. Clin. Med.* **2019**, *8*, 2027. [CrossRef] [PubMed]
126. Romejko, K.; Rymarz, A.; Szamotulska, K.; Bartoszewicz, Z.; Niemczyk, S. Relationships between Sclerostin, Leptin and Metabolic Parameters in Non-Dialysis Chronic Kidney Disease Males. *J. Pers. Med.* **2022**, *13*, 31. [CrossRef] [PubMed]

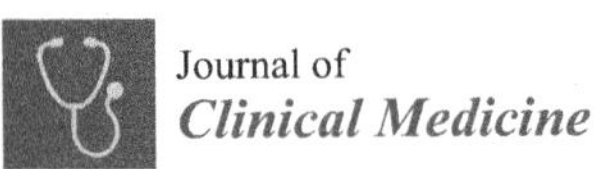

Journal of
Clinical Medicine

Review

Interleukin-23 Involved in Fibrotic Autoimmune Diseases: New Discoveries

Margherita Sisto * and Sabrina Lisi

Department of Translational Biomedicine and Neuroscience (DiBraiN), Section of Human Anatomy and Histology, University of Bari "Aldo Moro", 70123 Bari, Italy; sabrina.lisi@uniba.it
* Correspondence: margherita.sisto@uniba.it; Tel.: +39-080-547-8315

Abstract: Interleukin (IL)-23 is a central pro-inflammatory cytokine with a broad range of effects on immune responses. IL-23 is pathologically linked to the induction of the production of the pro-inflammatory cytokines IL-17 and IL-22, which stimulate the differentiation and proliferation of T helper type 17 (Th17) cells. Recent discoveries suggest a potential pro-fibrotic role for IL-23 in the development of chronic inflammatory autoimmune diseases characterized by intense fibrosis. In this review, we summarized the biological features of IL-23 and gathered recent research on the role of IL-23 in fibrotic autoimmune conditions, which could provide a theoretical basis for clinical targeting and drug development.

Keywords: IL-23; autoimmunity; inflammation; fibrosis

Citation: Sisto, M.; Lisi, S. Interleukin-23 Involved in Fibrotic Autoimmune Diseases: New Discoveries. *J. Clin. Med.* **2023**, *12*, 5699. https://doi.org/10.3390/jcm12175699

Academic Editor: Eugen Feist

Received: 3 August 2023
Revised: 29 August 2023
Accepted: 30 August 2023
Published: 1 September 2023

1. Introduction

Multiple autoimmune diseases are a group of clinically heterogeneous conditions that show common inflammatory signaling pathways arising from aberrant immune responses [1]. Some of these disorders are characterized by intense and severe fibrotic processes as the result of a complex interplay between different immune cell types following persistent inflammatory activity [2,3]. Autoimmune diseases, traditionally characterized by chronic inflammation, present tissue damage that often evolves towards fibrosis. This represents a serious clinical problem because it causes organ failure. The fibrotic evolution of autoimmune diseases presents an excessive release of pro-fibrotic factors as a result of the activation of molecular cascades depending on chronic inflammation. In recent years, researchers' efforts have focused on identifying molecular bridges that can connect the various fibrotic pathways identified so far [2,3]. Several cytokines have been well studied for their ability to generate inflammatory loops through positive feedback mechanisms [4]. Breaking these loops through cytokine neutralization has proved that inflammation attenuates and ameliorates the disease [5]. One of these cytokines is interleukin (IL)-23, a multifunctional pro-inflammatory cytokine that is involved in a variety of biological processes [6]. Although the role of IL-23 in the immune response during bacterial and viral infections has recently been evaluated, demonstrating its central role [7], its deregulation has been demonstrated to aggravate chronic inflammatory status, contributing to the development of autoimmune diseases [8,9]. As shown by several authors, IL-23 is involved in the pathogenesis of several autoimmune diseases [10–13]. The importance of IL-23 implicated in the evolution of autoimmune pathologies was demonstrated by analyzing the susceptibility of IL-12- or IL-23-deficient mice [10,11]. Indeed, mice that have a deletion of IL-23 were protected from disease in several experimental models of autoimmunity. Importantly, treatment of mice with anti-IL-23 prevents the development of autoimmune conditions [12].

In this review, we provide an overview of the most recent discoveries, focusing on the role of IL-23 in fibrotic pathways and its role in the pathogenesis of inflammatory autoimmune diseases characterized by fibrotic evolution.

2. Structure of IL-23 and Its Receptor

IL-23 is a heterodimeric member with pro-inflammatory characteristics that belongs to the special IL-12 family, and it is constituted of two different subunits: p19 and p40 [14]. The p40 subunit is a glycosylated type I soluble protein that has a molecular weight of 34.7 kDa and is positioned on the 11q1.3 chromosome [15,16]. The p19 subunit is a non-glycosylated protein with a molecular weight of 18.7 kDa located on chromosome 12q13.2 [8]. Both subunits are linked by a disulphide bond, and they are attached only if they are synthesized in the same cell [8,14]. Specifically, IL-23 is expressed and secreted by activated macrophages and dendritic cells located in several tissues, such as the skin, intestinal mucosa, joints, and lungs (Figure 1).

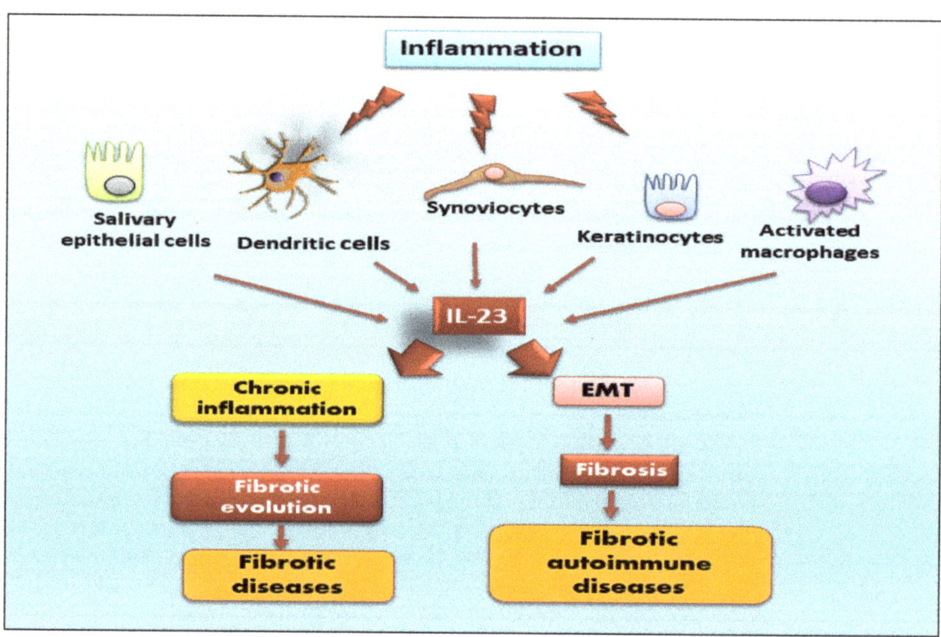

Figure 1. IL-23 is expressed and secreted by activated macrophages and dendritic cells located in different tissues and by non-immune cells, such as keratinocytes, synoviocytes, and salivary gland epithelial cells. IL-23, through several signaling pathways, provokes, on one side, the activation of the epithelial–mesenchymal transition (EMT) mechanism, inducing fibrotic processes in autoimmune diseases, and, on the other side, chronic inflammation that determines severe fibrotic evolution in several diseases.

Interestingly, it is also secreted by non-immune cells, such as keratinocytes, synoviocytes, and salivary gland epithelial cells [17–19]. The IL-23 signaling pathway occurs through a link with its receptor. IL-23 receptor (IL-23R) is a heterodimeric structure that consists of two subunits: a heterodimer with the IL-12Rβ1 subunit and its unique IL-23R subunit, positioned on human chromosome 19 and encoding the gene that constitutes the IL-12Rβ1 subunit, and on human chromosome 1, encoding the gene that forms the IL-23R subunit [20]. The IL-12Rβ1 subunit is principally expressed on T cells, monocytes/macrophages, natural killer T cells, and dendritic cells [7,21], with minor expression on B cells and lymphoid cells [22] (Figure 2).

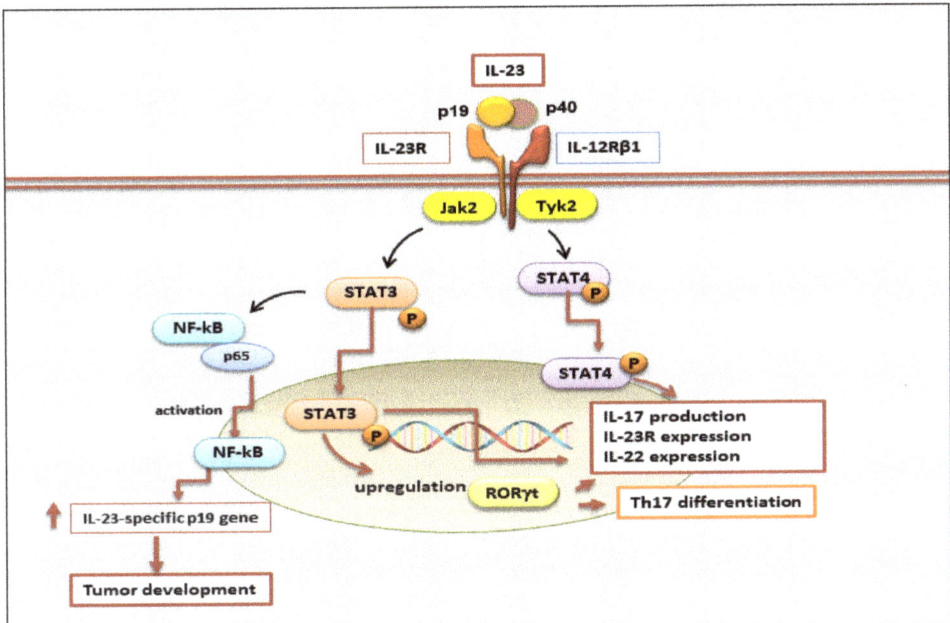

Figure 2. IL-23 is a heterodimeric cytokine composed of p40 and p19 subunits. It binds to its IL-23 receptor complex, composed of IL-12Rb1 and IL-23R subunits, which are linked to Jak2 and Tyk2, respectively. Active phosphorylated Jak2/Tyk2 leads to phosphorylation of STAT3 and STAT4. Phospho-STAT3 and phospho-STAT4 translocate into the nucleus, inducing transcription of cytokines, such as IL-17 and IL-22, and differentiation of T helper 17. STAT3 plus RORγt cooperate to increase IL23R, IL-17, and IL-22 expression and to stabilize the Th17 phenotype. The binding of IL-23 to its receptor through NF-κB/p65 activation leads to tumor progression. Jak2, Janus kinase 2; RORγt, RAR-related orphan receptor gamma; Tyk2, tyrosine kinase 2.

3. Regulation of IL-23 Signaling

Since its discovery, IL-23 has received widespread attention, and although it has a similar structure to IL-12, its role is totally different. Indeed, in spite of the protective function addressed by IL-23 against bacterial, fungal, and viral infections, extensive knowledge sustains the contribution of its alteration in triggering chronic inflammation and autoimmunity, providing a solid substrate for the development of several autoimmune diseases, like psoriasis, systemic lupus erythematosus (SLE), rheumatoid arthritis (RA), Sjögren's syndrome (SS), and multiple sclerosis (MS) [8,11,23,24].

Currently, the IL-23 signaling pathway remains largely uncharacterized. IL-23 involves the activation of members of the Janus family of tyrosine kinases (JAKs), their downstream factors, and the signal transducers and activators of transcription (STATs) family [25]. In particular, IL-23, through binding to its IL-23 receptor, provokes phosphorylation and activation of JAK/STAT signaling molecules (Jak2, Tyk2), promoting STAT3 and STAT4 phosphorylation and activation [25]. Subsequently, active STAT3 up-regulates the expression of the transcription factor RORγt, which is critical for IL-17 production [26]. Indeed, STAT3 plus RORγt cooperate to facilitate a positive loop that increases IL23R, IL-17, and IL-22 expression and that stabilizes the Th17 phenotype. Thus, STAT4 phosphorylation and activation promote upregulation of IL23R, IL-17, and IL-22 expression and the increase of Th17 [26]. However, other IL-23-regulated mechanisms are involved in the evolution of disease. For example, STAT3 activation is not restricted to IL-23 because other cytokines, such as IL-6, IL-21, IL-10, or IL-27, induce STAT3 activation without triggering adverse effects; rather, in some cases, it exerts anti-inflammatory events [25] (Figure 2).

To date, multiple cytokines play complex roles in IL-23 regulation. IL-23 was shown to be upregulated in fibroblast-like synoviocytes in response to IL-1β and Tumor Necrosis Factor (TNF)-α [27,28], while TNF-α receptor 1 can decrease IL-23 expression by downregulating subunit p40 [29]. Likewise, the cytokine IL-10, which has an anti-inflammatory role, can also diminish IL-23 expression [30].

A mounting number of studies have evidenced [23,31] that the key role of IL-23 is to drive the differentiation of T CD4+ naive cells into Th17 cells [32,33]. This leads to enhanced IL-17 production, considered a crucial player in the pathogenesis of inflammatory and autoimmune diseases [34,35]. Thus, IL-23/IL-17 axis activation leads to the onset of several inflammatory autoimmune diseases, and results obtained from experimental mouse models confirm the crucial role of the IL-23/IL-17 axis in the pathogenesis of various autoimmune conditions, such as arthritis [36]. Consequently, suppressing the trigger of the IL-23/IL-17 axis improves the inflammatory condition and is considered a promising therapeutic approach in patients with these disorders [34].

Recent advances have reported that IL-23 induction can also occur through Toll-like receptor (TLR, TLRs) signaling. It has been demonstrated that Theiler's murine encephalomyelitis virus (TMEV), which leads to infection of central nervous system microglia and macrophages in mice, provoking a disorder similar to MS in humans, stimulates the expression of IL-23 via binding to TLR3 and TLR7, contributing to the development of experimental autoimmune MS [37]. Additionally, other research findings have reported that IL-23 induction can also occur through TLR9 or cooperatively with other TLRs [37,38].

More recently, IL-23 has been demonstrated to be regulated during tumor-promoting development and to have protumor immunity [39]. An interesting study has demonstrated that Stat3 induces expression of IL-23, which is mainly secreted by macrophages in the tumor microenvironment via transcriptional activation of the IL-23/p19 gene and through NF-κB/p65 activation, promoting tumor development. In contrast, Stat3 also inhibits NF-kappaB/c-Rel-dependent IL-12/p35 gene expression in cancer-linked dendritic cells. Furthermore, tumor-associated regulatory T cells (Tregs) express the IL-23 receptor, which stimulates the expression of Stat3 in dendritic cells, leading to upregulation of the Treg-specific transcription factor Foxp3 and the immunosuppressive cytokine IL-10. These results demonstrate that Stat3 induces IL-23-mediated tumorigenes [40]. However, findings of IL-23's antitumorigenic and antimetastatic characteristics demonstrated that IL-23 induced long-term regression of tumors similar to that of IL-12-transduced cancers. Other studies have also shown that CD40 ligand expression on lung tumor cells activates the immune response, determining increased transcription of p19 and p40 subunits and influencing the regression of the tumors [41,42].

It has been suggested, based largely on in vitro observations, that IL-23 stimulation increases the number of already-differentiated Th-17 cells and maintains IL-17 production from Th17 cells. For example, the addition of IL-23 during the culture of activated or memory T cells results in an increase in their proliferation and the frequency of IL-17+ T cells produced [43]; IL-23 is also required during restimulation of Th17 cells (i.e., cells previously stimulated with TGF-β and IL-6 to maintain IL-17 production from the Th-17 cells) [44]. Similarly, it has been suggested that IL-23 may stabilize the phenotype of Th17 cells through mechanisms dependent on the transcription factor STAT3 [45,46]. Two other cytokines thought to be involved in Th17 differentiation, IL-6 and IL-21, also share the STAT3-dependent signaling pathway with IL-23.

Emerging evidence has highlighted that IL-23 can be considered a survival factor for Th17 cells [35]. These data are confirmed by the observation of reduced frequencies of Th17 cells in mice lacking the IL-23 gene [43].

Finally, several findings have highlighted the profibrogenic role of IL-23 as a promoter of the epithelial–mesenchymal transition (EMT) process, an aberrant pro-fibrotic response to repetitive injury of epithelia, and the acquisition of a mesenchymal phenotype. High levels of IL-23 have been found in some chronic inflammatory autoimmune disorders characterized by fibrosis [13,14,28].

4. Role of IL-23 in the Fibrotic Process

IL-23 is known to mediate inflammatory conditions through the induction of Th17 cells, which produce the pro-inflammatory IL-17 [12]. Because the prevailing hypothesis is that the fibrotic evolution of diseases is preceded by chronic inflammation, therapeutic strategies blocking IL-23 were suggested as a promising approach, though the specific role of IL-23 in fibrosis needs to be clarified. This section summarizes the most recent findings regarding the role of IL-23 in fibrotic diseases.

4.1. Idiopathic Pulmonary Fibrosis

Idiopathic pulmonary fibrosis (IPF) is characterized by chronic progressive fibrosis of the lung [47]. In pulmonary fibrosis, in vitro experiments have demonstrated that treatment with an anti-interleukin-23-specific antibody attenuated airway inflammation and reduced fibrosis by blocking interleukin-17A and -22 release. The role of IL-23 in the pathophysiology of respiratory diseases is attracting increasing attention from researchers. An important role of IL-23 in the pathological features of pulmonary emphysema was demonstrated [48], and the involvement of IL-23 in the pathogenesis of a lipopolysaccharide-induced animal model of acute respiratory distress syndrome was also demonstrated [49]. Also, in the overall accepted bleomycin or IL-1β-induced pulmonary fibrosis, both IL-23 and IL-17A play a significant role in this context. The data collected suggest that IL-23 and IL-17A are essential for fibrosis pathway activation [50]. Moreover, the data seem to point towards a priority role for IL-23, which would also be responsible for the consequent secretion of IL-17 and the acute exacerbation of pulmonary fibrosis; in fact, by blocking the secretion of IL-23, the release of IL-17 is also decreased [50]. In addition, IL-22, IL-23, and IL-17 were significantly increased in the serum of lung cancer patients associated with IPF; the levels of these cytokines found in the serum show such significant values that they represent a parameter used to discriminate between lung cancer patients and the lung-cancer-associated IPF group; finally, the expression of IL-22, IL-23, and IL-17 was positively correlated with the degree of differentiation and tumor metastasis [51].

4.2. Inflammatory Bowel Diseases

Idiopathic inflammatory bowel diseases (IBD) represent chronic inflammatory diseases of the gastro-intestinal tract characterized by a strong inflammatory component, often on an autoimmune basis, against the intestinal microbiome; the main diseases that fall into this group are Crohn's disease and ulcerative colitis [52,53]. Intestinal fibrosis is a severe complication of IBD. With the establishment of a fibrotic evolution, the intestinal wall undergoes substantial structural modifications that lead to stiffness and a reduction in caliber. These phenomena, in the long run, seriously compromise the quality of life of patients. Chronic inflammation is certainly a factor that predisposes to fibrotic evolution. Furthermore, currently, there are no drugs that have shown efficacy in blocking intestinal fibrosis or improving the pathological condition. For these reasons, surgical treatment remains the only intervention strategy in cases of intestinal fibrosis and stenosis. Interleukin (IL)-12 and IL-23, with their structural similarities, are important cytokines in the pathogenesis of IBD. Recent data reported the efficacy of p40 peptide-based vaccines on intestinal inflammation in a colitis model made in a laboratory [54]. The results demonstrate that the administration of the vaccine reduces the clinical symptoms, slows down the fibrotic process with a significant attenuation of the inflammatory parameters, and reduces the release of pro-inflammatory cytokines, leading to an improvement in intestinal conditions in the mouse model used. In addition, in the intestinal lamina propria and in the local lymph nodes, a high ratio of Treg/Th1 and Treg/Th17 cells was detected [54]; furthermore, in CD11c+ dendritic cells, the vaccine stimulates the release of IL-10, which is critical to controlling small intestinal immune homeostasis by limiting the reactivation of local memory T cells and so attenuating excessive immune responses [54]. These data confirm a key role for IL-23 in the modulation of the activation of Th17 cells involved in fibrosis pathway activation.

4.3. Liver Fibrosis

Non-alcoholic fatty liver disease (NAFLD) is a condition in which the liver has an excess of fat deposits [55]. Two types of NAFLD are non-alcoholic fatty liver (NAFL) and non-alcoholic steatohepatitis (NASH). People generally develop one form of NAFLD, but a good percentage appear to be predisposed to developing the second form in the long run as well. NAFL and NASH are constantly increasing around the world [56]. NASH is currently considered the progressive step of NAFLD. It is described in liver steatosis, inflammation, and fibrosis with different severity [57]. A predominant role in the inflammatory condition characterizing NASH is played by Th17 cells, which express high levels of IL-17 in response to IL-23. A vital transcription factor for Th17 is the retinoic acid receptor-related orphan receptor γt (RORγt), whose enhanced expression and nuclear translocation are correlated with IL-23-dependent phosphorylation and dimerization of the signal transducer and activator of transcription 3 (STAT3) [58]. Because no targeted therapies have been identified for NAFLD/NASH, any factor that attenuates the inflammatory process and the related fibrotic process is evaluated experimentally in order to test its efficacy in these complex diseases [59]. In this respect, it is useful for scientists to hold in high regard the fact that hepatic IL-17-producing cells promote liver inflammation and dysfunction [60]. However, the genetic analysis carried out in subjects at risk of developing the NASH disease but who do not yet show clinical signs has not yet given certain data regarding a possible alteration of the gene that synthesizes IL-23, and the candidacy of the IL-17/IL-23 axis in NASH is yet to be fully established. Experimental data obtained using a mouse model with a double mutation in the IL-23 gene have, however, shown that protection against chronic inflammation and fibrotic development is moderate but not total, and this seems to suggest that although the IL-17/IL-23 axis is involved, it is probably related to the activation of other inflammatory pathways, and targeting IL-23 signaling activation may not be the only therapeutic approach for NASH [61].

5. Novel Role of IL-23 in Autoimmune Fibrotic Diseases

IL-23 is a factor involved in the development of autoimmune diseases, such as multiple sclerosis (MS), rheumatoid arthritis (RA), and systemic lupus erythematosus; it carries out its activity by stimulating and activating the pathogenic Th17 cells. Therefore, IL-23 is a potential target for modulating autoimmune responses and pathogenic Th17 cell effects. Recently developed clinical trials have shown the beneficial effects of blocking the IL-23/Th17 pathway in chronic inflammatory autoimmune diseases characterized by fibrotic damage to the organs. Here, we report the most recent and pioneering discoveries in this field.

5.1. Rheumatoid Arthritis

The role of IL-23 in RA has been extensively studied in a co-morbidity that affects approximately 15% of RA patients that is termed RA interstitial lung disease (RA-ILD) [62]. How much an excessive or altered immune response mediated by Th17 activation is involved in this pathology remains to be demonstrated. Recently, insight on the direct role of IL-23 in lung fibrosis was obtained by experimentally investigating the responsiveness of lung fibroblasts to IL-23 stimulation. The induction of CCR2 expression that regulates monocyte chemotaxis and the increased fibroblast migration suggest a direct role for IL-23 in fibrotic lung disease associated with a Th17-biased immune response [63]. In this context, a process strictly correlated with fibrotic evolution [2,3] plays a role, represented by EMT, which seems to be activated in the lung by chronic inflammatory stimuli and tissue damage. The EMT process creates an environment that facilitates fibrosis when alveolar epithelial cells are injured. In this scenario, IL-23 exerts its profibrogenic role on somatic alveolar type I (ATI) epithelial cells [63]. Primary ATI cells, after prolonged culture on rigid culture dishes, clearly show signs of a gradual transformation towards a mesenchymal phenotype characterized by the loss of epithelial proteins, such as caveolin-1, and by a reorganization of the F-actin cytoskeleton, indicating the initiation of the EMT process. IL-23 appears to be actively involved in this process because the mesenchymal transformation process is accelerated by in vitro stimulation with this cytokine, which results in the loss of the epithelial marker caveolin-1 and increased expression of mesenchymal markers, such as α-smooth muscle actin (α-SMA) and collagen I/III protein. Furthermore, IL-23 significantly promotes cell migration and regulates apoptotic resistance in IL-23-transitioning-treated ATI cells [63]. IL-23-induced EMT seems to be activated and regulated by the Target of Rapamycin (mTOR)/S6 signaling pathway, which has already been demonstrated to be the pathway involved in the pro-fibrotic activity of IL-23 [64]. The hypothesis of an involvement of IL-23 in the pathogenesis of RA-ILD exerted by promoting mTOR/S6 signaling-dependent EMT in alveolar epithelial cells was supported by transcriptional sequencing analysis of human lung fibrosis biopsy tissue [63], which detected a significant increase in IL-23 mRNA expression in RA-ILD lung sections positively correlated with transitioning ATI epithelial cell [63] (Figure 3).

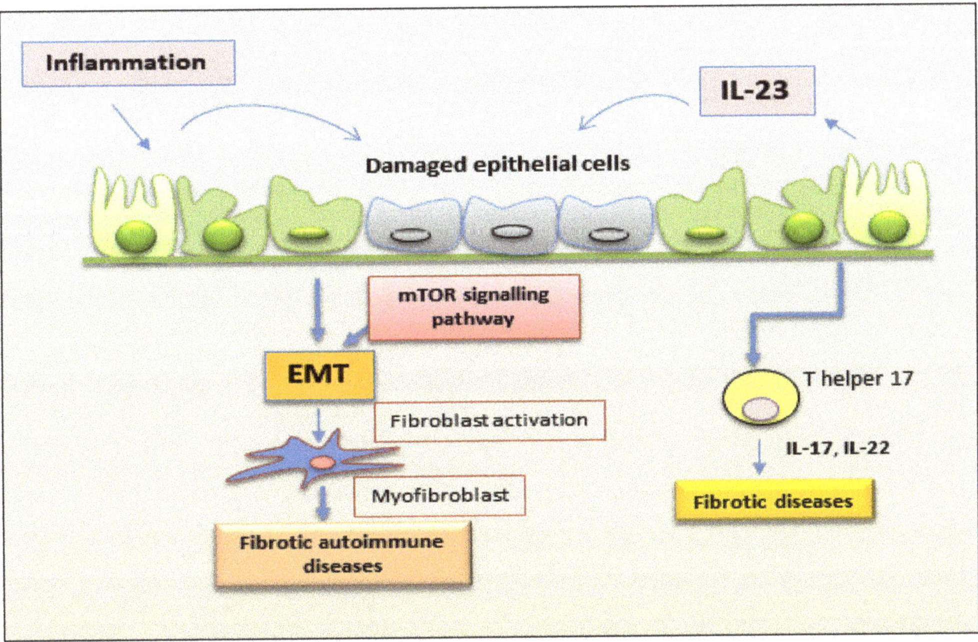

Figure 3. Schematic representation of a proposed mechanism by which IL-23 mediates EMT in epithelial cells. Inflammation promotes repetitive injury to epithelial cells that leads to the secretion of IL-23, inducing the EMT process. Injured cells start transforming into mesenchymal cells, and IL-23 amplifies the EMT process. On binding to its receptor, IL-23 activates the kinase mTOR and promotes the expression of mesenchymal markers. This process induces fibrosis in autoimmune diseases. (EMT, epithelial–mesenchymal transition; mTOR, mammalian target of rapamycin).

5.2. Crohn's Disease

Intestinal fibrosis is an important complication of Crohn's disease (CD) characterized by exaggerated proliferation of myofibroblasts and increased deposition of collagen in response to prolonged injury or chronic inflammation typical of IBD [65,66]. The mechanism underlying this hyperproliferation of myofibroblasts in CD seems to be linked, as in other pathological conditions mentioned above, to an involvement of mTOR. Experimental data report that the inhibition of mTOR determines a decreased production of IL-23, which, in turn, negatively regulates IL-22 expression and determines an improvement in the general conditions of the mouse model and a slowdown in the fibrotic evolution [66]. This inhibition of IL-23 expression is associated with elevated autophagy activity in intestinal Cx3cr1+ mononuclear phagocytes. This result paves the way to identifying a new molecular pathway that can explain the intestinal fibrotic progression in CD. The autophagy gene Atg7 knockdown determines, in fact, increased IL-23 expression and, consequently, induces the release of IL-22, triggering the fibrotic molecular events' activation [65]. This evidence suggests, once again, a correlation between the production of IL-23 and IL-22 and identifies a new activation pathway of the fibrotic process that originates in Cx3cr1+ mononuclear phagocytes, in which the mTOR/autophagy pathway regulates the IL-23/IL-22 axis-dependent fibrosis. The synergistic action performed by IL-23 and IL-22 is elucidated and confirmed by the fact that the double inhibition of the release of both cytokines determines a decrease in all the parameters characterizing fibrosis [65] (Figure 3).

5.3. Autoimmune Myocarditis

Recent observations have correlated IL-23 levels with the regulation of T cells' function in autoimmune myocarditis, thus confirming the role of IL-23 in the regulation of inflammatory processes [67]. Using mice mutated for the IL-23 gene and unable to produce a functional interleukin, IL23a−/− mice, it was demonstrated that IL-23 is necessary for the induction of cardiac inflammation in experimentally induced autoimmune myocarditis (EAM) [68]. EAM has been considered a disease characterized by the altered function of CD4+ T cells [67]. In addition, transfection experiments demonstrated that IL-23 was able to restore pathogenicity to CD4+ T cells lacking the IL-23 gene. These results support the hypothesis of a direct involvement of IL-23 in the autoimmune reactions of the heart, which could occur either thanks to the action of IL-23 on the activity of T helper cells or by inducing the secretion by the T helpers of a combination of cytokines capable of triggering autoimmune responses [69]. Both hypotheses seem to be valid and have found scientific evidence; in fact, continuous stimulation through IL-23 is necessary to determine the production of IL-17A by T helper lymphocytes. On the other hand, even a temporary stimulation by IL-23 seems to be sufficient to determine a pathogenic activation of the T helper. Confirming this, the lack of IL-23 does not compromise the establishment of an EAM condition when the T helpers have become autoreactive [68]. Based on this evidence, because high levels of IL-23 were found in patients with autoimmune myocarditis, which proceeded to stimulate T helper cells, determining an increased production and release of IL-17A, a therapy against IL-23 could be effective in blocking or delaying the fibrotic progression of the disease [68]. Moreover, elevated fibrosis and impaired heart function were detected in IL-23−/− mice but not in mice lacking the IL-12 gene at the chronic stage of the disease; this underlines the importance of IL-23-dependent T cell activation in the resolution phase of the acute stage of autoimmune myocarditis.

5.4. Sjögren's Syndrome

Sjögren's syndrome (SS) is an autoimmune disease characterized by a chronic inflammatory response that causes a morphological and functional alteration of the exocrine glands, in particular the salivary and lacrimal glands, and this seriously compromises the quality of life of these patients [2,3]. "Primary" SS is defined as a standalone entity occurring in the absence of another systemic autoimmune disease, whereas "secondary" disease is associated with the presence of other autoimmune conditions, such as RA, SLE, or systemic sclerosis (SSc). Currently, the data relating to the involvement of IL-23 in the pathogenesis of SS are still few, although very promising. Previous research revealed that IL-17/IL-23 expression was increased in mouse models of SS, highlighting that Th17 participates in lymphocytic infiltration of salivary glands and leads to lesion formation [70,71]. Another experimental study demonstrated that both protein and mRNA levels of IL-22, IL-23, and IL-17 were enhanced in the peripheral blood of patients affected by SS [72], assuming that the IL-23/IL-17/IL-22 axis could be one of the key mediators in the pathogenesis of primary SS [70,72–74]. Interestingly, in the absence of certain evidence of primary SS, the immunohistochemical detection of IL-17/IL-23 would classify these patients as involved in a Th17 reaction and lead to the selection of patients to be referred for subsequent periodic diagnostic screening. Based on this assumption, the use of IL-17/IL-23 immunohistochemical detection could be employed to improve the identification of SS patients with a possible diagnosis in all cases that do not fully meet the American–European criteria for pSS, in particular when the germinal center is not present at histopathological analysis and anti-SSA and anti-SSB antibodies are undetectable in the serum [19]. Recently, a role for the synergetic interaction between IL-23 and TLR was demonstrated in SS; TLR2 ligation induces the production of IL-23 and IL-17 via IL-6, STAT3, and the NF-kB pathway in primary SS. Therefore, therapeutic strategies directed against the TLR/IL-17 pathway might be valid candidates for the treatment of SS [75]. In recent years, a thriving research sector has demonstrated that SS is often accompanied by fibrotic phenomena affecting the salivary glands mediated by the activation of the EMT program, triggered by the chronic inflammation that characterizes the disease [2,3]. Therefore, based on the attribution of an important role for IL-23 in the exacerbation of the disease, there are all the premises to identify a correlation between IL-23 expression, chronic inflammation, and fibrosis in SS.

5.5. Systemic Sclerosis

Systemic sclerosis (SSc) is a heterogeneous chronic, autoimmune, multisystem connective tissue disorder characterized by vasculopathy, inflammation, and progressive fibrosis of the skin and internal organs [76]. Interstitial lung disease (ILD) is a major common complication, along with pulmonary arterial hypertension, which is the leading cause of morbidity and mortality in scleroderma patients [77]. The finding of pulmonary fibrosis in patients with elevated IL-23 levels had a higher frequency when compared with subjects showing normal IL-23 levels [78]. The increased release of IL-23 showed a correlation with the initial stages of the disease and with the simultaneous presence of pulmonary fibrosis; it was not associated with other clinical manifestations of SSc [78]. IL-23 has been demonstrated to be abnormally expressed in autoimmunity, including Experimental autoimmune encephalomyelitis (EAE), collagen-induced arthritis, and inflammatory bowel disease [79]. In SSc, chronic T cell activation certainly occurs, contributing to the exacerbation of tissue inflammation [76]. Recent studies imply that IL-23 may determine the differentiation of activated T cells into effector T cells in SSc [78,80]. Based on these considerations, it is possible that Th17 cells, induced by IL-23, release IL-17, which can be implicated in molecular processes leading to vascular lesions, fibrosis, and autoimmunity in patients with SSc, exploiting the binding with the IL-17 receptor expressed on fibroblasts and endothelial cells [81]. Recently, a strong correlation between the onset of the disease, the initiation of pulmonary fibrosis, and the increase of IL-23 expression has been demonstrated, suggesting that Th17, stimulated by IL-23, is involved in the onset of SSc, but not in disease progression [78]. This hypothesis has also recently found radiological confirmation because, in SSc patients, there was a statistically significant difference as regards serum concentration of IL-23 in patients with pulmonary fibrosis by chest X-ray [82].

5.6. Multiple Sclerosis

MS is a chronic autoimmune disorder affecting an estimated two million people worldwide. The pathological hallmarks of MS include perivascular T-cell inflammation and disseminated demyelinating lesions [83]. Experimental autoimmune encephalomyelitis (EAE) is an inflammatory autoimmune pathology that can be induced in mice and, in addition, presents many similarities with human MS [79]. EAE is a complex disease in which the interaction between several immunopathological and neuropathological events determines an approximation of the pathological characteristics of MS manifested morphologically by inflammation, demyelination, axonal loss, and gliosis [79]. The main characteristic of the EAE condition is a fibrotic scar that determines an inhibitory environment hindering the remyelination; thus, anti-fibrotic drugs may serve as novel therapeutic targets for MS. As in MS, aberrant T lymphocytes traffic against the brain and spinal cord, causing disruption of the myelin sheath integrity of the central nervous system (CNS), leading to paresthesia, paraparesis, neuritis, and ataxia [84]. Because EAE presents clinical features similar to human MS, it could be used as a model to identify the clinical efficacy of targeting the IL-23 immune pathway. Indeed, specific anti-IL-23p19 antibodies were produced to test whether blocking the functionality of IL-23 reduced the clinical symptoms of EAE and whether it could also be used in human disease [85]. The treatment of anti-IL-23p19 diminishes the serum level of IL-17 as well as the expression of IFN-γ, IP-10, IL-17, IL-6, and TNF in the CNS, thus inhibiting multiple inflammatory signaling pathways that drive CNS autoimmune inflammation. In addition, the therapeutic efficacy of the anti-IL-23p19 antibody was demonstrated to prevent disease relapse [85]. Recently, the wealth of knowledge in this field has been enriched with new discoveries that have demonstrated IL-23 as a key factor driving inflammatory processes in the CNS [86]. In particular, a transgenic mouse with astrocyte-specific expression of IL-23 developed an ataxic phenotype and cerebellar infiltrates with high amounts of B lymphocytes. In these mice, in which EAE was induced, it was demonstrated that the local IL-23 production in the CNS determines the aggravation of the disease course with severe paraparesis and an ataxic phenotype, leading to the enhancement of gliosis and neuroinflammation in the CNS [86,87]. Certainly, further studies will be necessary to identify the mechanisms that explain the key role of IL-23 in MS, but the premises are very interesting, and the preliminary results are very intriguing.

6. New Therapeutic Challenges

6.1. IL-23 Blocking Agents

In the last two decades, several biological agents have been developed to ameliorate the knowledge of the interactions between the immune system and related cytokines, which affect the entire pathologic condition process. Some of these agents inhibit specific molecular pathways involved in the pathogenesis of autoimmune diseases, specifically in those characterized by severe fibrosis. Biological drugs targeting IL-23, either specifically (anti-p19) or in conjunction with IL-12 (anti-p40), have displayed a wide range of antagonistic activities because IL-23 is an important upstream regulator of pathways involved in fibrotic autoimmune diseases [88]. Since their approval, several real-life studies have been published on IL-23 inhibitors use in routine clinical practice, and real-life results of anti-IL-23 seem to confirm the promising findings of IL-23 demonstrated by clinical trials, highlighting the efficacy and safety profiles of this new class of biologic agents also in clinical practice [89]. Therefore, growing evidence supports the idea that drugs targeting IL-23 have shown promising efficacy in inflammatory bowel disease. Indeed, they were approved for the treatment of Crohn's disease (CD) and, recently, for ulcerative colitis as well. Guselkumab, risankizumab, and tildrakizumab represent the latest biologic agents accepted for the treatment of psoriasis with varying degrees of severity and have ameliorated the perception of patients' quality of life affected by fibrotic diseases [89]. In particular, Guselkumab, in which the mechanism of action occurs through selective inhibition of IL-23 via binding to its p19 subunit, demonstrated greater efficacy and durability of response in the treatment of plaque-type psoriasis compared with a placebo [90]. Therefore, emerging studies have observed a good therapeutic effect after treatment with Guselkumab of patients affected by psoriasis vulgaris complicated by SSc, improving each symptom of SSc, such as immune abnormalities, fibrosis, and vasculopathy [91]. Unfortunately, the administration of anti-IL-23 agents has not had positive effects in all patients, and they can cause undesirable immunological and non-immunological adverse events. However, these inhibitors tend to be well tolerated, with good safety profiles [92]. Ustekinumab, for example, already accepted for psoriatic arthritis, has shown promising data in SLE, but its evaluation in clinical trials has led to very contradictory results [93].

In conclusion, the recent evaluations on the therapeutic use of IL-23 seem to have two advantages: on the one hand, the possibility that IL-23 could represent a valid marker for the initial stages of autoimmune diseases, and, on the other, the possibility of identifying pharmacological treatments that specifically modulate the T helper's immune response [94].

6.2. Epigenetics in the Control of IL-23 Expression in Autoimmune Diseases

Epigenetics studies how stress, age, and exposure to environmental factors, including physical and chemical agents, diet, and physical activity, can modify gene expression without modifying the DNA sequence. Epigenetic modifications of DNA regulate physiological processes, but recent data indicate that they play a role in the onset of diseases. A key factor in the development of autoimmunity is the impaired function of Treg cells. The identification and correction of diet, environmental, or stress factors improves the activity of Treg cells, and these considerations represent the epigenetic approach to autoimmune diseases [95]. Over the last few years, the field of epigenetics has been revolutionized by various innovative technologies aimed at determining these modifications (epimutations) through the analysis of DNA methylation, non-coding RNA expression, histone, and nucleosome modifications [95]. These data underline how the study of the genome and, even more, of the epigenome, helps to trace an individual profile that shows intra-individual variability. In this regard, epigenomics is also acquiring an important role in determining susceptibility to various diseases. The epigenetic study of IL-23 regulation, conducted in very recent times, has led to very intriguing results. The regulatory mechanism carried out via mTOR responsible for histone methylation mentioned above, e.g., in RA, represents an epigenetic modification that may regulate the IL-23-mediated process of EMT-dependent fibrosis [64]. In addition, Jin et al. report an epigenetic mechanism for the regulation of the gene Zranb1 (Zinc Finger RANBP2-Type Containing 1) responsible for the coding of the deubiquitinase Trabid, which seems to be involved in the regulation of IL-23 and correlated IL-12 expression in autoimmunity [96]. Deletion of Zranb1 in dendritic cells inhibits the expression of IL-12 and IL-23 by TLRs, impairing the differentiation of Treg and protecting mice from autoimmune inflammation. The role of Trabid takes place through the TLR-induced histone modifications at the IL-12 and IL-23 gene promoters, which involve deubiqutination. Another study conducted in SLE patients demonstrated the involvement of IL-23 in the STAT3-mediated alteration of the loci of RORγt at STAT binding sites, resulting in an exacerbated inflammatory function of Th17 in SLE [97]. Furthermore, evidence that an epigenetic mechanism involving TNF and the neural Wiskott–Aldrich syndrome protein (N-WASP) controls IL-23 expression in psoriatic keratinocytes has been provided by Li et al. [98]. Keratinocyte-restricted deletion of the N-WASP gene revealed an important function for N-WASP corresponding to increased TGF-β signaling, a potent pro-fibrotic cytokine. The loss of N-WASP in keratinocytes provokes IL-23 over-expression in keratinocytes, acting through the control of histone methylation mediated by IL-17 and TLRs. Once again, this evidence suggests that different independently studied pathways can converge in order to identify molecular bridges that can lead to a unique and complex mechanism of activation in autoimmune diseases.

Can epigenetics clarify which factors can determine the fibrotic evolution of autoimmune diseases? Or could epigenetics help identify common mechanisms that drive the chronic inflammation that characterizes multiple autoimmune diseases and that appears to be responsible for fibrosis? The answer seems to be far from being identified, but researchers engaged in this field of investigation are making giant strides and promising new perspectives for effective therapies.

7. Conclusions

Recent discoveries place IL-23 in a prominent position in the modulation of the immune response mediated by T helper lymphocytes. This has given rise to a series of investigations on the ability of IL-23 to modulate autoimmune processes characterized by chronic inflammation, which, frequently, evolve towards fibrotic processes. Although the mechanisms underlying the pro-fibrotic activity of IL-23 are not clear, some underlying mechanisms common to several fibrotic and autoimmune diseases have been identified.

This suggests that we are on the right track and that, soon, therapies that block the activity or the release of IL-23 could represent a valid therapeutic alternative in the course of autoimmune fibrotic diseases.

Author Contributions: All authors were involved in drafting the article or revising it critically for important intellectual content. M.S. and S.L. had full access to the data collected in the review, take responsibility for their integrity, and performed a critical reading. All authors have read and agreed to the published version of the manuscript.

Funding: This research received no external funding.

Institutional Review Board Statement: Not applicable.

Informed Consent Statement: Not applicable.

Data Availability Statement: Not applicable.

Conflicts of Interest: The authors declare no conflict of interest.

References

1. Pisetsky, D.S. Pathogenesis of autoimmune disease. *Nat. Rev. Nephrol.* **2023**, *19*, 509–524. [CrossRef] [PubMed]
2. Sisto, M.; Ribatti, D.; Lisi, S. Organ Fibrosis and Autoimmunity: The Role of Inflammation in TGFβ-Dependent EMT. *Biomolecules* **2021**, *11*, 310. [CrossRef]
3. Sisto, M.; Lisi, S. Immune and Non-Immune Inflammatory Cells Involved in Autoimmune Fibrosis: New Discoveries. *J. Clin. Med.* **2023**, *12*, 3801. [CrossRef] [PubMed]
4. Liu, C.; Chu, D.; Kalantar-Zadeh, K.; George, J.; Young, H.A.; Liu, G. Cytokines: From Clinical Significance to Quantification. *Adv. Sci.* **2021**, *8*, e2004433. [CrossRef] [PubMed]
5. Karki, R.; Kanneganti, T.D. The 'cytokine storm': Molecular mechanisms and therapeutic prospects. *Trends Immunol.* **2021**, *42*, 681–705. [CrossRef] [PubMed]
6. Duvallet, E.; Semerano, L.; Assier, E.; Falgarone, G.; Boissier, M.C. Interleukin-23: A key cytokine in inflammatory diseases. *Ann. Med.* **2011**, *43*, 503–511. [CrossRef] [PubMed]
7. Gaffen, S.L.; Jain, R.; Garg, A.V.; Cua, D.J. The IL-23-IL-17 immune axis: From mechanisms to therapeutic testing. *Nat. Rev. Immunol.* **2014**, *14*, 585–600. [CrossRef] [PubMed]
8. Oppmann, B.; Lesley, R.; Blom, B.; Timans, J.C.; Xu, Y.; Hunte, B.; Vega, F.; Yu, N.; Wang, J.; Singh, K.; et al. Novel p19 protein engages IL-12p40 to form a cytokine, IL-23, with biological activities similar as well as distinct from IL-12. *Immunity* **2000**, *13*, 715–725. [CrossRef]
9. Croxford, A.L.; Mair, F.; Becher, B. IL-23: One cytokine in control of autoimmunity. *Eur. J. Immunol.* **2012**, *42*, 2263–2273. [CrossRef]
10. Sherlock, J.P.; Cua, D.J. Interleukin-23 in perspective. *Rheumatology* **2021**, *60*, iv1–iv3. [CrossRef]
11. Abdo, A.I.K.; Tye, G.J. Interleukin 23 and autoimmune diseases: Current and possible future therapies. *Inflamm. Res.* **2020**, *69*, 463–480. [CrossRef] [PubMed]
12. Bianchi, E.; Vecellio, M.; Rogge, L. Editorial: Role of the IL-23/IL-17 Pathway in Chronic Immune-Mediated Inflammatory Diseases: Mechanisms and Targeted Therapies. *Front. Immunol.* **2021**, *12*, 770275. [CrossRef] [PubMed]
13. Senoo, S.; Taniguchi, A.; Itano, J.; Oda, N.; Morichika, D.; Fujii, U.; Guo, L.; Sunami, R.; Kanehiro, A.; Tokioka, F.; et al. Essential role of IL-23 in the development of acute exacerbation of pulmonary fibrosis. *Am. J. Physiol. Lung Cell. Mol. Physiol.* **2021**, *321*, L925–L940. [CrossRef] [PubMed]
14. Tang, C.; Chen, S.; Qian, H.; Huang, W. Interleukin-23: As a drug target for autoimmune inflammatory diseases. *Immunology* **2012**, *135*, 112–124. [CrossRef] [PubMed]
15. Gubler, U.; Chua, A.O.; Schoenhaut, D.S.; Dwyer, C.M.; McComas, W.; Motyka, R.; Nabavi, N.; Wolitzky, A.G.; Quinn, P.M.; Familletti, P.C. Coexpression of two distinct genes is required to generate secreted bioactive cytotoxic lymphocyte maturation factor. *Proc. Natl. Acad. Sci. USA* **1991**, *88*, 4143–4147. [CrossRef] [PubMed]
16. Shimozato, O.; Ugai, S.; Chiyo, M.; Takenobu, H.; Nagakawa, H.; Wada, A.; Kawamura, K.; Yamamoto, H.; Tagawa, M. The secreted form of the p40 subunit of interleukin (IL)-12 inhibits IL-23 functions and abrogates IL-23-mediated antitumour effects. *Immunology* **2006**, *117*, 22–28. [CrossRef] [PubMed]
17. McKenzie, B.S.; Kastelein, R.A.; Cua, D.J. Understanding the IL-23/IL-17 immune pathway. *Trends Immunol.* **2006**, *27*, 17–23. [CrossRef] [PubMed]
18. Brentano, F.; Ospelt, C.; Stanczyk, J.; Gay, R.E.; Gay, S.; Kyburz, D. Abundant expression of the interleukin (IL)23 subunit p19, but low levels of bioactive IL23 in the rheumatoid synovium: Differential expression and Toll-like receptor-(TLR) dependent regulation of the IL23 subunits, p19 and p40, in rheumatoid arthritis. *Ann. Rheum. Dis.* **2009**, *68*, 143–150. [CrossRef]

19. Fusconi, M.; Musy, I.; Valente, D.; Maggi, E.; Priori, R.; Pecorella, I.; Mastromanno, L.; Di Cristofano, C.; Greco, A.; Armeli, F.; et al. Immunohistochemical detection of IL-17 and IL-23 improves the identification of patients with a possible diagnosis of Sjogren's syndrome. *Pathol. Res. Pract.* **2020**, *216*, 153137. [CrossRef]
20. Zhu, C.; Nan, L.; Wu, K.; Zhai, J. Research progress on the role and therapeutic significance of IL-23/Th17 in the pathogenesis of inflammatory bowel disease. *J. Liaoning Med. Coll.* **2016**, *37*, 103–106.
21. Pahan, K.; Jana, M. Induction of lymphotoxin-alpha by interleukin-12 p40 homodimer, the so-called biologically inactive molecule, but not IL-12 p70. *Immunology* **2009**, *127*, 312–325.
22. Chognard, G.; Bellemare, L.; Pelletier, A.N.; Dominguez-Punaro, M.C.; Beauchamp, C.; Guyon, M.J.; Charron, G.; Morin, N.; Sivanesan, D.; Kuchroo, V.; et al. The dichotomous pattern of IL-12r and IL-23R expression elucidates the role of IL-12 and IL-23 in inflammation. *PLoS ONE* **2014**, *9*, 89092. [CrossRef]
23. Curtis, M.M.; Way, S.S. Interleukin-17 in host defence against bacterial, mycobacterial and fungal pathogens. *Immunology* **2009**, *126*, 177–185. [CrossRef] [PubMed]
24. Korta, A.; Kula, J.; Gomułka, K. The Role of IL-23 in the Pathogenesis and Therapy of Inflammatory Bowel Disease. *Int. J. Mol. Sci.* **2023**, *24*, 10172. [CrossRef] [PubMed]
25. Salamero, A.C.; Castillo-González, R.; Pastor-Fernández, G.; Mariblanca, I.R.; Pino, J.; Cibrian, D.; Navarro, M.N. IL-23 signaling regulation of pro-inflammatory T-cell migration uncovered by phosphoproteomics. *PLoS Biol.* **2020**, *18*, e3000646.
26. Venken, K.; Jacques, P.; Mortier, C.; Labadia, M.E.; Decruy, T.; Coudenys, J.; Hoyt, K.; Wayne, A.L.; Hughes, R.; Turner, M.; et al. RORγt inhibition selectively targets IL-17 producing iNKT and γδ-T cells enriched in Spondyloarthritis patients. *Nat. Commun.* **2019**, *10*, 9. [CrossRef] [PubMed]
27. Noack, M.; Miossec, P. Synoviocytes and skin fibroblasts show opposite effects on IL-23 production and IL-23 receptor expression during cell interactions with immune cells. *Arthritis Res. Ther.* **2022**, *24*, 220. [CrossRef] [PubMed]
28. Goldberg, M.; Nadiv, O.; Luknar-Gabor, N.; Agar, G.; Beer, Y.; Katz, Y. Synergism between tumor necrosis factor α and interleukin-17 to induce IL-23 p19 expression in fibroblast-like synoviocytes. *Mol. Immunol.* **2009**, *46*, 1854–1859. [CrossRef]
29. Zakharova, M.; Ziegler, H.K. Paradoxical anti-inflammatory actions of TNF-alpha: Inhibition of IL-12 and IL-23 via TNF receptor 1 in macrophages and dendritic cells. *J. Immunol.* **2005**, *175*, 5024–5033. [CrossRef]
30. Mills, K.H.G. IL-17 and IL-17-producing cells in protection versus pathology. *Nat. Rev. Immunol.* **2023**, *23*, 38–54. [CrossRef]
31. Aggarwal, S.; Ghilardi, N.; Xie, M.H.; de Sauvage, F.J.; Gurney, A.L. Interleukin-23 promotes a distinct CD4 T cell activation state characterized by the production of interleukin-17. *J. Biol. Chem.* **2003**, *278*, 1910–1914. [CrossRef] [PubMed]
32. Boniface, K.; Blom, B.; Liu, Y.J.; de Waal Malefyt, R. From interleukin-23 to T-helper 17 cells: Human T-helper cell differentiation revisited. *Immunol. Rev.* **2008**, *226*, 132–146. [CrossRef] [PubMed]
33. Maddur, M.S.; Miossec, P.; Kaveri, S.V.; Bayry, J. Th17 cells: Biology, pathogenesis of autoimmune and inflammatory diseases, and therapeutic strategies. *Am. J. Pathol.* **2012**, *181*, 8–18. [CrossRef] [PubMed]
34. Schinocca, C.; Rizzo, C.; Fasano, S.; Grasso, G.; La Barbera, L.; Ciccia, F.; Guggino, G. Role of the IL-23/IL-17 Pathway in Rheumatic Diseases: An Overview. *Front. Immunol.* **2021**, *12*, 637829. [CrossRef] [PubMed]
35. Bunte, K.; Beikler, T. Th17 Cells and the IL-23/IL-17 Axis in the Pathogenesis of Periodontitis and Immune-Mediated Inflammatory Diseases. *Int. J. Mol. Sci.* **2019**, *20*, 3394. [CrossRef] [PubMed]
36. Tsukazaki, H.; Kaito, T. The Role of the IL-23/IL-17 Pathway in the Pathogenesis of Spondyloarthritis. *Int. J. Mol. Sci.* **2020**, *21*, 6401. [CrossRef] [PubMed]
37. Al-Salleeh, F.; Petro, T.M. TLR3 and TLR7 are involved in expression of IL-23 subunits while TLR3 but not TLR7 is involved in expression of IFN-beta by Theiler's virus-infected RAW264.7 cells. *Microbes Infect.* **2007**, *9*, 1384–1392. [CrossRef]
38. Bhan, U.; Ballinger, M.N.; Zeng, X.; Newstead, M.J.; Cornicelli, M.D.; Standiford, T.J. Cooperative interactions between TLR4 and TLR9 regulate interleukin 23 and 17 production in a murine model of gram negative bacterial pneumonia. *PLoS ONE* **2010**, *5*, e9896. [CrossRef]
39. Yan, J.; Smyth, M.J.; Teng, M.W.L. Interleukin (IL)-12 and IL-23 and Their Conflicting Roles in Cancer. *Cold Spring Harb. Perspect. Biol.* **2018**, *10*, a028530. [CrossRef]
40. Kortylewski, M.; Xin, H.; Kujawski, M.; Lee, H.; Liu, Y.; Harris, T.; Drake, C.; Pardoll, D.; Yu, H. Regulation of the IL-23 and IL-12 balance by Stat3 signaling in the tumor microenvironment. *Cancer Cell* **2009**, *15*, 114–123. [CrossRef]
41. Weiss, J.M.; Subleski, J.J.; Wigginton, J.M.; Wiltrout, R.H. Immunotherapy of cancer by IL-12-based cytokine combinations. *Expert Opin. Biol. Ther.* **2007**, *7*, 1705–1721. [CrossRef] [PubMed]
42. Cheng, E.M.; Tsarovsky, N.W.; Sondel, P.M.; Rakhmilevich, A.L. Interleukin-12 as an in situ cancer vaccine component: A review. *Cancer Immunol. Immunother.* **2022**, *71*, 2057–2065. [CrossRef] [PubMed]
43. Langrish, C.L.; Chen, Y.; Blumenschein, W.M.; Mattson, J.; Basham, B.; Sedgwick, J.D.; Mc Clanahan, T.; Kastelein, R.A.; Cua, D.J. IL-23 drives a pathogenic T cell population that induces autoimmune inflammation. *J. Exp. Med.* **2005**, *201*, 233–240. [CrossRef] [PubMed]
44. Veldhoen, M.; Hocking, R.J.; Atkins, C.J.; Locksley, R.M.; Stockinger, B. TGF beta in the context of an inflammatory cytokine milieu supports de novo differentiation of IL-17-producing T cells. *Immunity* **2006**, *24*, 179–189. [CrossRef] [PubMed]
45. Yang, X.O.; Panopoulos, A.D.; Nurieva, R.; Chang, S.H.; Wang, D.; Watowich, S.S.; Dong, C. STAT3 regulates cytokine-mediated generation of inflammatory helper T cells. *J. Biol. Chem.* **2007**, *282*, 9358–9363. [CrossRef] [PubMed]

46. Zhou, L.; Ivanov, I.I.; Spolski, R.; Min, R.; Shenderov, K.; Egawa, T.; Levy, D.E.; Leonard, W.J.; Littman, D.R. IL-6 programs T(H)-17 cell differentiation by promoting sequential engagement of the IL-21 and IL-23 pathways. *Nat. Immunol.* **2007**, *8*, 967–974. [CrossRef] [PubMed]
47. Morena, D.; Fernández, J.; Campos, C.; Castillo, M.; López, G.; Benavent, M.; Izquierdo, J.L. Clinical Profile of Patients with Idiopathic Pulmonary Fibrosis in Real Life. *J. Clin. Med.* **2023**, *12*, 1669. [CrossRef]
48. Fujii, U.; Miyahara, N.; Taniguchi, A.; Waseda, K.; Morichika, D.; Kurimoto, E.; Koga, H.; Kataoka, M.; Gelfand, E.W.; Cua, D.J.; et al. IL-23 is essential for the development of elastase-induced pulmonary inflammation and emphysema. *Am. J. Respir. Cell Mol. Biol.* **2016**, *55*, 697–707. [CrossRef]
49. Sakaguchi, R.; Chikuma, S.; Shichita, T.; Morita, R.; Sekiya, T.; Ouyang, W.; Ueda, T.; Seki, H.; Morisaki, H.; Yoshimura, A. Innate-like function of memory Th17 cells for enhancing endotoxin-induced acute lung inflammation through IL-22. *Int. Immunol.* **2016**, *28*, 233–243. [CrossRef]
50. Gasse, P.; Riteau, N.; Vacher, R.; Michel, M.L.; Fautrel, A.; di Padova, F.; Fick, L.; Charron, S.; Lagente, V.; Eberl, G.; et al. IL-1 and IL-23 mediate early IL-17A production in pulmonary inflammation leading to late fibrosis. *PLoS ONE* **2011**, *6*, e23185. [CrossRef]
51. Zhao, Y.; Jia, S.; Zhang, K.; Zhang, L. Serum cytokine levels and other associated factors as possible immunotherapeutic targets and prognostic indicators for lung cancer. *Front. Oncol.* **2023**, *13*, 1064616. [CrossRef] [PubMed]
52. Davis, J.; Kellerman, R. Gastrointestinal Conditions: Inflammatory Bowel Disease. *FP Essent.* **2022**, *516*, 23–30. [PubMed]
53. Rodríguez-Lago, I.; Blackwell, J.; Mateos, B.; Marigorta, U.M.; Barreiro-de Acosta, M.; Pollok, R. Recent Advances and Potential Multi-Omics Approaches in the Early Phases of Inflammatory Bowel Disease. *J. Clin. Med.* **2023**, *12*, 3418. [CrossRef] [PubMed]
54. Guan, Q.; Weiss, C.R.; Wang, S.; Qing, G.; Yang, X.; Warrington, R.J.; Bernstein, C.N.; Peng, Z. Reversing Ongoing Chronic Intestinal Inflammation and Fibrosis by Sustained Block of IL-12 and IL-23 Using a Vaccine in Mice. *Inflamm. Bowel Dis.* **2018**, *24*, 1941–1952. [CrossRef]
55. Kosmalski, M.; Frankowski, R.; Ziółkowska, S.; Różycka-Kosmalska, M.; Pietras, T. What's New in the Treatment of Non-Alcoholic Fatty Liver Disease (NAFLD). *J. Clin. Med.* **2023**, *12*, 1852. [CrossRef] [PubMed]
56. Banini, B.A.; Sanyal, A.J. Nonalcoholic Fatty Liver Disease: Epidemiology, Pathogenesis, Natural History, Diagnosis, and Current Treatment Options. *Clin. Med. Insights Ther.* **2016**, *8*, 75–84. [CrossRef] [PubMed]
57. Méndez-Sánchez, N.; Valencia-Rodríguez, A.; Coronel-Castillo, C.; Vera-Barajas, A.; Contreras-Carmona, J.; Ponciano-Rodríguez, G.; Zamora-Valdés, D. The cellular pathways of liver fibrosis in non-alcoholic steatohepatitis. *Ann. Transl. Med.* **2020**, *8*, 400. [CrossRef]
58. Rau, M.; Schilling, A.K.; Meertens, J.; Hering, I.; Weiss, J.; Jurowich, C.; Kudlich, T.; Hermanns, H.M.; Bantel, H.; Beyersdorf, N.; et al. Progression from Nonalcoholic Fatty Liver to Nonalcoholic Steatohepatitis Is Marked by a Higher Frequency of Th17 Cells in the Liver and an Increased Th17/Resting Regulatory T Cell Ratio in Peripheral Blood and in the Liver. *J. Immunol.* **2016**, *196*, 97–105. [CrossRef]
59. Albhaisi, S.; Noureddin, M. Current and Potential Therapies Targeting Inflammation in NASH. *Front. Endocrinol.* **2021**, *12*, 767314. [CrossRef]
60. Meng, F.; Wang, K.; Aoyama, T.; Grivennikov, S.I.; Paik, Y.; Scholten, D.; Cong, M.; Iwaisako, K.; Liu, X.; Zhang, M.; et al. Interleukin-17 signaling in inflammatory, Kupffer cells, and hepatic stellate cells exacerbates liver fibrosis in mice. *Gastroenterology* **2012**, *143*, 765–776. [CrossRef]
61. Heredia, J.E.; Sorenson, C.; Flanagan, S.; Nunez, V.; Jones, C.; Martzall, A.; Leong, L.; Martinez, A.P.; Scherl, A.; Brightbill, H.D.; et al. IL-23 signaling is not an important driver of liver inflammation and fibrosis in murine non-alcoholic steatohepatitis models. *PLoS ONE* **2022**, *17*, e0274582. [CrossRef] [PubMed]
62. Laria, A.; Lurati, A.M.; Zizzo, G.; Zaccara, E.; Mazzocchi, D.; Re, K.A.; Marrazza, M.; Faggioli, P.; Mazzone, A. Interstitial Lung Disease in Rheumatoid Arthritis: A Practical Review. *Front. Med.* **2022**, *9*, 837133. [CrossRef] [PubMed]
63. Zhang, C.; Wang, S.; Lau, J.; Roden, A.C.; Matteson, E.L.; Sun, J.; Luo, F.; Tschumperlin, D.J.; Vassallo, R. IL-23 amplifies the epithelial-mesenchymal transition of mechanically conditioned alveolar epithelial cells in rheumatoid arthritis-associated interstitial lung disease through mTOR/S6 signaling. *Am. J. Physiol. Lung Cell. Mol. Physiol.* **2021**, *321*, L1006–L1022. [CrossRef] [PubMed]
64. Chen, F.; Cao, A.; Yao, S.; Evans-Marin, H.L.; Liu, H.; Wu, W.; Carlsen, E.D.; Dann, S.M.; Soong, L.; Sun, J.; et al. mTOR Mediates IL-23 Induction of Neutrophil IL-17 and IL-22 Production. *J. Immunol.* **2016**, *196*, 4390–4399. [CrossRef] [PubMed]
65. Mathur, R.; Alam, M.M.; Zhao, X.F.; Liao, Y.; Shen, J.; Morgan, S.; Huang, T.; Lee, H.; Lee, E.; Huang, Y.; et al. Induction of autophagy in Cx3cr1+ mononuclear cells limits IL-23/IL-22 axis-mediated intestinal fibrosis. *Mucosal Immunol.* **2019**, *12*, 612–623. [CrossRef] [PubMed]
66. Wang, Y.; Huang, B.; Jin, T.; Ocansey, D.K.W.; Jiang, J.; Mao, F. Intestinal Fibrosis in Inflammatory Bowel Disease and the Prospects of Mesenchymal Stem Cell Therapy. *Front. Immunol.* **2022**, *13*, 835005. [CrossRef] [PubMed]
67. Vdovenko, D.; Wijnen, W.J.; Zarak Crnkovic, M.; Blyszczuk, P.; Bachmann, M.; Costantino, S.; Paneni, F.; Camici, G.G.; Luescher, T.F.; Eriksson, U. IL-23 promotes T-cell mediated cardiac inflammation but protects the heart from fibrosis. *Eur. Heart J.* **2020**, *41*, ehaa946.3725. [CrossRef]

68. Wu, L.; Diny, N.L.; Ong, S.; Barin, J.G.; Hou, X.; Rose, N.R.; Talor, M.V.; Čiháková, D. Pathogenic IL-23 signaling is required to initiate GM-CSF-driven autoimmune myocarditis in mice. *Eur. J. Immunol.* **2016**, *46*, 582–592. [CrossRef]
69. Burkett, P.R.; Meyer, G.; Kuchroo, V.K. Pouring fuel on the fire: Th17 cells, the environment, and autoimmunity. *J. Clin. Investig.* **2015**, *125*, 1–9. [CrossRef]
70. Nguyen, C.Q.; Hu, M.H.; Li, Y.; Stewart, C.; Peck, A.B. Salivary gland tissue expression of interleukin-23 and interleukin-17 in sjogren's syndrome: Findings in humans and mice. *Arthritis Rheum.* **2008**, *58*, 734–743. [CrossRef]
71. Luo, D.; Chen, Y.; Zhou, N.; Li, T.; Wang, H. Blockade of Th17 response by IL-38 in primary sjogren's syndrome. *Mol. Immunol.* **2020**, *127*, 107–111. [CrossRef] [PubMed]
72. Ciccia, F.; Guggino, G.; Rizzo, A.; Ferrante, A.; Raimondo, S.; Giardina, A.; Dieli, F.; Campisi, G.; Alessandro, R.; Triolo, G. Potential involvement of IL-22 and IL-22-producing cells in the inflamed salivary glands of patients with Sjogren's syndrome. *Ann. Rheum. Dis.* **2012**, *71*, 295–301. [CrossRef] [PubMed]
73. Zhan, Q.; Zhang, J.; Lin, Y.; Chen, W.; Fan, X.; Zhang, D. Pathogenesis and treatment of Sjogren's syndrome: Review and update. *Front. Immunol.* **2023**, *14*, 1127417. [CrossRef] [PubMed]
74. Soypaçacı, Z.; Gümüş, Z.Z.; Çakaloğlu, F.; Özmen, M.; Solmaz, D.; Gücenmez, S.; Gercik, Ö.; Akar, S. Role of the mTOR pathway in minor salivary gland changes in Sjogren's syndrome and systemic sclerosis. *Arthritis Res. Ther.* **2018**, *20*, 170. [CrossRef]
75. Kwok, S.K.; Cho, M.L.; Her, Y.M.; Oh, H.J.; Park, M.K.; Lee, S.Y.; Woo, Y.J.; Ju, J.H.; Park, K.S.; Kim, H.Y.; et al. TLR2 ligation induces the production of IL-23/IL-17 via IL-6, STAT3 and NF-kB pathway in patients with primary Sjogren's syndrome. *Arthritis Res. Ther.* **2012**, *14*, R64. [CrossRef]
76. Truchetet, M.E.; Brembilla, N.C.; Chizzolini, C. Current Concepts on the Pathogenesis of Systemic Sclerosis. *Clin. Rev. Allergy Immunol.* **2023**, *64*, 262–283. [CrossRef]
77. Mendoza, F.A.; Allawh, T.; Jimenez, S.A. Pharmacological treatment of systemic sclerosis-associated interstitial lung disease: An updated review and current approach to patient care. *Clin. Exp. Rheumatol.* **2023**, *41*, 1704–1712. [CrossRef] [PubMed]
78. Komura, K.; Fujimoto, M.; Hasegawa, M.; Ogawa, F.; Hara, T.; Muroi, E.; Takehara, K.; Sato, S. Increased serum interleukin 23 in patients with systemic sclerosis. *J. Rheumatol.* **2008**, *35*, 120–125. [CrossRef]
79. Constantinescu, C.S.; Farooqi, N.; O'Brien, K.; Gran, B. Experimental autoimmune encephalomyelitis (EAE) as a model for multiple sclerosis (MS). *Br. J. Pharmacol.* **2011**, *164*, 1079–1106. [CrossRef]
80. Kastelein, R.A.; Hunter, C.A.; Cua, D.J. Discovery and biology of IL-23 and IL-27: Related but functionally distinct regulators of inflammation. *Annu. Rev. Immunol.* **2007**, *25*, 221–242. [CrossRef]
81. Kurasawa, K.; Hirose, K.; Sano, H.; Endo, H.; Shinkai, H.; Nawata, Y.; Takabayashi, K.; Iwamoto, I. Increased interleukin-17 production in patients with systemic sclerosis. *Arthritis Rheum* **2000**, *43*, 2455–2463. [CrossRef] [PubMed]
82. Hammad, G.A.; Eltanawy, R.M.; Fawzy, R.M.; Gouda, T.M.; Eltohamy, M.A. Serum interleukin 23 and its associations with interstitial lung disease and clinical manifestations of scleroderma. *Egypt. J. Bronchol.* **2018**, *12*, 69–75.
83. Khan, Z.; Gupta, G.D.; Mehan, S. Cellular and Molecular Evidence of Multiple Sclerosis Diagnosis and Treatment Challenges. *J. Clin. Med.* **2023**, *12*, 4274. [CrossRef] [PubMed]
84. El Behi, M.; Dubucquoi, S.; Lefranc, D.; Zéphir, H.; De Seze, J.; Vermersch, P.; Prin, L. New insights into cell responses involved in experimental autoimmune encephalomyelitis and multiple sclerosis. *Immunol Lett.* **2005**, *96*, 11–26. [CrossRef] [PubMed]
85. Chen, Y.; Langrish, C.L.; McKenzie, B.; Joyce-Shaikh, B.; Stumhofer, J.S.; McClanahan, T.; Blumenschein, W.; Churakovsa, T.; Low, J.; Presta, L.; et al. Anti-IL-23 therapy inhibits multiple inflammatory pathways and ameliorates autoimmune encephalomyelitis. *J. Clin. Investig.* **2006**, *116*, 1317–1326. [CrossRef] [PubMed]
86. Cua, D.J.; Sherlock, J.; Chen, Y.; Murphy, C.A.; Joyce, B.; Seymour, B.; Lucian, L.; To, W.; Kwan, S.; Churakova, T.; et al. Interleukin-23 rather than interleukin-12 is the critical cytokine for autoimmune inflammation of the brain. *Nature* **2003**, *421*, 744–748. [CrossRef] [PubMed]
87. Ahern, P.P.; Schiering, C.; Buonocore, S.; McGeachy, M.J.; Cua, D.J.; Maloy, K.J.; Powrie, F. Interleukin-23 drives intestinal inflammation through direct activity on T cells. *Immunity* **2010**, *33*, 279–288. [CrossRef]
88. Parigi, T.L.; Iacucci, M.; Ghosh, S. Blockade of IL-23: What is in the Pipeline? *J. Crohns Colitis* **2022**, *16*, ii64–ii72. [CrossRef]
89. Ruggiero, A.; Picone, V.; Martora, F.; Fabbrocini, G.; Megna, M. Guselkumab, Risankizumab, and Tildrakizumab in the Management of Psoriasis: A Review of the Real-World Evidence. *Clin. Cosmet. Investig. Dermatol.* **2022**, *15*, 1649–1658. [CrossRef]
90. Nogueira, M.; Torres, T. Guselkumab for the treatment of psoriasis—Evidence to date. *Drugs Context* **2019**, *8*, 212594. [CrossRef]
91. Armstrong, A.W.; Fitzgerald, T.; McLean, R.R.; Teeple, A.; Uy, J.P.; Olurinde, M.; Rowland, K.; Guo, L.; Shan, Y.; Callis Duffin, K. Effectiveness of Guselkumab Therapy among Patients with Plaque Psoriasis with Baseline IGA Score $\geq$ 2 in the CorEvitas Psoriasis Registry. *Dermatol. Ther.* **2023**, *13*, 487–504. [CrossRef]
92. Ru, Y.; Ding, X.; Luo, Y.; Li, H.; Sun, X.; Zhou, M.; Zhou, Y.; Kuai, L.; Xing, M.; Liu, L.; et al. Adverse events associated with anti-IL-23 agents: Clinical evidence and possible mechanisms. *Front. Immunol.* **2021**, *12*, 670398. [CrossRef] [PubMed]
93. Vukelic, M.; Laloo, A.; Kyttaris, V.C. Interleukin 23 is elevated in the serum of patients with SLE. *Lupus* **2020**, *29*, 1943–1947. [CrossRef]
94. Xiong, D.K.; Shi, X.; Han, M.M.; Zhang, X.M.; Wu, N.N.; Sheng, X.Y.; Wang, J.N. The regulatory mechanism and potential application of IL-23 in autoimmune diseases. *Front. Pharmacol.* **2022**, *13*, 982238. [CrossRef] [PubMed]

95. Huang, B.; Jiang, C.; Zhang, R. Epigenetics: The language of the cell? *Epigenomics* **2014**, *6*, 73–88. [CrossRef]
96. Jin, J.; Xie, X.; Xiao, Y.; Hu, H.; Zou, Q.; Cheng, X.; Sun, S.C. Epigenetic regulation of the expres-sion of Il12 and Il23 and autoimmune inflammation by the deubiquitinase Trabid. *Nat. Immunol.* **2016**, *17*, 259–268. [CrossRef] [PubMed]
97. Lee, S.; Nakayamada, S.; Kubo, S.; Yamagata, K.; Yoshinari, H.; Tanaka, Y. Interleukin-23 drives expansion of Thelper 17 cells through epigenetic regulation by signal transducer and activators of transcription 3 in lupus patients. *Rheumatology* **2020**, *59*, 3058–3069. [CrossRef]
98. Li, H.; Yao, Q.; Mariscal, A.G.; Wu, X.; Hülse, J.; Pedersen, E.; Helin, K.; Waisman, A.; Vinkel, C.; Thomsen, S.F.; et al. Epigenetic control of IL-23 expression in keratinocytes is important for chronic skin inflammation. *Nat. Commun.* **2018**, *9*, 1420. [CrossRef]

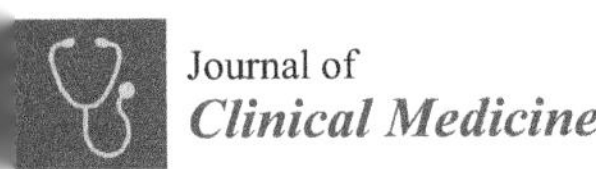
Journal of
Clinical Medicine

Immune and Non-Immune Inflammatory Cells Involved in Autoimmune Fibrosis: New Discoveries

Margherita Sisto * and Sabrina Lisi

Department of Translational Biomedicine and Neuroscience (DiBraiN), Section of Human Anatomy and Histology, University of Bari "Aldo Moro", 70124 Bari, Italy; sabrina.lisi@uniba.it
* Correspondence: margherita.sisto@uniba.it; Tel.: +39-080-547-8315; Fax: +39-080-547-8327

Abstract: Fibrosis is an important health problem and its pathogenetic activation is still largely unknown. It can develop either spontaneously or, more frequently, as a consequence of various underlying diseases, such as chronic inflammatory autoimmune diseases. Fibrotic tissue is always characterized by mononuclear immune cells infiltration. The cytokine profile of these cells shows clear proinflammatory and profibrotic characteristics. Furthermore, the production of inflammatory mediators by non-immune cells, in response to several stimuli, can be involved in the fibrotic process. It is now established that defects in the abilities of non-immune cells to mediate immune regulation may be involved in the pathogenicity of a series of inflammatory diseases. The convergence of several, not yet well identified, factors results in the aberrant activation of non-immune cells, such as epithelial cells, endothelial cells, and fibroblasts, that, by producing pro-inflammatory molecules, exacerbate the inflammatory condition leading to the excessive and chaotic secretion of extracellular matrix proteins. However, the precise cellular mechanisms involved in this process have not yet been fully elucidated. In this review, we explore the latest discoveries on the mechanisms that initiate and perpetuate the vicious circle of abnormal communications between immune and non-immune cells, responsible for fibrotic evolution of inflammatory autoimmune diseases.

Keywords: autoimmunity; inflammation; fibrosis

Citation: Sisto, M.; Lisi, S. Immune and Non-Immune Inflammatory Cells Involved in Autoimmune Fibrosis: New Discoveries. *J. Clin. Med.* **2023**, *12*, 3801. https://doi.org/10.3390/jcm12113801

Academic Editor: Eugen Feist

Received: 26 April 2023
Revised: 27 May 2023
Accepted: 30 May 2023
Published: 31 May 2023

1. Introduction

Fibrotic autoimmune disorders are a group of chronic pathologies characterized by a damage in self-tolerance to a broad variety of autoantigens in which fibrosis develops as the end-result of a chronic inflammatory process [1]. The pathogenesis of autoimmunity involves dysfunction of the entire immune system, including neutrophils among the innate immune cells, B and T cells of the adaptive immunity, dendritic cells, and macrophages [2]. Within the various cell types related to fibrotic autoimmune diseases' pathogeneses, non-immune cells, such as epithelial cells, endothelial cells, and fibroblasts, are considered to be key players in the occurrence and progression of these diseases [3]. Based on these premises, immune and non-immune inflammatory cells are considered to be accountable for tissue failure in a wide range of fibrotic autoimmune disorders such as rheumatoid arthritis (RA), systemic lupus erythematosus (SLE), primary Sjögren's syndrome (pSS), and systemic sclerosis (SSc) [4]. Indeed, a plethora of recent advances has documented the functional role of inflammatory cells as therapeutic targets in autoimmune disorders [5]. However, major questions and controversies in the field remain and the comprehension of the different mechanisms that trigger fibrosis in autoimmune diseases is a challenge for many researchers. This review collects the latest advances in understanding how an alteration in the delicate balance between immune and non-immune cells is at the basis of the fibrotic evolution that is observed in various autoimmune diseases. A list of autoantigens associated with autoimmune fibrosis was reported in Table 1.

Table 1. Autoantigens associated with autoimmune fibrosis. (RF = rheumatoid factor; RNP = ribonucleoprotein).

Antigen Location	Antigen	Fibrosis Autoimmune Diseases
Nuclear	Ro-RNP complex	Systemic lupus erythematosus, Sjögren's syndrome
	La antigen	Systemic lupus erythematosus, Sjögren's syndrome
	Small nuclear RNP	Systemic lupus erythematosus, Idiopathic pulmonary fibrosis
	Chromatin	Autoimmune hepatitis, Systemic sclerosis
	dsDNA	Systemic lupus erythematosus, Autoimmune hepatitis
	Topoisomerase I	Systemic sclerosis
	Centromere	Systemic sclerosis
Modified proteins	Citrullinated proteins	Rheumatoid arthritis, Idiopathic pulmonary fibrosis
	Carbamylated proteins	Rheumatoid arthritis
Extracellular	RF (IgG)	Rheumatoid arthritis

2. The Role of Immune and Non-Immune Inflammatory Cells in Fibrotic Autoimmune Diseases: New Discoveries

Inflammatory process is considered to be one of the main steps leading to fibrosis in autoimmune diseases [6]. Numerous studies have demonstrated that the pathophysiology of fibrosis in autoimmune diseases involves an aberrant interplay between the immune and non-immune systems [7]. Both immune and non-immune responses play an essential role in the early events of fibrosis. Dysregulation of these processes comprises inflammatory changes, including proliferation of ECM-producing cells and the occurrence of mononuclear cell inflammatory infiltrates. In this context, both immune and non-immune cells have been implicated as important active participants in inflammatory processes involving fibrotic autoimmune diseases [8]. This section will review new insights on the role of immune and non-immune inflammatory cell types in fibrotic autoimmune diseases.

2.1. Current Understanding of the Involvement of Immune Cells in Fibrotic Autoimmune Diseases

Both innate and adaptive immunity are involved in fibrogenesis of autoimmune diseases and, interestingly, altered orchestration of the immune system might be an early event of fibrosis [7]. Dysregulation of these processes results in autoimmune responses triggered by T lymphocytes, macrophages, or dendritic cells [2]. These activated immune cells highly secrete factors that modulate inflammatory process and rapidly promote progressive fibrosis, involving the activation of resident fibroblasts and their transformation in myofibroblasts [2,7,8]. The following paragraphs report the recent discoveries on the role of immune cells in the fibrotic evolution of autoimmune pathologies.

2.1.1. Update on the Correlated Pro-Fibrotic Role of CD4+ and CD8+ T Cells

Traditionally, B lymphocytes and CD4+ T lymphocytes are considered to be key cells in the immunopathogenesis of autoimmune diseases and they have already been widely studied and are well recognized [9]. However, more recently, studies have demonstrated the increasing evidence that CD8+ T cells, infiltrating inflamed tissues, cooperate to induce tissue fibrosis in autoimmune diseases [10]. Emerging studies reported that CD8+ T cells infiltrate the lesioned skin of patients with SSc, predominantly in the early stage of the disease and exert a pro-inflammatory and pro-fibrotic activity through the induction of tissue damage [11,12]. Of particular note, key pro-fibrotic mediators, such as interleukin (IL)-6, through their signal activate CD8+ T cells and promote their interactions with fibroblasts, leading to the deposition of extracellular matrix (ECM) and contributing to the perpetuation of the fibrotic process in SSc patients [13,14]. High levels of the profibrotic type 2 cytokine IL-13 were produced following activation of peripheral blood effector CD8+ T cells from patients with SSc as compared with healthy controls or with patients with RA. In contrast, CD4+ T cells showed a lower and more variable level of IL-13 production. This abnormality was correlated with the extent of fibrosis and with a high grade of cutaneous involvement [11]. The role of CD4+ T cells is controversial because, recently, Sakkas and collaborators demonstrated that in SSc a great number of T cells of TH2 type is detected, producing pro-fibrotic IL-4, IL-13, and IL-31; in addition, CD4+ cytotoxic T lymphocytes are increased in skin lesions, and cause fibrosis and endothelial cell apoptosis [15].

A key role for CD8+T cells was also demonstrated in SLE nephritis; Zhang and colleagues showed that tubule-interstitial CD8+ T cells correlate with clinic-histologic kidney impairment in SLE nephritis, determining an evident progression of interstitial fibrosis and, thus, tubular organ atrophy [16]. In addition, the expression of cytotoxic T cells is increased and the inactivation of CD4+ T cells induces fibrosis and injury of the liver tissue in patients affected by autoimmune hepatitis [17]. Autoimmune hepatitis is a progressive inflammatory liver disease characterized by chronic inflammation of the liver, circulating autoantibodies, hypergammaglobulinemia, and progressive liver fibrosis [18]. CD8+ T lymphocytes may have a significant influence on liver fibrosis and intravascular effects. After activation, CD8+ T cells usually differentiate into cytotoxic T lymphocytes, which represent effector cells that destroy tumor cells and infected cells. Actually, the function of CD8+ T lymphocytes in hepatic fibrosis needs further investigation because their role is unclear. In the liver, the activity of immune surveillance of the CD8+ T cells against virus-infected cells seems to be reduced in mice with liver fibrosis caused by HBV infection [19]. Additionally, in an experimental mice model of carbon tetrachloride-induced liver fibrosis, the transfer of splenic CD8+ T cells into the mice had the effect of exacerbating fibrosis, a process that can be prevented by IL-10 treatment [20]. On the contrary, a reduction of the number of CD8+ T cells had little effect on the progression of hepatic fibrosis in carbon tetrachloride-treated animals [21]. Given that spleen-derived CD8+ T cells induce liver fibrosis and that hepatic CD8+ T-cell depletion probably has no effect on liver fibrosis, various subtypes of CD8+ T-cell may be distributed differently in the spleen and liver of mice, playing distinct roles in liver fibrosis [22] (Figure 1).

CD8+ T lymphocytes are also crucial players in the mechanism of exocrine gland injury in pSS [23,24]. In fact, CD8+ T lymphocytes contribute to acinar injury in the salivary glands, triggering a worsening fibrotic event in pSS [12,23]. Joachims et al. [25] showed that expanded clones of memory CD4+ T cells in the salivary glands displayed sequence similarity both within expanded clones of the same individual and among different patients, indicating that these cells are able to recognize shared antigens. They also observed that an increased frequency of expanded clones in salivary glands was correlated with decreased salivary secretion and increased fibrosis. Although CD4+ cells are the majority of T cells within the glandular infiltrates of pSS patients, CD8+ T cells are also present. A percentage of these CD8+ T cells show an activated phenotype, as shown by a higher expression level of Human Leukocyte Antigen–DR isotype (HLA-DR, an MHC class II cell surface receptor). Increased proportions of HLA-DR$^+$ T cells were associated with higher disease severity [26]. Additionally, in the blood of pSS patients with anti-SSA positivity, the increased frequencies of HLA-DR-expressing activated CD4+ and CD8+ T cells in blood was correlated with the EULAR Sjögren's syndrome (SS) disease activity index (ESSDAI) scores [26]. Furthermore, the proportion of activated CD8+ T cells in blood was established by a multi-omic study based on whole blood transcriptomes, serum proteomes, and peripheral immunophenotyping, which identified pSS disease signatures dysregulated in widespread epigenomes, mRNAs, and proteins. [27]. For example, the expression of the chemokine receptor CXCR3 by activated CD8+ T cells in pSS patients may be important for their migration to the inflamed salivary glands and, as demonstrated in mice, the recruitment of activated CD8+ T cells to salivary gland tissue was dependent on CXCR3 [28]. We speculate that chronic antigen stimulation leading to systemic inflammation, reflected as higher ESSDAI scores, results in the activation of CD8+ T cells in secondary lymphoid organs, such as spleen, CXCR3 upregulation, and consequent migration to the salivary glands [29]. Whether CD8+ T cells, in turn, contribute to glandular dysfunction and fibrotic evolution or systemic disease activity is unknown (Figure 2).

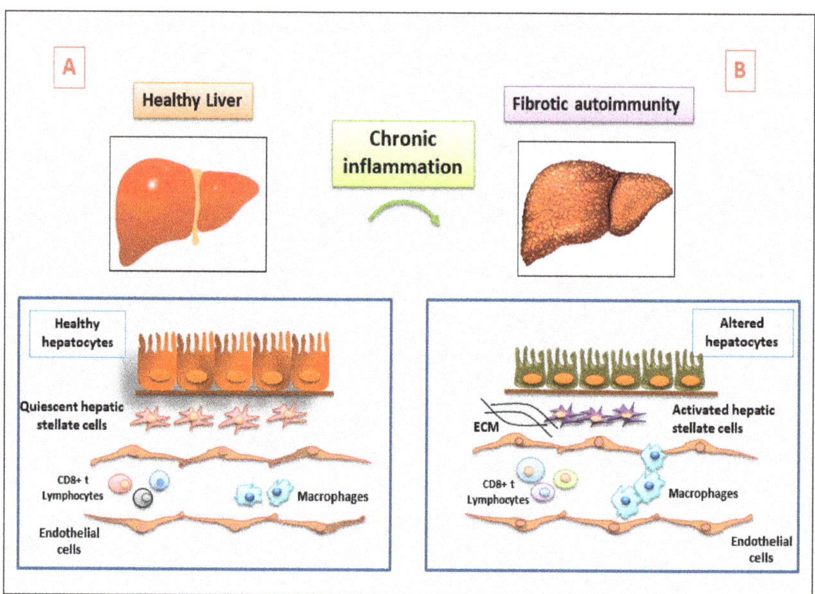

Figure 1. Schematic representation of the involvement of the immune cells in autoimmune hepatitis, derived from experimental mouse models (ECM = extracellular matrix) (A: Healthy liver; B: Fibrotic liver).

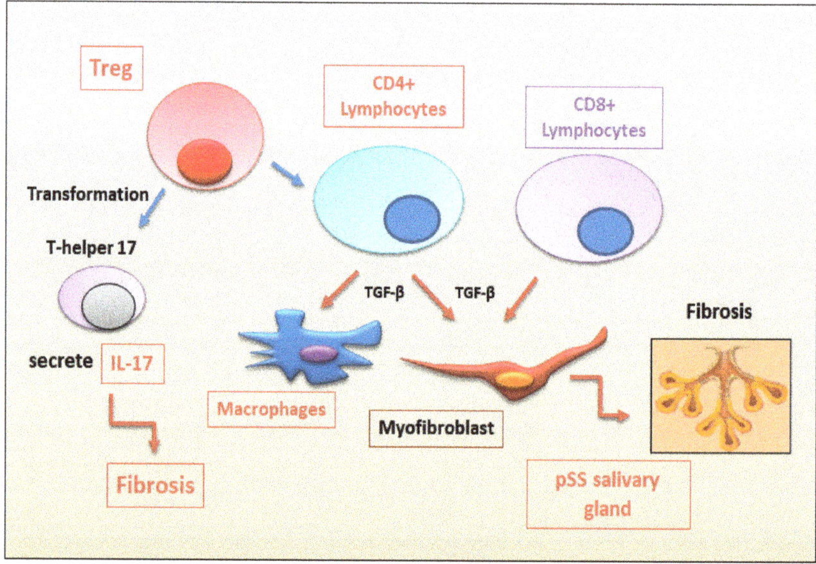

Figure 2. Immune cells involved in the fibrosis of salivary glands observed in the chronic inflammatory autoimmune diseases primary Sjögren's syndrome (pSS), according to the most recent findings. The figure highlights the role of TGF-β as pro-fibrotic factor (Treg = regulatory T lymphocytes; TGF-β = tumor growth factor beta).

2.1.2. Autoimmune Treg Pro-Fibrotic Role

Recently, an intriguing role identified for a functional T cell subset named regulatory T lymphocytes (Treg) in tissue fibrosis has also begun to emerge [30]. Treg are crucial keepers of the immune system, shaping the development of fibrosis and causing lethal organ dysfunction [31]. Although some investigations have highlighted a controversial role for the Treg cells depending on the disease model, in recent years the majority of reports demonstrated an increase in the number of Treg in patients at the early phase of SSc [32]. Treg seem to be able to secrete transforming growth factor-β (TGF-β), the major pro-fibrotic factor, which induces myofibroblast activation and fibrosis [33]. In addition, the dysfunction of Treg cells in the early phase of SSc leads to autoimmunity and inflammation [34]. Notably, Treg cells have the capacity to differentiate in T-helper17 (Th17) cells under inflammatory conditions. Th17 cells secrete IL-17A, which could also promote myofibroblast transformation and fibrosis and was related to vasculopathy by promoting *endothelial inflammation*. A transcriptomic comparison between the early and late phases of SSc revealed a differentiated gene expression exclusively in Treg cells. Using an RNA-seq analysis to compare early SSc vs. late SSc patients, it was also reported that, in the early phase of SSc, enhancement of the oxidative phosphorylation pathway was observed which represents a metabolic sign of differentiation of Treg to Th17 cells [34]. Therefore, an imbalance between Treg and Th17 cells seems to be implicated in the pathogenesis of the early SSc. The contribution of Treg cells to the pathophysiology of SSc has been explained by several mechanisms, sometimes conflicting. In a normal function, Treg cells release inhibitory cytokines, such as IL-10, TGF-β, and IL-35, which function as immunosuppressive factors [35]. First, in SSc the suppressive effect of Treg cells is limited, causing an altered immune response and leading to chronic inflammation and fibrosis. The decreased inhibitory ability of Treg cells in SSc patients is attributed to the decreased production of TGF-β and IL-10 [36]. On the other hand, it is now established that the promotion of fibrosis by pro-fibrotic cytokines is produced by Treg cells. For example, TGF-β contributes to fibrotic pathology through the proliferation of fibroblasts, promoting collagen production and ECM secretion, and also induces the epithelial–mesenchymal transition (EMT). In addition, Treg cells seem to be able to differentiate into Th2-like cells in SSc and to promote fibrosis through the production of IL-4 and IL-13 [36]. By these mechanisms, Treg cells are thought to be associated with several aspects of immune dysregulation and fibrosis during SSc pathogenesis.

Recent findings, based on the study of the dysfunction and imbalance of Treg cells in pSS, have demonstrated a significantly lower frequency of Treg positive for pSTAT5 in pSS patients after IL-2 stimulation, compared with healthy controls [37]. No differences were demonstrated in other T-cell populations, indicating a specific impact of Tregs in pSS pathogenesis which, of course, will need to be clarified [37] (Figure 2). A decreased number of Treg cells was also demonstrated, specifically, in the patients with SLE, psoriatic arthritis, juvenile idiopathic arthritis, and autoimmune liver disease [31,38]. In the liver, a dual role of Tregs in fibrogenesis was detected because they are responsible for fibrosis promotion or immunosuppression [39]. In fact, a large number of Tregs are revealed in the fibrotic microenvironment in patients with hepatocellular carcinoma, in which it was observed that a reduction in Tregs promoted the regression of fibrosis [40]. Conversely, in autoimmune hepatitis, hepatic stellate cells (HSCs) were activated, whose function is to produce and accumulate ECM, a pivotal event in liver fibrosis. Simultaneously, HSCs selectively promote the survival and the activity of Tregs in an IL-2–dependent manner. Tregs can both protect HSCs from NK cell attack and, on the contrary, exert an inhibitory effect on HSCs, confirming the dual role of Tregs in liver fibrogenesis and the importance of equilibrium. The balance between Tregs which could convert to Th17 cells, seems, once again, fundamental in maintaining homoeostasis and immunoregulation; this mechanism, for reasons that are still unclear, can deregulate and leads to the production of pro-inflammatory cytokine by Th17, such as IL-17 and IL-22 [39].

2.1.3. Emerging Pro-Fibrotic Role of T Follicular Helper Cells

T follicular helper (Tfh) cells have been identified as a distinct CD4+ helper T cell subset. They express a high level of surface markers, such as CXCR5, CD40L, inducible co-stimulator (ICOS), programmed cell death protein-1 (PD-1), and a downmodulation of C-C chemokine receptor type 7 (CCR7) [7,41]. Tfh cells are important modulators of B cell maturation and specialized to help B cells to produce high-affinity antibodies toward antigens and, thus, to develop an important humoral immune response [42,43]. Moreover, they are characterized by enhanced expression of IL-21 that promotes B cells' differentiation into plasma cells and Ig isotype switching and by elevated production of the nuclear transcriptional repressor B cell lymphoma 6 (Bcl-6), essential for B cell function [43]. Many investigations have found severe proliferation and/or activation of Tfh cells in multiple autoimmune disorders characterized by intense fibrosis [7]. A possible role played by Tfh cells in the pathogenesis of SS was known; indeed, increased percentages of circulating Tfh cells (cTfh) have been demonstrated in peripheral blood [44] and in salivary glands of SS patients [45]. Several lines of evidence also support a pathogenic role of Tfh cells and IL-21 in human SLE. The Tfh surface marker ICOS seems to be crucial for optimal IL-21 production [46]. Higher plasma levels of IL-21 are found in SLE patients correlating with the number of switched memory B cells and with several markers of disease severity [43,47]. Findings from the literature are instead conflicting regarding Tfh cells' frequencies in human RA. In some studies, augmented frequencies of cTfh cells in RA patients were observed, in particular in those with new-beginning disease [48]. On the role of Tfh in the fibrotic evolution of autoimmune diseases, few results are available in literature regarding the role of Tfh cells in SSc pathogenesis. A recent study provides evidence that Tfh cells induce skin fibrosis and correlate with dermal fibrosis [49] in SSc patients. Furthermore, it has been shown that the administration of both IL-21 and ICOS antibodies can effectively reduce skin fibrosis [50]. Moreover, an interesting recent report also evidenced that in patients with idiopathic pulmonary fibrosis (IPF), the levels of Tfh cells in the peripheral blood were increased [51]. Overall, from these data it can be deduced that Tfh cells may be involved in both immunological and fibrotic autoimmune disease, regulating autoreactive B cell expansion and fibroblast activation.

2.1.4. Macrophages, Dendritic Cells, Mast Cells

In the complexity of the immune scenario, macrophages—key cells that classically initiate and sustain chronic inflammation in a simultaneous or parallel manner—are now recognized as capable of secreting fibrotic factors once activated [52]. Monocytes'/macrophages' activation, due to the plasticity of these cells, could be an important step for the transition from the inflammatory to the fibrotic phase in SSc pathology. Through the release of fibro-proliferative factors, macrophages trigger the fibrotic process determining, for example, skin and lung SSc-related tissue fibrosis [52,53]. Consequently, an autocrine loop begins in which the release of fibrotic factors by macrophages drives the transformation of more monocytes/macrophages into cells with pro-fibrotic phenotype [52–54]. This cellular crosstalk occurs, clearly, in autoimmune hepatitis; hepatic resident macrophages have been shown to exert an intricate role in the initiation of inflammatory responses causing liver injury and can acquire a pro-fibrogenic phenotype that leads to aberrant tissue remodeling, culminating in liver and fibrosis and failure [55]. It is not possible to define exactly whether the macrophages involved in liver fibrosis belong to the M1 or M2 type. A switch between M1 and M2 phenotypes probably occurs because of their plasticity. M2 macrophages can be activated through IL-4Rα signaling, which determines liver inflammation and fibrosis. However, it has been demonstrated that the activation of M2-macrophages also represents a key event in viral-associated immune dysregulation and liver fibrosis [55].

Interestingly, in line with this concept, studies have highlighted that dendritic cells also display high plasticity after injury, driving pro-fibrotic inflammatory mechanisms in autoimmune diseases. Functional alterations of dendritic cells assist the immune processes favoring the altered T cell polarization and pro-fibrotic inflammation in the SSc [56]. DCs are commonly categorized into three major populations: the conventional DC (cDC)1, cDC2, and the plasmacytoid DC (pDC) [57]. pDCs are the subtype that appears to be more relevant for the development of fibrosis in SSc pathogenesis [56,58]. In patients with SSc, pDCs are mainly found in the skin and lungs [59], correlated with the severity of SSc disease [59]. Importantly, pDCs play a direct role in causing and maintaining fibrosis, as their depletion has been shown to improve skin and lung fibrosis. Furthermore, the presence of pDCs in the lungs appears to be a feature of pulmonary fibrosis, since their frequency in the lungs is similar in both SSc-interstitial lung disease (ILD) and idiopathic pulmonary fibrosis patients [60]. A key role in the pro-fibrotic activity of pDCs is done by CXCL4, secreted from pDCs of SSc patients, which creates an inflammatory environment in the tissues that they infiltrate. CXCL4 plays a central role in a feedback loop that contributes to increased inflammation and fibrosis [61]. It can directly promote the differentiation of different cell types into myofibroblasts, increasing the collagen and ECM component production and contributing to fibrosis [62]. Furthermore, increased levels of CXCL4 are found in the blood and skin of SSc patients [63], correlated with disease complications, such as ILD and pulmonary hypertension (PH). The production of CXCL4 from pDCs of SSc patients was also stimulated by TLR8, aberrantly expressed in this disease [64]. TLR8 induces the production of CXCL4 [64]. Additionally, TLR8 expression leads to an increased infiltration of pDCs into the tissues, exacerbating the disease and resulting in worse skin fibrosis [64].

Mast cells are immune cells mainly found in connective tissues with a well-established role in allergy and anaphylaxis. However, a great deal of evidence underlines their active role in tissue healing, angiogenesis, and exacerbation of chronic inflammation that characterizes autoimmune diseases [65]. Leehan and collaborators have recently investigated the role of mast cells in salivary gland fibrosis which is a pathological feature of pSS and positively correlates with high focus scores, but not with the age of the patients [66]. They demonstrated that mast cells are strongly associated with fibrosis and fatty infiltration of salivary glands that represent a biological response to gland injury. It is hypothesized that they promote fibrosis by interacting with local fibroblasts and producing enzymes responsible for cleavage and activation of metalloproteinases, which are important mediators of tissue injury and repair [66]. A schematic comprehensive overview of the involvement of immune cells in autoimmune-related fibrosis is reported in Figure 3.

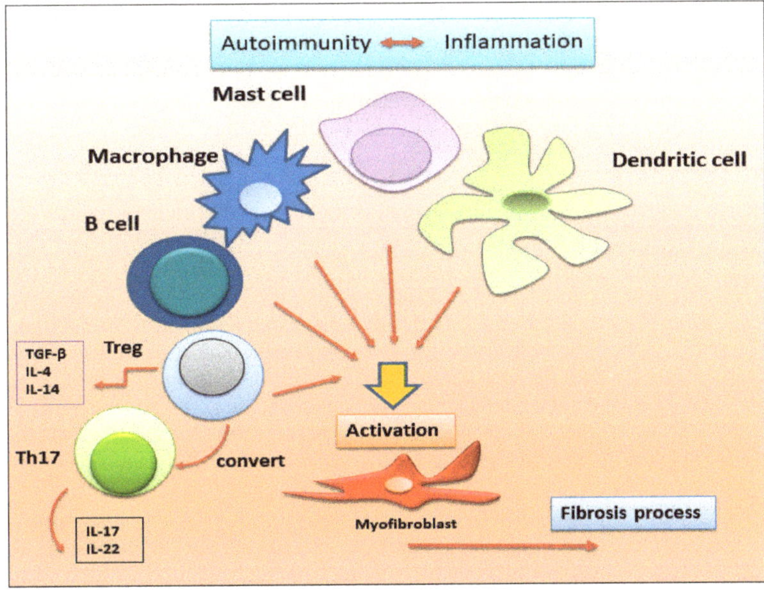

Figure 3. Immune cells recently linked to the fibrotic evolution of autoimmune diseases. In a condition

of chronic inflammation, many immune cell populations with diverse functions are activated to produce multiple cytokines that lead to the proliferation and activation of myofibroblasts, directly involved in the development of fibrosis in various autoimmune diseases (Th17 = T helper 17; Treg = regulatory T lymphocytes).

2.2. Non-Immune Cells in Fibrotic Autoimmune Diseases

Recently, it has been proposed that also the non-immune cells, such as epithelial cells, endothelial cells, and fibroblasts may contribute to inflammation, autoimmunity, as well as fibrosis. Non-immune cells, when damaged or activated, release molecules involved in the regulation of several types of immune responses. Furthermore, the de novo production of bioactive factors by non-immune cells, in response to several stimuli, can influence immunological processes. Therefore, defects in the abilities of non-immune cells to mediate immune regulation may be involved in the pathogenicity of a series of inflammatory autoimmune diseases which often show a fibrotic organ evolution. This section will review the main non-immune cell types involved in fibrotic autoimmune diseases.

2.2.1. Epithelial Cells

Epithelium includes various highly specialized cells that play critical roles in almost all biological processes, and they are considered essential to maintain tissue homeostasis in many organs. In this context, several studies have begun to examine the active role of epithelial cells in several autoimmune disorders characterized by fibrosis. The EMT program, under pathological conditions, can lead to the reduction of normal epithelial cells, destroying tissue architecture, inducing pathogenic activation of fibroblasts, and driving organ failure [8]. The knowledge of the molecular mechanisms that occur in the EMT program has demonstrated that the epithelial state of the cells initially considered immutable can undergo important changes in gene expression and post-translational regulation, leading to the repression of the epithelial characteristics and to the acquisition of mesenchymal characteristics displaying fibroblast-like morphology and cytoarchitecture [67]. Recently, considerable attention has been paid to chronic inflammatory disorders pSS in which the inflammatory status is often associated with pathological EMT-dependent salivary gland fibrosis [68]. Emerging evidence suggests that epithelial cells are also an important source of myofibroblasts in organ fibrosis [69], and this trans-differentiation is evaluated as a tightly specialized system of the EMT process that may be a central event in the salivary gland fibrosis [68]. The implications of these findings were very important and the recent explosion of knowledge in the biology of cellular differentiation has highlighted, for example, that differentiated cell type, such as a tubular or acinar salivary gland epithelial cell in pSS, with a wide set of glandular characteristics, such as secretion and transport, could radically change their transcriptional process, transcribing genes characteristic of the mesenchymal cell type [68–71]. Supporting this opinion, recent evidence highlights that salivary gland epithelial cells derived from healthy biopsies, when exposed to TGF-β1 stimulation, acquired a more fibroblast-like morphology [68,72,73]. Additionally, in SSc, recent studies have demonstrated anomalous phenotypes of the skin epithelium [74]. Indeed, phenotypically altered epithelial cells possibly explain the selective organ fibroses in the skin, oesophagus, and lung that occur in SSc [74]. In this context, several studies have begun to examine the functional role of tubular epithelial cells in the pathogenesis of lupus nephritis [75]. Renal tubular epithelial cells actively participate in the tubulointerstitial pathology of lupus nephritis through the expression of cytokines, chemokines, and pro-fibrotic factors, and play a crucial crosstalk with infiltrating cells of the immune system [75,76]. Findings suggest that anti-dsDNA antibodies that bind to the surface of renal tubular epithelial cells, but without cellular uptake and cytoplasmic/nuclear translocation, can promote tubule interstitial fibrosis and subsequently kidney dysfunction [77]. Yung et al. reported that anti-dsDNA antibodies derived from lupus nephritis patients induce a significant increase in the fibronectin expression in human renal tubular epithelial cells, a process dependent, in part, on the secretion of such fibrogenic factors as TGF-β [77]. These data suggest that fibrosis development in lupus nephritis is initiated and amplified via complex signaling pathways involving anti-dsDNA antibodies, fibronectin, and TGF-β in renal tubular epithelial cells [75]. A recent study has identified a key role for IL-23 as a pro-fibrotic molecule in RA-associated interstitial lung disease through the induction of the EMT-dependent transformation of somatic alveolar type I epithelial cells in fibroblast-like cells. The acquisition of a mesenchymal phenotype induced by IL-23 included increased deposition of ECM, the acquisition of invasiveness, and resistance to apoptosis—all events which may contribute to the formation of fibroblastic foci in fibrotic ILD, especially in the context of autoimmune pathology such as RA [78] (Figure 4).

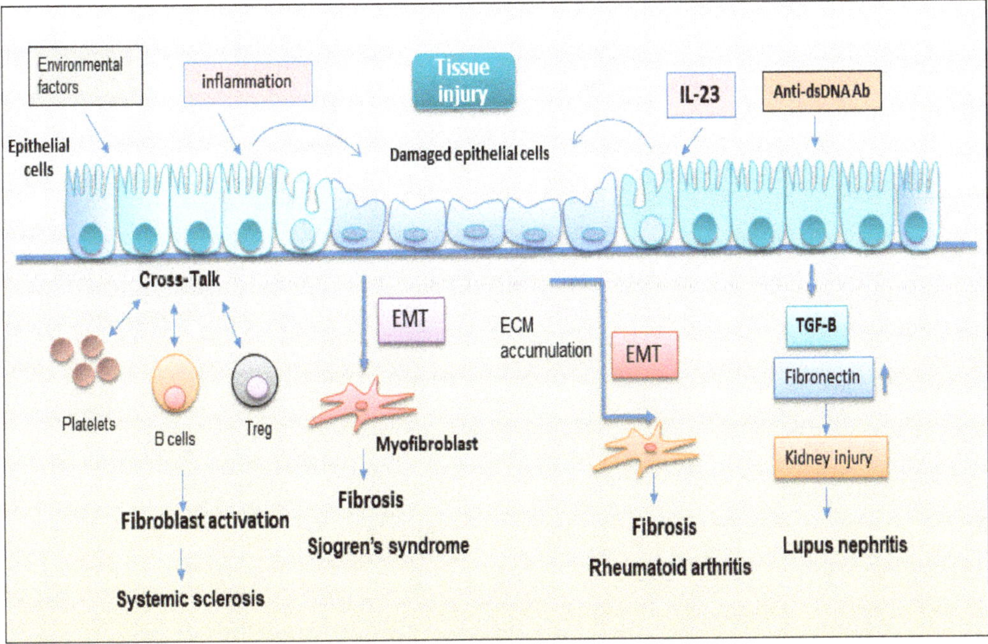

Figure 4. Representation of the hypothetical role of epithelial cells in the activation of the fibrotic program in various autoimmune diseases (anti-ds DNA Ab = anti-double-stranded DNA antibody; ECM = extracellular matrix; EMT = epithelial to mesenchymal transformation; TGF-β = tumor growth factor beta; Treg = regulatory T lymphocytes).

2.2.2. EMT: New Player Regulating the Interplay between the Immunity and Fibrosis

In recent years, epithelial to mesenchymal transition (EMT) has been extensively studied as a possible therapeutic target for fibrosis [72,73,79] and, therefore, a brief refresher in this area is needed. A better understanding of the crosstalk between chronic inflammation, autoimmunity, fibrosis, and EMT may represent an opportunity for the development of a broadly effective anti-fibrotic therapy in autoimmune diseases. Cells of multicellular organisms hire several phenotypes that have different functions, morphologies, and gene expression patterns, and, drastically, can undergo specific changes when subjected to determinants stimuli and microenvironments [80]. The inflammatory cells secrete crucial regulatory proteins, such as pro-fibrotic cytokines, chemokines, and growth factors, which can trigger the EMT process [81]. EMT is a highly dynamic process that often gives rise to a series of intermediate phenotypic states in which the cells progressively acquire mesenchymal markers without a concomitant complete loss of epithelial markers [82]. The expression of both mesenchymal and epithelial markers reflects the plasticity of cells depending on their environment [83]. Importantly, EMT leads to the early development of pathological organ fibrosis through paracrine signaling from the epithelium to potential fibroblasts [84]. The fibrotic process affects a variety of organs and tissues through the activation of specific molecular pathways [84]. However, two common hallmarks are evidenced: the critical role of the TGF-β and the implication of the inflammatory process, which are essential for initiating the fibrotic degeneration [72,79]. EMT is tightly related to fibrosis development in several organs and fibrogenesis represents the common response of organs and tissues to virtually all chronic repetitive injuries in multiple autoimmune disorders [72,73,79]. During chronic autoimmune diseases, inflammatory and epithelial cells produce fibrogenic mediators. In this context, TGF-β1 emerged as a crucial factor regulating interactions between epithelial and mesenchymal cells and fibroblasts proliferation [85]. One of the hallmarks of excessive pathological fibrogenesis is the acquisition by resident fibroblasts of a myofibroblasts contractile phenotype expressing high levels of α-Smooth muscle actin (α-SMA). Additional immune cells are recruited into the fibrotic tissue, amplifying the fibrotic response by the secretion of chemokines, cytokines, and growth factors responsible for the differentiation of other myofibroblasts implicated in ECM deposition [86]. The principal EMT pathway is mediated by Smad and we can indicate it as TGF-β1/SMAD/Snail pathway; it is a particularly interesting system active in the EMT-dependent fibrotic process in a number of diseases [72,87]. Alternatively, or parallel to Smads pathways, TGF-β1 also utilizes a multitude of intracellular non-canonical, non-Smads TGF-β-mediated cascade triggered by the binding of ligands different from TGF-β family members to tyrosine kinase receptors [88,89]. This may suggest that the therapeutic use of TGF-β signaling inhibitors, actually used in cancer, may also be hypothetically extended to the treatment of inflammatory autoimmune disorders, but future investigations are needed to prove this hypothesis.

2.2.3. Endothelial Cell

Dysregulation of endothelial cell function is proposed as a crucial start event, leading to vascular remodeling linked to fibroproliferative vasculopathy. Impaired angiogenesis may be induced by the massive proliferation of fibroblasts observed in some autoimmune diseases characterized by intense pathological fibrosis. New insights have evidenced that myofibroblasts involved in tissue fibrosis can still derive from endothelial cells through a process known as EndoMT [90,91]. It is a non-malignant phenomenon of cellular transdifferentiation in which endothelial cells undergo a phenotypical change where they lose vascular epithelial factors and acquire mesenchymal cell markers [92]. Among systemic autoimmune diseases, endothelial dysfunction has been extensively studied in SLE. In SLE patients, endothelial dysfunction is the main factor of vascular aging and pre-clinical atherosclerosis that leads to vascular fibrosis, contributing to the early onset of cardiovascular disease and cardiovascular mortality [93]. Interesting studies have highlighted that endothelial dysfunction also occurs in patients with pSS. Recent epidemiologic data indicate an increase in cardiovascular risk in patients with pSS and endothelial dysregulation may cause vascular fibrosis, leading to arterial stiffness, which precedes the development of high blood pressure [94]. This study demonstrates that patients with pSS, without clinically evident cardiovascular disease or without concomitant cardiovascular risk factors, have an altered endothelial function and a massive proliferation of fibroblasts, which suggest a higher susceptibility to the development of vascular fibrosis [94]. Therefore, induction of pro-inflammatory cytokines, such as TNFα and IL-6, involved in atherosclerotic damage, in combination with IFNγ and IL-17, reduces the number of smooth muscle cells, increases collagen production, and favors fibrosis development, with subsequent formation of fibrous atherosclerotic plaque [95]. In this intriguing scenario, the evidence that circulating biomarkers of inflammation predict future cardiovascular events in patients with pSS further reinforces the strict interplay between chronic inflammation and atherosclerosis. Furthermore, subclinical cardiovascular involvement is directly related to elevated inflammatory injury, postulating that inflammation and disease activity are cardiovascular disease risk factors in patients with pSS [94]. In the case of SSc, recent reports have evidenced that this disease was characterized by a massive accumulation of fibroblasts and myofibroblasts and by an abnormal production of interstitial collagens and extracellular matrix components, and was identified by the dysregulation of endothelial cell activity as a pivotal event that contribute to vasculopathy in SSc [92,96] (Figure 5).

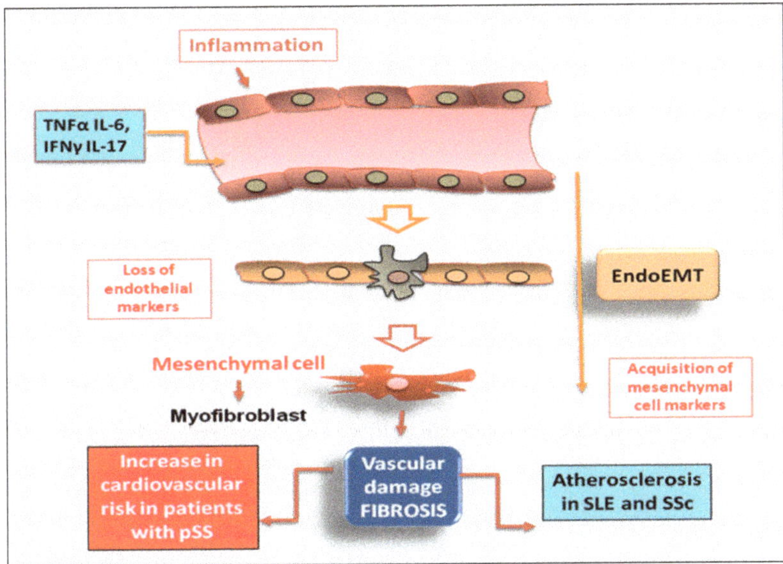

Figure 5. In chronic autoimmune diseases, endothelial cells are often the primary site of inflammation that triggers the downstream molecular events of fibrosis. The activation of myofibroblasts in various autoimmune diseases such as SLE (Systemic Lupus Erythematosus) and SSc (systemic sclerosis) may result from the phenotypic conversion of endothelial cells into activated mesenchymal cells, a process known as endothelial to mesenchymal transition (EndoMT) (IFN-γ = interferon gamma; pSS = primary Sjögren's syndrome; TNF-α = tumor necrosis factor-alpha).

2.2.4. Fibroblasts

Traditionally, fibroblasts were considered the main contributory cells to the structural integrity of tissues; only recently have they been recognized as cells that exhibit a dynamic role in physiological or pathological processes [97,98] and are considered active producers of inflammatory cytokines and chemokines. An emerging concept, derived from experimental research on fibroblasts in inflammatory and fibrotic diseases, is that their differentiation is maintained by extrinsic and intrinsic danger signals and local microenvironment-derived morphogens [99,100]. Moreover, fibroblasts can initiate the early molecular processes leading to inflammatory events [100] and, consequently, can be involved with a prominent role in the pathogenesis of fibrotic autoimmune conditions [100].

An interesting paper by Wang, W. et al. [101] demonstrated an incisive role of fibroblasts in systemic sclerosis. In this study, fibroblasts isolated from skin and lung biopsies of patients with systemic sclerosis was analyzed and an altered expression of the A20 gene was detected; A20 is a gene strongly linked with disease susceptibility and fibrotic manifestations [101]. According to some reports it was demonstrated that A20 expression in fibroblasts can inhibit the fibrotic process, whereas its negative transcriptional regulator, called DREAM (downstream regulatory element antagonist modulator), promotes fibrotic processes [102]. The authors proposed that the upregulation of DREAM in systemic sclerosis fibroblasts underlies suppression of A20, which in turn contributes to unchecked pro-fibrotic signaling in stimulated fibroblasts [101]. Interestingly, targeting the

A20–DREAM regulatory network could represent a novel therapeutic approach in systemic sclerosis [102].

New reports have documented that the immunomodulatory role of the fibroblasts derived from salivary glands was discovered in a primary site affected by the pSS [103]. Interestingly, these specific clusters of fibroblasts constitute the formation of tertiary lymphoid structures, which are linked to severe disease and can determine a risk factor for the development of lymphoma in pSS [103]. Recent advances in single-cell profiling techniques have demonstrated the presence of fibroblasts in inflamed salivary glands tissue, providing evidence of the existence of inflammation-associated fibroblasts in chronically inflamed tissues [104]. Clusters of fibroblasts were identified as key players in the development of renal fibrosis and, in particular, in lupus nephritis [105].

New discoveries highlighted as myofibroblasts are the main actors involved in renal fibrogenesis. Interestingly, the differentiation of fibroblasts to myofibroblasts is a key cellular event in many autoimmune fibrotic disorders [106].

Single-cell sequencing has demonstrated that myofibroblasts have different gene expression profiles with dynamic changes in fibrosis of different organs [107]. Myofibroblasts, armed with myosin and smooth muscle actin (α-SMA), become able to secrete TGFβ, VEGF, CTGF, IL-1, IL-6, and IL-8 [108].

It has been suggested that myofibroblasts localized in renal fibrotic tissue may derive from different precursor resident cells, including fibroblasts and epithelial cells [109]. Moreover, myofibroblasts not only contribute to deposition of ECM, but they can produce radical oxygen species and, through their intrinsic contractile properties, can alter renal tissue architecture [109]. Their pathogenic role in renal fibrosis has been discovered in different murine models in which the removal of myofibroblasts can reduce fibrogenesis [98]. Moreover, myofibroblasts are considered as one of the principal participants in the final point of EMT. After an acute insult, a temporary activation of the EMT process is considered of fundamental importance in renal repair [105,110]. The identification of key morphogen signals that regulate fibroblast differentiation could provide a therapeutic opportunity (Figure 6).

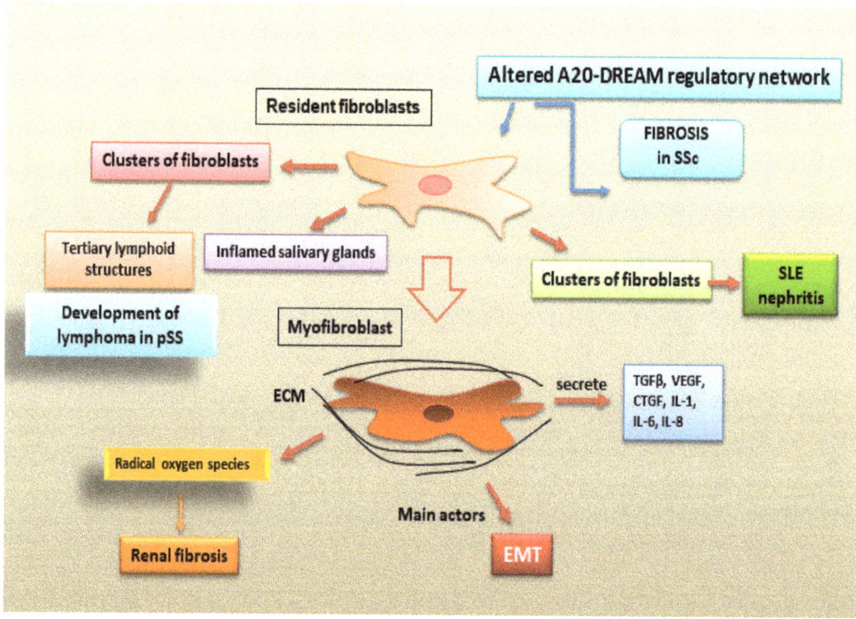

Figure 6. Recent advances in the pro-fibrotic role of fibroblasts in autoimmune diseases. The traditional

view that fibroblasts represent purely structural elements has been gradually replaced by the acknowledgement that they are dynamic cells actively involved in the evolution from inflammatory states to fibrosis (A20-DREAM = A20-downstream regulatory element antagonist modulator; CTGF = connective tissue growth factor; ECM = extracellular matrix; EMT = epithelial to mesenchymal transition; Il: interleukin; pSS = primary Sjögren's syndrome; SLE = Systemic Lupus Erythematosus; SSc = systemic sclerosis; TGF-β = tumor growth factor beta; VEGF = vascular endothelial growth factor).

3. Conclusions

The fibrotic consequences of various primary autoimmune diseases, characterized by tissue damage resulting from chronic inflammatory conditions, remain a major unsolved diagnostic and therapeutic challenge. From experimental experience, it seems that all fibrotic tissues derived from autoimmune patients display signs of chronic immunologically mediated inflammation during the earliest periods of fibrosis. In these initial stages of fibrotic evolution, a predominant role is certainly played by immune cells, although some questions remain open about the specificity of lymphocyte subtypes occurring in fibrotic tissue, as well as about a possible imbalance of pro- and anti-fibrotic factors produced by components of the immune cells infiltrate. For example, the precise mechanism underlying the immune reaction in fibrogenesis mediated by Tregs, probably depending on different immune microenvironments and molecular pathways, is still unclear and will require further investigation. Actually, there is accumulating evidence showing that non-immune cells, such as epithelial cells, endothelial cells, and fibroblasts are cells with important immunomodulatory properties, play a pivotal role in the switch to chronic inflammation. Determining the exact contribution of these mechanisms remains a challenge, as they are at the cross-point of multiple regulatory networks also involving immune and non-immune cells and this, in an autoimmune condition in which the immune system works in an altered way, makes the scenario even more complex. For example, whether EMT activation may interfere with the crosstalk between epithelial cells, mesenchymal cells, and immune cells, stimulating fibrotic evolution, remains elusive. Since valid biomarkers for the diagnosis and staging of autoimmune-related fibrosis are not yet available, more detailed knowledge on the cellular and molecular basis of fibrogenesis is urgently needed. From this point of view, a better knowledge of the non-immune cells contribution to autoimmune fibrosis should help to appreciate the reasons underlying the actual clinical failures and design more effective therapies.

Author Contributions: All authors were involved in drafting the article or revising it critically for important intellectual content, and all authors approved the final version for publication. M.S. and S.L. had full access to the data collected in the review, take responsibility for their integrity, and performed a critical reading. All authors have read and agreed to the published version of the manuscript.

Funding: This research received no external funding.

Institutional Review Board Statement: Not applicable.

Informed Consent Statement: Not applicable.

Data Availability Statement: Not applicable.

Conflicts of Interest: The authors declare no conflict of interest.

References

1. Duan, L.; Rao, X.; Sigdel, K.R. Regulation of Inflammation in Autoimmune Disease. *J. Immunol. Res.* **2019**, *2019*, 7403796. [CrossRef] [PubMed]
2. Frizinsky, S.; Haj-Yahia, S.; Machnes Maayan, D.; Lifshitz, Y.; Maoz-Segal, R.; Offengenden, I.; Kidon, M.; Agmon-Levin, N. The innate immune perspective of autoimmune and autoinflammatory conditions. *Rheumatology* **2019**, *58*, vi1–vi8. [CrossRef] [PubMed]

3.   Lai, Y.; Wei, X.; Ye, T.; Hang, L.; Mou, L.; Su, J. Interrelation Between Fibroblasts and T Cells in Fibrosing Interstitial Lung Diseases. *Front. Immunol.* **2021**, *12*, 747335. [CrossRef]
4.   Fu, X.; Liu, H.; Huang, G.; Dai, S.S. The emerging role of neutrophils in autoimmune-associated disorders: Effector, predictor, and therapeutic targets. *MedComm* **2021**, *2*, 402–413. [CrossRef]
5.   Jung, S.M.; Kim, W.U. Targeted Immunotherapy for Autoimmune Disease. *Immune Netw.* **2022**, *22*, e9. [CrossRef]
6.   Distler, J.H.W.; Gyorfi, A.H.; Ramanujam, M.; Whitfield, M.L.; Konigshoff, M.; Lafyatis, R. Shared and distinct mechanisms of fibrosis. *Nat. Rev. Rheumatol.* **2019**, *15*, 705–730. [CrossRef]
7.   Zhang, M.; Zhang, S. T Cells in Fibrosis and Fibrotic Diseases. *Front. Immunol.* **2020**, *11*, 1142. [CrossRef]
8.   Zhao, X.; Chen, J.; Sun, H.; Zhang, Y.; Zou, D. New insights into fibrosis from the ECM degradation perspective: The macrophage-MMP-ECM interaction. *Cell Biosci.* **2022**, *12*, 117. [CrossRef] [PubMed]
9.   Raphael, I.; Joern, R.R.; Forsthuber, T.G. Memory CD4$^+$ T Cells in Immunity and Autoimmune Diseases. *Cells* **2020**, *9*, 531. [CrossRef]
10.   Deng, Q.; Luo, Y.; Chang, C.; Wu, H.; Ding, Y.; Xiao, R. The Emerging Epigenetic Role of CD8+T Cells in Autoimmune Diseases: A Systematic Review. *Front. Immunol.* **2019**, *10*, 856. [CrossRef]
11.   Fuschiotti, P. Current perspectives on the role of CD8+ T cells in systemic sclerosis. *Immunol. Lett.* **2018**, *195*, 55–60. [CrossRef] [PubMed]
12.   Kaneko, N.; Chen, H.; Perugino, C.A.; Maehara, T.; Munemura, R.; Yokomizo, S.; Sameshima, J.; Diefenbach, T.J.; Premo, K.R.; Chinju, A.; et al. Cytotoxic CD8$^+$ T cells may be drivers of tissue destruction in Sjögren's syndrome. *Sci. Rep.* **2022**, *12*, 15427. [CrossRef] [PubMed]
13.   Shima, Y. Cytokines Involved in the Pathogenesis of SSc and Problems in the Devel-opment of Anti-Cytokine Therapy. *Cells* **2021**, *10*, 1104. [CrossRef]
14.   Valenzi, E.; Tabib, T.; Papazoglou, A.; Sembrat, J.; Trejo Bittar, H.E.; Rojas, M.; Lafyatis, R. Disparate Interferon Signaling and Shared Aberrant Basaloid Cells in Single-Cell Profiling of Idiopathic Pulmonary Fibrosis and Systemic Sclerosis-Associated Interstitial Lung Disease. *Front. Immunol.* **2021**, *12*, 595811. [CrossRef] [PubMed]
15.   Sakkas, L.I.; Bogdanos, D.P. The Role of T Cells in SSc: An Update. *Immuno* **2022**, *2*, 534–547. [CrossRef]
16.   Zhang, T.; Wang, M.; Zhang, J.; Feng, X.; Liu, Z.; Cheng, Z. Association between tubulointerstitial CD8+T cells and renal prognosis in lupus nephritis. *Int. Immunopharmacol.* **2021**, *99*, 107877. [CrossRef] [PubMed]
17.   Vuerich, M.; Wang, N.; Kalbasi, A.; Graham, J.J.; Longhi, M.S. Dysfunctional Immune Regulation in Autoimmune Hepatitis: From Pathogenesis to Novel Therapies. *Front. Immunol.* **2021**, *12*, 746436. [CrossRef]
18.   Covelli, C.; Sacchi, D.; Sarcognato, S.; Cazzagon, N.; Grillo, F.; Baciorri, F.; Fanni, D.; Cacciatore, M.; Maffeis, V.; Guido, M. Pathology of autoimmune hepatitis. *Pathologica* **2021**, *113*, 185–193. [CrossRef] [PubMed]
19.   Guidotti, L.G.; Inverso, D.; Sironi, L.; Di Lucia, P.; Fioravanti, J.; Ganzer, L.; Fiocchi, A.; Vacca, M.; Aiolfi, R.; Sammicheli, S.; et al. Immunosurveillance of the liver by intravascular effector CD8(+) T. *Cell* **2015**, *161*, 486–500. [CrossRef]
20.   Safadi, R.; Ohta, M.; Alvarez, C.E.; Fiel, M.I.; Bansal, M.; Mehal, W.Z.; Friedman, S.L. Immune stimulation of hepatic fibrogenesis by CD8 cells and attenuation by transgenic interleukin-10 from hepatocytes. *Gastroenterology* **2004**, *127*, 870–882. [CrossRef]
21.   Novobrantseva, T.I.; Majeau, G.R.; Amatucci, A.; Kogan, S.; Brenner, I.; Casola, S.; Shlomchik, M.J.; Koteliansky, V.; Hochman, P.S.; Ibraghimov, A. Attenuated liver fibrosis in the absence of B cells. *J. Clin. Investig.* **2005**, *115*, 3072–3082. [CrossRef]
22.   Sun, R.; Xiang, Z.; Wu, B. T cells and liver fibrosis. *Portal Hypertens. Cirrhosis* **2022**, *1*, 125–132. [CrossRef]
23.   Zhou, H.; Yang, J.; Tian, J.; Wang, S. CD8+ T Lymphocytes: Crucial Players in Sjögren's Syndrome. *Front. Immunol.* **2021**, *11*, 602823. [CrossRef]
24.   Chihaby, N.; Orliaguet, M.; Le Pottier, L.; Pers, J.O.; Boisramé, S. Treatment of Sjögren's Syndrome with Mesenchymal Stem Cells: A Systematic Review. *Int. J. Mol. Sci.* **2021**, *22*, 10474. [CrossRef] [PubMed]
25.   Joachims, M.L.; Leehan, K.M.; Lawrence, C.; Pelikan, R.C.; Moore, J.S.; Pan, Z.; Rasmussen, A.; Radfar, L.; Lewis, D.M.; Grundahl, K.M.; et al. Single-cell analysis of glandular T cell receptors in Sjögren's syndrome. *JCI Insight* **2016**, *1*, e85609. [CrossRef] [PubMed]
26.   Mingueneau, M.; Boudaoud, S.; Haskett, S.; Reynolds, T.L.; Nocturne, G.; Norton, E.; Zhang, X.; Constant, M.; Park, D.; Wang, W.; et al. Cytometry by time-of-flight immunophenotyping identifies a blood Sjögren's signature correlating with disease activity and glandular inflammation. *J. Allergy Clin. Immunol.* **2016**, *137*, 1809–1821.e12. [CrossRef] [PubMed]
27.   Tasaki, S.; Suzuki, K.; Nishikawa, A.; Kassai, Y.; Takiguchi, M.; Kurisu, R.; Okuzono, Y.; Miyazaki, T.; Takeshita, M.; Yoshimoto, K.; et al. Multiomic disease signatures converge to cytotoxic CD8 T cells in primary Sjögren's syndrome. *Ann. Rheum. Dis.* **2017**, *76*, 1458–1466. [CrossRef]
28.   Caldeira-Dantas, S.; Furmanak, T.; Smith, C.; Quinn, M.; Teos, L.Y.; Ertel, A.; Kurup, D.; Tandon, M.; Alevizos, I.; Snyder, C.M. The Chemokine Receptor CXCR3 Promotes CD8$^+$ T Cell Accumulation in Uninfected Salivary Glands but Is Not Necessary after Murine Cytomegalovirus Infection. *J. Immunol.* **2018**, *200*, 1133–1145. [CrossRef]
29.   Verstappen, G.M.; Kroese, F.G.M.; Bootsma, H. T cells in primary Sjögren's syndrome: Targets for early intervention. *Rheumatology* **2021**, *60*, 3088–3098. [CrossRef]
30.   Lee, J.; Kim, D.; Min, B. Tissue Resident Foxp3$^+$ Regulatory T Cells: Sentinels and Saboteurs in Health and Disease. *Front. Immunol.* **2022**, *13*, 865593. [CrossRef]
31.   Rajendeeran, A.; Tenbrock, K. Regulatory T cell function in autoimmune disease. *J. Transl. Autoimmun.* **2021**, *4*, 100130. [CrossRef]

32. Miao, M.; Hao, Z.; Guo, Y.; Zhang, X.; Zhang, S.; Luo, J.; Zhao, X.; Zhang, C.; Liu, X.; Wu, X.; et al. Short-term and low-dose IL-2 therapy restores the Th17/Treg balance in the peripheral blood of patients with primary Sjogren's syndrome. *Ann. Rheum. Dis.* **2018**, *77*, 1838–1840. [CrossRef] [PubMed]

33. Frantz, C.; Auffray, C.; Avouac, J.; Allanore, Y. Regulatory T Cells in Systemic Sclerosis. *Front. Immunol.* **2018**, *9*, 2356. [CrossRef] [PubMed]

34. Kobayashi, S.; Nagafuchi, Y.; Shoda, H.; Fujio, K. The Pathophysiological Roles of Regulatory T Cells in the Early Phase of SSc. *Front. Immunol.* **2022**, *24*, 900638. [CrossRef] [PubMed]

35. Vignali, D.A.; Collison, L.W.; Workman, C.J. How regulatory T cells work. *Nat. Rev. Immunol.* **2008**, *8*, 523–532. [CrossRef]

36. MacDonald, K.G.; Dawson, N.A.J.; Huang, Q.; Dunne, J.V.; Levings, M.K.; Broady, R. Regulatory T cells produce profibrotic cytokines in the skin of patients with systemic sclerosis. *J. Allergy Clin. Immunol.* **2015**, *135*, 946–955.e9. [CrossRef] [PubMed]

37. Keindl, M.; Davies, R.; Bergum, B.; Brun, J.G.; Hammenfors, D.; Jonsson, R.; Lyssenko, V.; Appel, S. Impaired activation of STAT5 upon IL-2 stimulation in Tregs and elevated sIL-2R in Sjögren's syndrome. *Arthritis Res. Ther.* **2022**, *24*, 101. [CrossRef]

38. Uchida, K. Recent progress on the Roles of Regulatory T Cells in IgG4-Related Disease. *Immuno* **2022**, *2*, 430–442. [CrossRef]

39. Wu, K.J.; Qian, Q.F.; Zhou, J.R.; Sun, D.L.; Duan, Y.F.; Zhu, X.; Sartorius, K.; Lu, Y.J. Regulatory T cells (Tregs) in liver fibrosis. *Cell Death Discov.* **2023**, *9*, 53. [CrossRef]

40. Ormandy, L.A.; Hillemann, T.; Wedemeyer, H.; Manns, M.P.; Greten, T.F.; Korangy, F. Increased populations of regulatory T cells in peripheral blood of patients with hepatocellular carcinoma. *Cancer Res.* **2005**, *65*, 2457–2464. [CrossRef]

41. Liu, X.; Nurieva, R.I.; Dong, C. Transcriptional regulation of follicular T-helper (Tfh) cells. *Immunol. Rev.* **2013**, *252*, 139–145. [CrossRef] [PubMed]

42. Breitfeld, D.; Ohl, L.; Kremmer, E.; Ellwart, J.; Sallusto, F.; Lipp, M.; Förster, R. Follicular B helper T cells express CXC chemokine receptor 5, localize to B cell follicles, and support immunoglobulin production. *J. Exp. Med.* **2000**, *192*, 1545–1552. [CrossRef] [PubMed]

43. Gensous, N.; Charrier, M.; Duluc, D.; Contin-Bordes, C.; Truchetet, M.E.; Lazaro, E.; Duffau, P.; Blanco, P.; Richez, C. T Follicular Helper Cells in Autoimmune Disorders. *Front. Immunol.* **2018**, *9*, 1637. [CrossRef]

44. Li, X.; Wu, Z.; Ding, J.; Zheng, Z.; Li, X.; Chen, L.; Zhu, P. Role of the frequency of blood CD4(+) CXCR5(+) CCR6(+) T cells in autoimmunity in patients with Sjögren's syndrome. *Biochem. Biophys. Res. Commun.* **2012**, *422*, 238–244. [CrossRef] [PubMed]

45. Jin, L.; Yu, D.; Li, X.; Yu, N.; Li, X.; Wang, Y.; Wang, Y. CD4+CXCR5+ follicular helper T cells in salivary gland promote B cells maturation in patients with primary Sjogren's syndrome. *Int. J. Clin. Exp. Pathol.* **2014**, *7*, 1988–1996.

46. Vogelzang, A.; McGuire, H.M.; Yu, D.; Sprent, J.; Mackay, C.R.; King, C. A fundamental role for interleukin-21 in the generation of T follicular helper cells. *Immunity* **2008**, *29*, 127–137. [CrossRef]

47. Yang, X.; Yang, J.; Chu, Y.; Xue, Y.; Xuan, D.; Zheng, S.; Zou, H. T follicular helper cells and regulatory B cells dynamics in systemic lupus erythematosus. *PLoS ONE* **2014**, *9*, e88441. [CrossRef]

48. Zhang, Y.; Li, Y.; Lv, T.T.; Yin, Z.J.; Wang, X.B. Elevated circulating Th17 and follicular helper CD4(+) T cells in patients with rheumatoid arthritis. *APMIS* **2015**, *123*, 659–666. [CrossRef]

49. Taylor, D.K.; Mittereder, N.; Kuta, E.; Delaney, T.; Burwell, T.; Dacosta, K.; Zhao, W.; Cheng, L.I.; Brown, C.; Boutrin, A.; et al. T follicular helper-like cells contribute to skin fibrosis. *Sci. Transl. Med.* **2018**, *431*, 5307. [CrossRef]

50. Papadimitriou, T.I.; van Caam, A.; van der Kraan, P.M.; Thurlings, R.M. Therapeutic Options for Systemic Sclerosis: Current and Future Perspectives in Tackling Immune-Mediated Fibrosis. *Biomedicines* **2022**, *10*, 316. [CrossRef]

51. Asai, Y.; Chiba, H.; Nishikiori, H.; Kamekura, R.; Yabe, H.; Kondo, S.; Miyajima, S.; Shigehara, K.; Ichimiya, S.; Takahashi, H. Aberrant populations of circulating T follicular helper cells and regulatory B cells underlying idiopathic pulmonary fibrosis. *Respir Res.* **2019**, *20*, 244. [CrossRef]

52. Al-Adwi, Y.; Westra, J.; van Goor, H.; Burgess, J.K.; Denton, C.P.; Mulder, D.J. Macrophages as determinants and regulators of fibrosis in systemic sclerosis. *Rheumatology* **2023**, *62*, 535–545. [CrossRef] [PubMed]

53. Ross, E.A.; Devitt, A.; Johnson, J.R. Macrophages: The Good, the Bad, and the Gluttony. *Front. Immunol.* **2021**, *12*, 708186. [CrossRef] [PubMed]

54. Hoeft, K.; Schaefer, G.J.L.; Kim, H.; Schumacher, D.; Bleckwehl, T.; Long, Q.; Klinkhammer, B.M.; Peisker, F.; Koch, L.; Nagai, J.; et al. Platelet-instructed SPP1$^+$ macrophages drive myofibroblast activation in fibrosis in a CXCL4-dependent manner. *Cell Rep.* **2023**, *42*, 112131. [CrossRef]

55. Cheng, D.; Chai, J.; Wang, H.; Fu, L.; Peng, S.; Ni, X. Hepatic macrophages: Key players in the development and progression of liver fibrosis. *Liver Int.* **2021**, *41*, 2279–2294. [CrossRef] [PubMed]

56. Choreño-Parra, J.A.; Cervantes-Rosete, D.; Jiménez-Alvarez, L.A.; Ramírez-Martínez, G.; Márquez-García, J.E.; Cruz-Lagunas, A.; Magaña-Sanchez, A.Y.; Lima, G.; López-Maldonado, H.; Gaytán-Guzmán, E.; et al. Dendritic cells drive profibrotic inflammation and aberrant T cell polarization in systemic sclerosis. *Rheumatology* **2022**, *62*, 1687–1698. [CrossRef]

57. Guilliams, M.; Ginhoux, F.; Jakubzick, C.; Naik, S.H.; Onai, N.; Schraml, B.U.; Segura, E.; Tussiwand, R.; Yona, S. Dendritic cells, monocytes and macrophages: A unified nomenclature based on ontogeny. *Nat. Rev. Immunol.* **2014**, *4*, 571–578. [CrossRef]

58. Silva, I.S.; Ferreira, B.H.; Almeida, C.R. Molecular Mechanisms Behind the Role of Plasmacytoid Dendritic Cells in Systemic Sclerosis. *Biology* **2023**, *12*, 285. [CrossRef]

59. Kafaja, S.; Valera, I.; Divekar, A.A.; Saggar, R.; Abtin, F.; Furst, D.E.; Khanna, D.; Singh, R.R. pDCs in lung and skin fibrosis in a bleomycin-induced model and patients with systemic sclerosis. *JCI Insight.* **2018**, *3*, e98380. [CrossRef]

60. Khedoe, P.; Marges, E.; Hiemstra, P.; Ninaber, M.; Geelhoed, M. Interstitial Lung Disease in Patients With Systemic Sclerosis: Toward Personalized-Medicine-Based Prediction and Drug Screening Models of Systemic Sclerosis-Related Interstitial Lung Disease (SSc-ILD). *Front Immunol.* **2020**, *11*, 1990. [CrossRef]

61. Lande, R.; Mennella, A.; Palazzo, R.; Pietraforte, I.; Stefanantoni, K.; Iannace, N.; Butera, A.; Boirivant, M.; Pica, R.; Conrad, C.; et al. Anti-CXCL4 Antibody Reactivity Is Present in Systemic Sclerosis (SSc) and Correlates with the SSc Type I Interferon Signature. *Int. J. Mol. Sci.* **2020**, *21*, 5102. [CrossRef]

62. Affandi, A.J.; Carvalheiro, T.; Ottria, A.; de Haan, J.J.; Brans, M.A.D.; Brandt, M.M.; Tieland, R.G.; Lopes, A.P.; Fernández, B.M.; Bekker, C.P.J.; et al. CXCL4 drives fibrosis by promoting several key cellular and molecular processes. *Cell Rep.* **2022**, *38*, 110189. [CrossRef]

63. van Bon, L.; Affandi, A.J.; Broen, J.; Christmann, R.B.; Marijnissen, R.J.; Stawski, L.; Farina, G.A.; Stifano, G.; Mathes, A.L.; Cossu, M.; et al. Proteome-wide analysis and CXCL4 as a biomarker in systemic sclerosis. *N. Engl. J. Med.* **2014**, *370*, 433–443. [CrossRef]

64. Ah Kioon, M.D.; Tripodo, C.; Fernandez, D.; Kirou, K.A.; Spiera, R.F.; Crow, M.K.; Gordon, J.K.; Barrat, F.J. Plasmacytoid dendritic cells promote systemic sclerosis with a key role for TLR8. *Sci. Transl. Med.* **2018**, *10*, eaam8458. [CrossRef]

65. Conti, P.; Stellin, L.; Caraffa, A.; Gallenga, C.E.; Ross, R.; Kritas, S.K.; Frydas, I.; Younes, A.; Di Emidio, P.; Ronconi, G. Advances in Mast Cell Activation by IL-1 and IL-33 in Sjogren's Syndrome: Promising Inhibitory Effect of IL-37. *Int. J. Mol. Sci.* **2020**, *21*, 4297. [CrossRef] [PubMed]

66. Leehan, K.M.; Pezant, N.P.; Rasmussen, A.; Grundahl, K.; Moore, J.S.; Radfar, L.; Lewis, D.M.; Stone, D.U.; Lessard, C.J.; Rhodus, N.L.; et al. Minor salivary gland fibrosis in Sjogren's syndrome is elevated, associated with focus score and not solely a consequence of aging. *Clin. Exp. Rheumatol.* **2018**, *36*, 80–88. [PubMed]

67. Lamouille, S.; Xu, J.; Derynck, R. Molecular mechanisms of epithelial-mesenchymal transition. *Nat. Rev. Mol. Cell. Biol.* **2014**, *15*, 178–196. [CrossRef] [PubMed]

68. Sisto, M.; Ribatti, D.; Lisi, S. Sjögren's Syndrome-Related Organs Fibrosis: Hypotheses and Realities. *J. Clin. Med.* **2022**, *11*, 3551. [CrossRef] [PubMed]

69. Wynn, T.A.; Ramalingam, T.R. Mechanisms of fibrosis: Therapeutic translation for fibrotic disease. *Nat. Med.* **2012**, *18*, 1028–1040. [CrossRef]

70. Wendt, M.K.; Allington, T.M.; Schiemann, W.P. Mechanisms of the epithelial-mesenchymal transition by TGF-beta. *Future Oncol.* **2009**, *5*, 1145–1168. [CrossRef]

71. Kuppe, C.; Ibrahim, M.M.; Kranz, J.; Zhang, X.; Ziegler, S.; Perales-Patón, J.; Jansen, J.; Reimer, K.C.; Smith, J.R.; Dobie, R.; et al. Decoding myofibroblast origins in human kidney fibrosis. *Nat. Cell Biol.* **2021**, *589*, 281–286. [CrossRef]

72. Sisto, M.; Ribatti, D.; Lisi, S. Organ Fibrosis and Autoimmunity: The Role of Inflammation in TGFβ-Dependent EMT. *Biomolecules.* **2021**, *11*, 310. [CrossRef] [PubMed]

73. Sisto, M.; Ribatti, D.; Lisi, S. Molecular Mechanisms Linking Inflammation to Autoimmunity in Sjögren's Syndrome: Identification of New Targets. *Int. J. Mol. Sci.* **2022**, *23*, 13229. [CrossRef]

74. Asano, Y.; Takahashi, T.; Saigusa, R. Systemic sclerosis: Is the epithelium a missing piece of the pathogenic puzzle? *J. Dermatol. Sci.* **2019**, *94*, 259–265. [CrossRef] [PubMed]

75. Hong, S.; Healy, H.; Kassianos, A.J. The Emerging Role of Renal Tubular Epithelial Cells in the Immunological Pathophysiology of Lupus Nephritis. *Front. Immunol.* **2020**, *11*, 578952. [CrossRef] [PubMed]

76. Ruiz-Ortega, M.; Rayego-Mateos, S.; Lamas, S.; Ortiz, A.; Rodrigues-Diez, R.R. Targeting the progression of chronic kidney disease. *Nat. Rev. Nephrol.* **2020**, *16*, 269–288. [CrossRef]

77. Yung, S.; Ng, C.Y.; Ho, S.K.; Cheung, K.F.; Chan, K.W.; Zhang, Q.; Chau, M.K.; Chan, T.M. Anti-dsDNA antibody induces soluble fibronectin secretion by proximal renal tubular epithelial cells and downstream increase of TGF-beta1 and collagen synthesis. *J. Autoimmun.* **2015**, *58*, 111–122. [CrossRef]

78. Zhang, C.; Wang, S.; Lau, J.; Roden, A.C.; Matteson, E.L.; Sun, J.; Luo, F.; Tschumperlin, D.J.; Vassallo, R. IL-23 amplifies the epithelial-mesenchymal transition of mechanically conditioned alveolar epithelial cells in rheumatoid arthritis-associated interstitial lung disease through mTOR/S6 signaling. *Am. J. Physiol. Lung Cell Mol. Physiol.* **2021**, *321*, L1006–L1022. [CrossRef]

79. Di Gregorio, J.; Robuffo, I.; Spalletta, S.; Giambuzzi, G.; De Iuliis, V.; Toniato, E.; Martinotti, S.; Conti, P.; Flati, V. The Epithelial-to-Mesenchymal Transition as a Possible Therapeutic Target in Fibrotic Disorders. *Front. Cell Dev. Biol.* **2020**, *8*, 607483. [CrossRef]

80. Wang, W.; Poe, D.; Yang, Y.; Hyatt, T.; Xing, J. Epithelial-to-mesenchymal transition proceeds through directional destabilization of multidimensional attractor. *eLife* **2022**, *11*, e74866. [CrossRef]

81. López-Novoa, J.M.; Nieto, M.A. Inflammation and EMT: An alliance towards organ fibrosis and cancer progression. *EMBO Mol. Med.* **2009**, *1*, 303–314. [CrossRef] [PubMed]

82. Marconi, G.D.; Fonticoli, L.; Rajan, T.S.; Pierdomenico, S.D.; Trubiani, O.; Pizzicannella, J.; Diomede, F. Epithelial-Mesenchymal Transition (EMT): The Type-2 EMT in Wound Healing, Tissue Regeneration and Organ Fibrosis. *Cells* **2021**, *10*, 1587. [CrossRef] [PubMed]

83. Zheng, X.; Dai, F.; Feng, L.; Zou, H.; Feng, L.; Xu, M. Communication Between Epithelial-Mesenchymal Plasticity and Cancer Stem Cells: New Insights Into Cancer Progression. *Front. Oncol.* **2021**, *11*, 617597. [CrossRef] [PubMed]

84. Lovisa, S. Epithelial-to-Mesenchymal Transition in Fibrosis: Concepts and Targeting Strategies. *Front. Pharmacol.* **2021**, *12*, 737570. [CrossRef]

85. Kim, K.K.; Sheppard, D.; Chapman, H.A. TGF-β1 signaling and tissue fibrosis. *Perspect. Biol.* **2018**, *10*, a022293. [CrossRef]

86. Li, M.O.; Wan, Y.Y.; Sanjabi, S.; Robertson, A.K.; Flavell, R.A. Transforming growth factor-beta regulation of immune responses. *Annu. Rev. Immunol.* **2006**, *24*, 99–146. [CrossRef]

87. Fabregat, I.; Moreno-Càceres, J.; Sánchez, A.; Dewidar, B.; Giannelli, G.; Ten Dijke, P. IT-LIVER Consortium. TGF-β signalling and liver disease. *FEBS J.* **2016**, *283*, 2219–2232. [CrossRef]

88. Willis, B.C.; Borok, Z. TGF-β-induced EMT: Mechanisms and implications for fibrotic lung disease. *Am. J. Physiol.* **2007**, *293*, L525–L534. [CrossRef]

89. Zhang, Y.E. Non-Smad pathways in TGF-beta signaling. *Cell Res.* **2009**, *19*, 128–139. [CrossRef]

90. Jimenez, S.A. Role of endothelial to mesenchymal transition in the pathogenesis of the vascular alterations in systemic sclerosis. *ISRN Rheumatol.* **2013**, *2013*, 835948. [CrossRef]

91. Ebmeier, S.; Horsley, V. Origin of fibrosing cells in systemic sclerosis. *Curr. Opin. Rheumatol.* **2015**, *27*, 555–562. [CrossRef]

92. Di Benedetto, P.; Ruscitti, P.; Berardicurti, O.; Vomero, M.; Navarini, L.; Dolo, V.; Cipriani, P.; Giacomelli, R. Endothelial-to-mesenchymal transition in systemic sclerosis. *Clin. Exp. Immunol.* **2021**, *205*, 12–27. [CrossRef]

93. Moschetti, L.; Piantoni, S.; Vizzardi, E.; Sciatti, E.; Riccardi, M.; Franceschini, F.; Cavazzana, I. Endothelial Dysfunction in Systemic Lupus Erythematosus and Systemic Sclerosis: A Common Trigger for Different Microvascular Diseases. *Front. Med.* **2022**, *9*, 849086. [CrossRef]

94. Łuczak, A.; Małecki, R.; Kulus, M.; Madej, M.; Szahidewicz-Krupska, E.; Doroszko, A. Cardiovascular Risk and Endothelial Dysfunction in Primary Sjogren Syndrome Is Related to the Disease Activity. *Nutrients* **2021**, *13*, 2072. [CrossRef] [PubMed]

95. Robert, M.; Miossec, P. Effects of Interleukin 17 on the cardiovascular system. *Autoimmun. Rev.* **2017**, *16*, 984–991. [CrossRef] [PubMed]

96. Mostmans, Y.; Cutolo, M.; Giddelo, C.; Decuman, S.; Melsens, K.; Declercq, H.; Vandecasteele, E.; De Keyser, F.; Distler, O.; Gutermuth, J.; et al. The role of endothelial cells in the vasculopathy of systemic sclerosis: A systematic review. *Autoimmun. Rev.* **2017**, *16*, 774–786. [CrossRef]

97. Plikus, M.V.; Wang, X.; Sinha, S.; Forte, E.; Thompson, S.M.; Herzog, E.L.; Driskell, R.R.; Rosenthal, N.; Biernaskie, J.; Horsley, V. Fibroblasts: Origins, definitions, and functions in health and disease. *Cell* **2021**, *184*, 3852–3872. [CrossRef]

98. LeBleu, V.S.; Taduri, G.; O'Connell, J.; Teng, Y.; Cooke, V.G.; Woda, C.; Sugimoto, H.; Kalluri, R. Origin and Function of Myofibroblasts in Kidney Fibrosis. *Nat. Med.* **2013**, *19*, 1047–1053. [CrossRef] [PubMed]

99. Wei, K.; Korsunsky, I.; Marshall, J.L.; Gao, A.; Watts, G.F.M.; Major, T.; Croft, A.P.; Watts, J.; Blazar, P.E.; Lange, J.K.; et al. Notch signalling drives synovial fibroblast identity and arthritis pathology. *Nature* **2020**, *582*, 259–264. [CrossRef]

100. Smith, T.J. Insights into the role of fibroblasts in human autoimmune diseases. *Clin. Exp. Immunol.* **2005**, *141*, 388–397. [CrossRef]

101. Wang, W.; Bale, S.; Wei, J.; Yalavarthi, B.; Bhattacharyya, D.; Yan, J.J.; Abdala-Valencia, H.; Xu, D.; Sun, H.; Marangoni, R.G.; et al. Fibroblast A20 governs fibrosis susceptibility and its repression by DREAM promotes fibrosis in multiple organs. *Nat. Commun.* **2022**, *13*, 6358. [CrossRef] [PubMed]

102. Onuora, S. Fibroblast A20 and its suppressor DREAM regulate fibrosis in SSc. *Nat. Rev. Rheumatol.* **2023**, *19*, 1. [CrossRef] [PubMed]

103. Klein, K. *Fibroblasts in Sjögren's Syndrome, Fibroblasts—Advances in Inflammation, Autoimmunity and Cancer*; Bertoncelj, M.F., Lakota, K., Eds.; IntechOpen: London, UK, 2021.

104. Lee, B.; Lee, S.H.; Shin, K. Crosstalk between fibroblasts and T cells in immune networks. *Front. Immunol.* **2023**, *13*, 1103823. [CrossRef]

105. Sciascia, S.; Cozzi, M.; Barinotti, A.; Radin, M.; Cecchi, I.; Fenoglio, R.; Mancardi, D.; Wilson Jones, G.; Rossi, D.; Roccatello, D. Renal Fibrosis in Lupus Nephritis. *Int. J. Mol. Sci.* **2022**, *23*, 14317. [CrossRef]

106. Tai, Y.; Woods, E.L.; Dally, J.; Kong, D.; Steadman, R.; Moseley, R.; Midgley, A.C. Myofibroblasts: Function, Formation, and Scope of Molecular Therapies for Skin Fibrosis. *Biomolecules* **2021**, *11*, 1095. [CrossRef]

107. Tabib, T.; Morse, C.; Wang, T.; Chen, W.; Lafyatis, R. SFRP2/DPP4 and FMO1/LSP1 Define Major Fibroblast Populations in Human Skin. *J. Investig. Dermatol.* **2018**, *138*, 802–810. [CrossRef]

108. van Caam, A.; Vonk, M.; van den Hoogen, F.; van Lent, P.; van der Kraan, P. Unraveling SSc Pathophysiology; The Myofibroblast. *Front. Immunol.* **2018**, *9*, 2452. [CrossRef]

109. Falke, L.L.; Gholizadeh, S.; Goldschmeding, R.; Kok, R.J.; Nguyen, T.Q. Diverse Origins of the Myofibroblast—Implications for Kidney Fibrosis. *Nat. Rev. Nephrol.* **2015**, *11*, 233–244. [CrossRef] [PubMed]

110. Schunk, S.J.; Floege, J.; Fliser, D.; Speer, T. WNT-β-Catenin Signalling—A Versatile Player in Kidney Injury and Repair. *Nat. Rev. Nephrol.* **2021**, *17*, 172–184. [CrossRef]

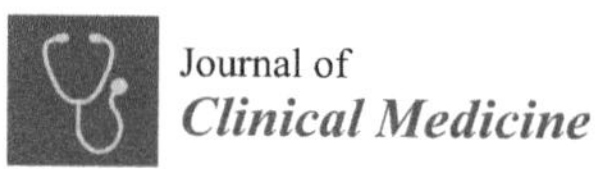

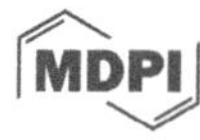

Brief Report

Anti-Interleukin-1 Therapy Does Not Affect the Response to SARS-CoV-2 Vaccination and Infection in Patients with Systemic Autoinflammatory Diseases

Leonie Geck [1,2,3,†], Koray Tascilar [1,2,3,†], David Simon [1,2], Arnd Kleyer [1,2], Georg Schett [1,2,3] and Jürgen Rech [1,2,3,*]

[1]   Department of Internal Medicine 3, Rheumatology and Immunology, Universitätsklinikum Erlangen, Friedrich-Alexander-University Erlangen-Nürnberg (FAU), 91054 Erlangen, Germany; leonie.geck@fau.de (L.G.); koray.tascilar@uk-erlangen.de (K.T.); simon.david@extern.uk-erlangen.de (D.S.); arnd.kleyer@extern.uk-erlangen.de (A.K.); georg.schett@uk-erlangen.de (G.S.)

[2]   Deutsches Zentrum Immuntherapie, Universitätsklinikum Erlangen, Friedrich-Alexander-University Erlangen-Nürnberg (FAU), 91054 Erlangen, Germany

[3]   Centre for Rare Diseases Erlangen, Universitätsklinikum Erlangen, Friedrich-Alexander-University Erlangen-Nürnberg (FAU), 91054 Erlangen, Germany

*   Correspondence: juergen.rech@uk-erlangen.de

†   These authors contributed equally to this work.

Abstract: Patients with systemic autoinflammatory diseases (sAIDs) are a section of the population at high risk of severe COVID-19 outcomes, but evidence on the efficacy of SARS-CoV-2 vaccination in this group of patients is scarce. To investigate the efficacy of SARS-CoV-2 vaccination in patients with sAIDs receiving interleukin-1 (IL-1) inhibition is important. Vaccination and infection responses from 100 sAID patients and 100 healthy controls (HCs) were analyzed. In total, 98% of patients were treated with IL-1 inhibitors at the time of vaccination ($n = 98$). After the second SARS-CoV-2 vaccination, sAID patients showed similar anti-SARS-CoV-2 antibody responses (mean (standard deviation (SD)): 6.7 (2.7)) compared to HCs (5.7 (2.4)) as well as similar neutralizing antibodies ($85.1 \pm 22.9\%$ vs. $82.5 \pm 19.7\%$). Anti-SARS-CoV-2 antibody responses and neutralizing antibodies were similar in sAID patients after SARS-CoV-2 infection and double vaccination. Furthermore, while antibodies increased after the first and second vaccination in sAID patients, they did not further increase after the third and fourth vaccination. No difference was found in antibody responses between anakinra and anti-IL-1 antibody treatment and the additional use of colchicine or other drugs did not impair vaccination responses. Primary and booster SARS-CoV-2 vaccinations led to protective antibody responses in sAID patients, which were at the same level of vaccination responses in HCs and in sAID patients after SARS-CoV-2 infection. Immunomodulatory treatments used in sAID do not seem to affect antibody responses to the SARS-CoV-2 vaccine.

Keywords: autoinflammatory diseases; SARS-CoV-2; vaccination; familial Mediterranean fever; adult-onset Still's disease; cryopyrin-associated periodic syndrome; systemic autoinflammatory diseases

Citation: Geck, L.; Tascilar, K.; Simon, D.; Kleyer, A.; Schett, G.; Rech, J. Anti-Interleukin-1 Therapy Does Not Affect the Response to SARS-CoV-2 Vaccination and Infection in Patients with Systemic Autoinflammatory Diseases. *J. Clin. Med.* **2023**, *12*, 7587. https://doi.org/10.3390/jcm12247587

Academic Editor: Ferdinando Nicoletti

Received: 13 October 2023
Revised: 23 November 2023
Accepted: 6 December 2023
Published: 8 December 2023

1. Background

Immune responses to vaccines depend on the quality of the vaccine used and the immune response of the host. In immune-mediated inflammatory diseases (IMIDs), the immune response of the host is altered due to intrinsic changes in the innate and adaptive immune system as well as the concomitant presence of immune-modulatory drugs [1]. Initial studies on the use of SARS-CoV-2 vaccines in patients with IMIDs were reassuring as to the efficacy of the vaccines despite the use of different immune-modulatory drugs such as cytokine inhibitors [2], nevertheless indicating a reduced longevity in overall humoral responses to SARS-CoV-2 vaccines [3]. However, patients with systemic autoinflammatory diseases (sAIDs) were not included or were highly underrepresented in these studies, which substantially limits our current knowledge on the efficacy of SARS-CoV-2 vaccines in these disease groups [4]. Notably, sAID patients receive different drugs than other patient groups from the IMID disease spectrum. Thus, interleukin-1 (IL-1) inhibitors and colchicine are widely used to treat sAIDs. As commonalities between sAIDs and COVID-19 infection have been observed, e.g., dysfunctional cytokine release [5], these medications have been used outside the sAID field in the treatment of COVID-19, but with little to no effect on adult hospitalized patients [6,7]. Furthermore, under certain circumstances, such as comorbidities and glucocorticoid use, sAID patients are at risk of developing severe COVID-19 [8]. This observation indicates that better knowledge about the response of sAID patients to SARS-CoV-2 vaccine is of utmost importance.

We therefore addressed anti-SARS-CoV-2 antibody responses in a larger group of sAID patients treated with IL-1 inhibitors to find out whether sAID patients are able to mount sufficient humoral immunity against the coronavirus. We thereby analyzed primary antibody responses and booster responses and compared them to data obtained from healthy controls (HCs). In addition, we analyzed whether the additional use of colchicine influenced the vaccination response.

2. Materials and Methods

2.1. Participants

After approval by the Research Ethics Committee of the Friedrich-Alexander-University Erlangen-Nürnberg (FAU), 100 consecutive sAID patients were recruited. The HC group was age- and gender-matched with the large COVID-19 study at the Deutsche Zentrum Immuntherapie (DZI), Universitätsklinikum Erlangen (UKER), established in February 2020. Patient demographic data (age, sex, body mass index, comorbidities, medication) and information on SARS-CoV-2 vaccination (date, type of vaccine) and infection (date, general symptoms, severity of symptoms) were obtained through telephone interviews and supplemented using a retrospective analysis of physician letters in the UKER electronic archive and document management system Soarian® (Soarin Clinicals, version 4.5.200, Bay Lake, FL, USA) until the end of July 2022.

2.2. Anti-SARS-CoV-2 Antibody Testing

Quantitative detection of specific antibodies of the IgG class against the SARS-CoV-2 spike protein was performed with the CE-marked version of the enzyme-linked immunosorbent assay (ELISA) kit from EUROIMMUN (Lübeck, Germany). The reagent vials were evaluated photometrically at an optical density (OD) of 450 nm with reference wavelength at 630 nm. The ratio was then determined by dividing the absorbances of the control or patient sample and the calibrator; a ratio ≥ 0.8 was considered positive.

The determination of SARS-CoV-2 neutralizing antibodies was performed with the CE-In Vitro Diagnostics (CE-IVD)-certified cPass surrogate virus neutralization assay from the manufacturer GenScript (Piscataway, NJ, USA). Per test run, neutralizing antibodies from 92 participants' sera can be determined on a microtiter plate with two negative and two positive controls. Photometric analysis was performed at 450 nm and a calculation formula was used to determine the inhibition percentage. A cut-off value of 30% was considered a positive test result and indicated the presence of neutralizing antibodies.

2.3. Statistical Analysis

Characteristics of the study groups were described using descriptive analyses—including mean, standard deviation (SD) and counts/percentages. We used the Wilcoxon rank-sum test to compare controls with the sAID group. Since on average, a longer time had elapsed between the second vaccination and sample collection, we used linear regression to adjust for this time difference. Separate models were fitted for the antibody and neutralizing antibody values as independent variables and OD ratio values from the antibody assay as the dependent variables. The visual image of an initial scatter plot in the analysis indicated that the use of a native scale did not adequately present the data, which is why the neutralizing antibodies were analyzed in the logit transformation and the SARS-CoV-2 antibody ratio in the log transformation. The freely available programming language "R v.4.01" (R Foundation for Statistical Computing, Vienna, Austria) was used for all statistical analyses. A p-value < 0.05 was considered statistically significant.

3. Results

3.1. Characteristics of Patients and Controls

A total of 100 sAID patients were analyzed, of whom 58 were female and 42 were male (Table 1). At the time of data collection in June and July 2022, the age (mean (min; max) $\pm$ SD) of sAID patients was 43 (18; 80) $\pm$ 16 years. The largest proportionally represented disease was familial Mediterranean fever (FMF), present in more than one third (37%) of the patients, followed by adult-onset Still's disease (AoSD; 25%), gout (15%), cryopyrin-associated periodic syndrome (CAPS; 7%), sAID of unclear etiology (7%), Behçet's disease (4%), tumor necrosis receptor-associated periodic syndrome (TRAPS; 4%) and Yao syndrome (1%).

Table 1. Demographics and characteristics of patients and controls.

	sAID	HC
n	100	100
Demographic characteristics		
Age, years	42.7 $\pm$ 16.0	42.7 $\pm$ 15.8
Females, n (%)	58 (58.0)	57 (57.0)
Body weight	77.7 $\pm$ 21.5	-
Current smokers, n (%)	22 (22.0)	-
Comorbidities, n (%)		
Diabetes	10 (10.0)	-
Hypertension	23 (23.0)	-
History of CV event	8 (8.0)	-
History of thrombotic event	7 (7.0)	-
Type of sAID, n (%)		
FMF	37 (37.0)	0
AoSD	25 (25.0)	0
Gout	15 (15.0)	0
CAPS	7 (7.0)	0
sAID of unclear etiology	7 (7.0)	0
Behçet's disease	4 (4.0)	0
TRAPS	4 (4.0)	0
Yao syndrome	1 (1.0)	0
COVID-19 vaccinations, n (%) *		
1st	96 (96.0)	100 (100.0)
2nd	95 (95.0)	100 (100.0)
3rd	82 (82.0)	-
4th	9 (9.0)	-
Immune-modulatory treatment, n (%)		
IL-1 inhibitors	98 (98.0)	0
Anakinra	48 (48.0)	0

Table 1. *Cont.*

	sAID	HC
Canakinumab	50 (50.0)	0
No IL-1 inhibitors	2 (2.0)	0
Colchicine	36 (36.0)	0
Glucocorticoids **	5 (5.0)	0
csDMARDs	4 (4.0)	0
MTX	3 (3.0)	0
Allopurinol	2 (2.0)	0
Febuxostat	2 (2.0)	0
COVID-19 infections, *n* (%)		
Total infected	43 (43.0)	-
Infected more than once	3 (3.0)	-

AoSD, Adult-onset Still's disease; CAPS, cryopyrin-associated periodic syndrome; csDMARDs, conventional synthetic disease-modifying antirheumatic drugs; CV, cardiovascular; FMF, familial Mediterranean fever; HC, healthy control; IL, interleukin; MTX, methotrexate; sAID, systemic autoinflammatory disease; TRAPS, tumor necrosis receptor-associated periodic syndrome. * For sAID patients: The majority of patients had received a mRNA-based, not a vector-based vaccine—more specifically, 89% of all patients who received the 1st vaccination (85 patients with a mRNA-based vaccine and 11 with a vector-based vaccine), 96% (91 and 4) for the 2nd, 100% (82 and 0) for the 3rd and 100% (9 and 0) for the 4th vaccination. ** Overall, five patients used glucocorticoids, for only one of whom the dose was >10 mg.

At the time of vaccination, 48 patients were treated with an IL-1 receptor antagonist (IL1RA) and 50 patients with an IL-1 inhibiting antibody, while two patients did not receive anti-IL1 treatment due to being in remission during the vaccination period. Three patients on treatment with anakinra received the IL1RA only on demand during a disease flare, whereas the remaining 95 patients received anti-IL1 treatment permanently. The mean dose was 104.17 mg (on average 6.6/days per week) for anakinra and 183 mg (once every 5.7 weeks) for canakinumab. The mean treatment duration before the first vaccination was 715 (SD: 1287) days for anakinra and 337 (511) days for canakinumab.

In addition to IL-1 inhibitors, colchicine was used in 36% of sAID patients. Glucocorticoids and methotrexate were infrequently used treatments. Four patients were treated with a dose of glucocorticoids lower than 10 mg per day, while one patient received a dose of 20 mg/day. By the end of July 2022, one patient had received only one shot of the COVID-19 vaccine, while 13 patients (13%) had received two, the vast majority (73%) had received three and 9% had received four vaccinations. Only four patients (4%) received no SARS-CoV-2 vaccination. In sAID patients, mRNA-based vaccines were by far the most frequently used, whereas only a minority of patients received a vector-based vaccine. The HC group (*n* = 100) had a similar age and sex distribution as the sAID patients and consisted of 57 females and 43 males with a mean age of 43 (18; 89) $\pm$ 16 years.

3.2. Anti-SARS-CoV-2 IgG and Neutralizing Antibodies Responses in sAID

All analyses of anti-SARS-CoV-2 IgG antibodies in sAID patients showed an increase from the first to the second vaccination (mean values in Table 2), with similar antibody levels after the second vaccination in sAID patients compared to HCs (Figure 1A). Further vaccinations did not increase anti-SARS-CoV-2 IgG antibody responses. Also, anti-SARS-CoV-2 IgG antibody levels after additional SARS-CoV-2 infection were comparable to the ones found after vaccination. The fact that HCs (5.7 (SD: 2.4)) had even lower anti-SARS-CoV-2 IgG levels than sAID patients (7 (2.7); *p* = 0.0017) after two vaccinations was due to the timing of sample collection after the second vaccination, which was 9.1 (7.5) weeks in the sAID group as compared to 21.9 (6.5) weeks in the control group. When we adjusted the sample collection time after the second vaccination, no difference in antibody levels between the HC and the sAID groups was found (adjusted mean between group difference

0.17; 95% CI −0.80 to 1.13, $p = 0.73$). The results for neutralizing antibodies were very similar, with an increase in neutralizing capacity from the first to the second vaccination, a peak after the second vaccination and no major differences between the vaccinations with and without additional SARS-CoV-2 infection, as well as between vaccinated HCs and sAID patients (Figure 1B).

Table 2. Mean anti-SARS-CoV-2 IgG and neutralizing antibodies.

		Anti-SARS-CoV-2 IgG		Neutralizing Antibodies in %	
Event	**Sex**	**sAID**	**HC**	**sAID**	**HC**
1st vacc.	F	3.3 ± 2.9 ($n = 37$) *	-	42.5 ± 30.2 ($n = 32$)	-
	M	3.4 ± 2.3 ($n = 23$)	-	40.2 ± 25.5 ($n = 20$)	-
	All	3.4 ± 2.7 ($n = 60$)	-	41.6 ± 28.2 ($n = 52$)	-
2nd vacc.	F	7.2 ± 2.2 ($n = 56$)	6.2 ± 2.2 ($n = 57$)	89.9 ± 15.5 ($n = 54$)	86.5 ± 17.6 ($n = 57$)
	M	6.0 ± 3.2 ($n = 38$)	5.1 ± 2.5 ($n = 43$)	77.2 ± 30.1 ($n = 33$)	77.3 ± 21.3 ($n = 43$)
	All	6.7 ± 2.7 ($n = 94$)	5.7 ± 2.4 ($n = 100$)	85.1 ± 22.9 ($n = 87$)	82.5 ± 19.7 ($n = 100$)
3rd vacc.	F	8.1 ± 1.7 ($n = 45$)	-	94.6 ± 5.3 ($n = 43$)	-
	M	7.2 ± 2.9 ($n = 35$)	-	85.3 ± 27.5 ($n = 33$)	-
	All	7.7 ± 2.3 ($n = 80$)	-	90.5 ± 19.1 ($n = 76$)	-
4th vacc.	F	7.3 ± 2.2 ($n = 3$)	-	92.4 ± 5.7 ($n = 2$)	-
	M	7.4 ± 1.7 ($n = 5$)	-	86.1 ± 20.6 ($n = 5$)	-
	All	7.4 ± 1.8 ($n = 8$)	-	87.9 ± 17.2 ($n = 7$)	-
1st infection	F	7.4 ± 2.4 ($n = 29$)	-	92.9 ± 9.8 ($n = 23$)	-
	M	7.3 ± 2.8 ($n = 13$)	-	90.7 ± 14.1 ($n = 12$)	-
	All	7.3 ± 2.5 ($n = 42$)	-	92.1 ± 11.3 ($n = 35$)	-
2nd infection	F	6.6 ± 0.8 ($n = 2$)	-	97.3 ± NA ($n = 1$)	-
	M	-	-	-	-
	All	6.6 ± 0.8 ($n = 2$)	-	97.3 ± NA ** ($n = 1$)	-

F, female; HC, healthy control; M, male; n, number; NA, not available; sAID, systemic autoinflammatory disease; vacc., vaccination. * The numbers (n) represent the number of results we have measured for each category, not necessarily the total number of individuals with 1st/2nd/3rd/4th vaccination or 1st/2nd infection in our study. ** We only had a serum from one patient to measure the neutralizing antibodies after 2nd infection, so there is no standard deviation (SD) here.

3.3. Relation between Anti-SARS-CoV-2 Antibody Levels and Neutralizing Capacity

We have also analyzed the association between anti-SARS-CoV-2 antibody levels and the neutralizing capacity. Figure 1C shows a descriptive plot showing the neutralizing antibody levels observed at each total antibody measurement. The regression lines fit separately for HCs and sAID patients, suggesting that at the lower range of antibody levels, HCs show higher levels of neutralizing capacity compared to sAID patients, and neutralizing capacity becomes similar with higher antibody levels. We have analyzed this relationship using a mixed-effects linear regression model with the logit-transformed neutralizing antibody levels as the dependent variable, log-transformed antibody levels and study groups as fixed effects and patient identifier and sample collection timepoint (i.e., vaccination or infection) as crossed random effects. By adding an interaction term between the study group and the log-transformed antibody levels, we tested the equality of the slopes between sAID and HC groups for the relationship between the antibody levels and neutralizing capacity. This interaction term was non-zero, indicating that the relationship between the total antibody levels and neutralizing antibody levels depended on the study group (p for interaction = 0.0051).

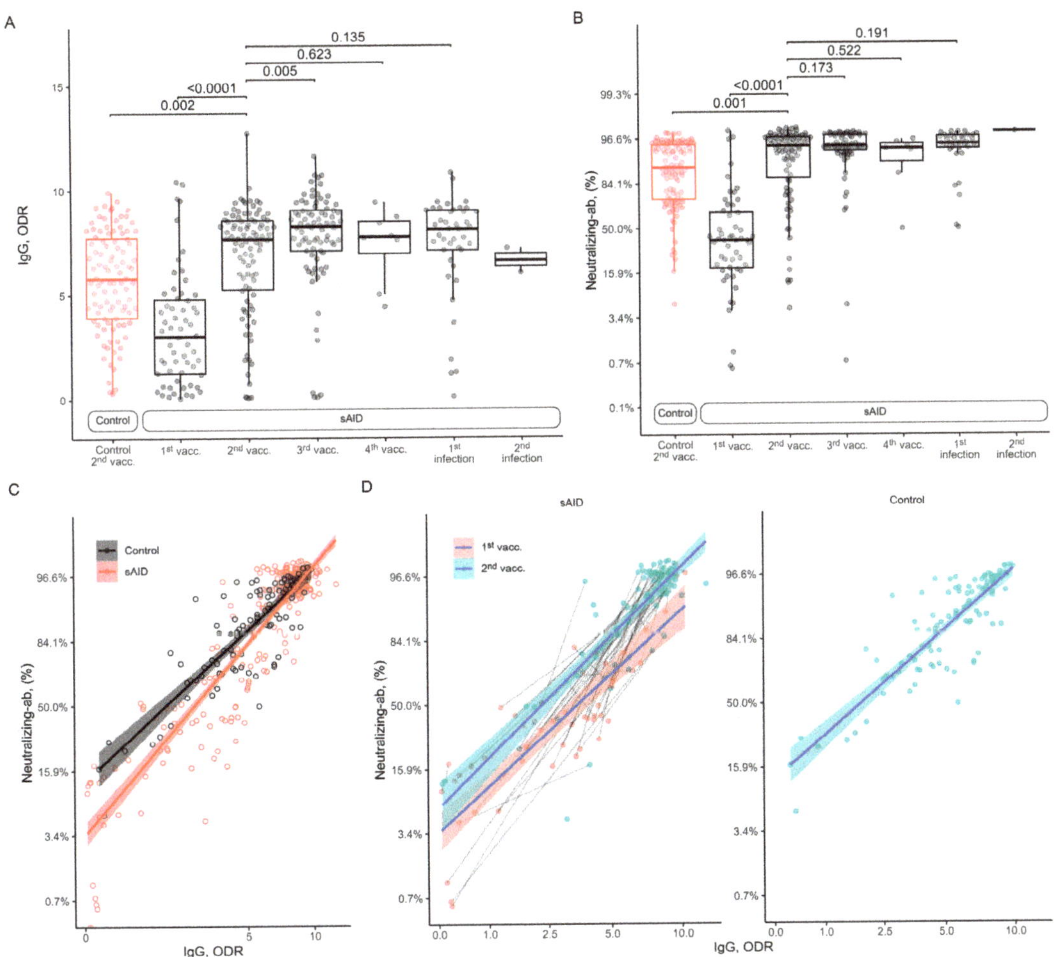

Figure 1. Association between anti-SARS-CoV-2 IgG and neutralizing antibodies in patients and healthy controls after COVID-19 vaccination and infection. (**A**) Anti-SARS-CoV-2 IgG antibodies and (**B**) SARS-CoV-2 neutralizing antibodies for sAID patients and HCs after COVID-19 vaccination and infection. (**C**) Anti-SARS-CoV-2 IgG and neutralizing antibodies in patients and HCs for all measured events. (**D**) Anti-SARS-CoV-2 IgG and neutralizing antibodies observed separately in patients after primary vaccination and in HCs after 2nd vaccination only. HC, healthy control; IgG (here), anti-SARS-CoV-2 IgG antibodies; Neutralizing-ab, neutralizing antibodies; ODR, optical density ratio; sAID, systemic autoinflammatory disease; vacc., vaccination.

3.4. Association between Immunomodulatory Treatment and Vaccination Response

We did not observe lower antibody levels in sAID patients compared to HCs, and since the vast majority of the sAID patients but none of the HCs received IL-1 inhibition, there seems to be no effect from IL-1 inhibitors on SARS-CoV-2 vaccination response. Accordingly, the few sAID patients who did not use IL-1 inhibitors did not show different vaccination responses compared to those using IL-1 inhibitors (Figure 2A,B). We next assessed whether additional therapies with colchicine, methotrexate or glucocorticoids affected vaccination responses in sAID patients but no major differences in anti-SARS-CoV-2 IgG antibodies or neutralizing antibodies were found. Only one patient receiving mycophenolate and tacrolimus treatment at different timepoints showed negative results in both ELISA tests at all time points.

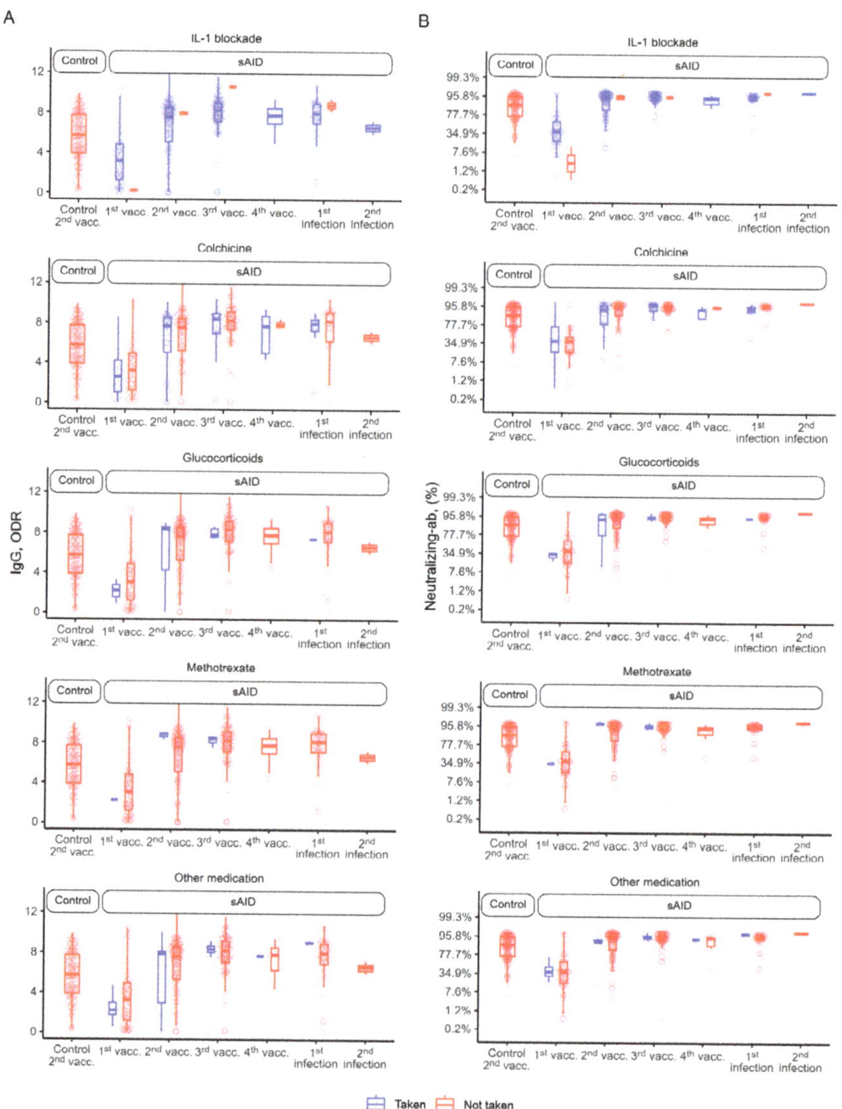

Figure 2. Distribution of antibody levels by type of treatment. "Not taken" here refers to the single drug considered. (**A**) Anti-SARS-CoV-2 IgG antibodies and (**B**) SARS-CoV-2 neutralizing antibodies for sAID patients and HCs after COVID-19 vaccination and disease. HC, healthy control; IgG (here), anti-SARS-CoV-2 IgG antibodies; Neutralizing-ab, neutralizing antibodies; ODR, optical density ratio; sAID, systemic autoinflammatory disease; vacc., vaccination.

4. Discussion

This study shows that SARS-CoV-2 vaccines trigger adequate humoral responses in sAID patients. Anti-SARS-CoV-2 IgG antibodies as well as neutralizing antibodies are already formed after primary vaccination and increase after the second vaccination to a level that is comparable to that of HCs. These results, acquired from a rather large sAID population treated with IL-1 inhibitors, confirm the initial data obtained in a smaller group of sAID patients [9].

One unexpected finding of this study was that antibody responses appeared to be even higher in sAID patients than in HCs. These differences, however, disappeared after adjusting for the time interval between vaccination and sample acquisition. On the other hand, we also found a slightly lower neutralizing antibody response in sAID patients for a given total antibody level at the lower range.

Whether vaccination protects sAID patients from severe COVID-19 is beyond the scope of our study. However, it was interesting to observe that a large proportion of sAID patients (79% of all infected persons) only contracted the virus during the "fifth Corona wave" (from calendar week 51/2021 on), when a majority of patients had already received triple vaccinations. The four unvaccinated patients only had low anti-SARS-CoV-2 IgG antibodies after infection. Whether a certain immunomodulatory treatment used for the treatment of sAIDs dampens vaccination responses is another important question: Our results suggest that therapy with an IL-1 inhibitor, which the vast majority of our patients received, did not have a negative impact on vaccination response. Also, further treatment with colchicine did not affect the vaccination response. Only one patient treated with a combination of mycophenolate showed low antibody titers across all measurement time points, which could be ascribed to the mycophenolate treatment as previously observed [10].

Our study has some limitations. Although the HC group had a similar age and sex distribution to the sAID group, we were only able to compare the sAIDs to HCs at different average time intervals after their second vaccination. We have addressed this issue with regression adjustments and observed that the apparently higher antibody levels in sAID patients were explained by this time difference in sample collection. Our findings on the non-uniform association between total and neutralizing antibody levels in controls vs. sAIDs could also have been affected for the same reason; therefore, this finding needs to be interpreted accordingly. In addition, we did not collect information on adverse events after vaccination as we focused on the analysis of antibody responses. However, a previous study on a large cohort of FMF patients presented reassuring results, as they did not report any relevant safety concern or an increasing number of flares after vaccination [11]. Finally, we did not have data on the persistence of the vaccination response in sAID patients.

5. Conclusions

Primary SARS-CoV-2 vaccination as well as booster vaccinations showed efficacy in sAID patients. In general, immunosuppressive therapy with IL-1 inhibitors could not be associated with a weakened immune response to the vaccination. One further research goal could be to investigate the long-term course of the antibody response. Hence, we do not see the necessity to control anti-SARS-CoV-2 antibody responses and neutralizing antibodies in sAID patients to ensure vaccination success.

The data provide the basis for recommendations and guidelines for the clinician in the consultation of sAID patients in vaccination planning.

Author Contributions: Conceptualization, J.R. and L.G.; data collection, validation and curation, L.G., J.R., D.S. and A.K.; writing—original draft preparation, L.G., K.T., G.S. and J.R.; visualization, L.G. and K.T.; writing—review and editing: K.T., G.S. and J.R.; visualization, L.G. and K.T. All authors have read and agreed to the published version of the manuscript.

Funding: The authors declare that no funds, grants, or other support were received during the preparation of this manuscript. The authors have no relevant financial or non-financial interests to disclose.

Institutional Review Board Statement: Based on ethics approval #157_20 B and the TARDA Database patient consent for publication.

Informed Consent Statement: Informed consent was obtained from all subjects involved in the study.

Data Availability Statement: All relevant data can be found in the manuscript.

Acknowledgments: The present work was performed in fulfillment of the requirements for obtaining the doctoral degree "Dr. med" for Leonie Geck at the Friedrich-Alexander-University Erlangen-Nürnberg (FAU).

Conflicts of Interest: The authors declare no conflict of interest.

References

1. Atagündüz, P.; Keser, G.; Soy, M. Interleukin-1 Inhibitors and Vaccination Including COVID-19 in Inflammatory Rheumatic Diseases: A Nonsystematic Review. *Front. Immunol.* **2021**, *12*, 734279. [CrossRef] [PubMed]
2. Geisen, U.M.; Berner, D.K.; Tran, F.; Sümbül, M.; Vullriede, L.; Ciripoi, M.; Reid, H.M.; Schaffarzyk, A.; Longardt, A.C.; Franzenburg, J.; et al. Immunogenicity and safety of anti-SARS-CoV-2 mRNA vaccines in patients with chronic inflammatory conditions and immunosuppressive therapy in a monocentric cohort. *Ann. Rheum. Dis.* **2021**, *80*, 1306–1311. [CrossRef] [PubMed]
3. Simon, D.; Tascilar, K.; Fagni, F.; Kleyer, A.; Krönke, G.; Meder, C.; Dietrich, P.; Orlemann, T.; Mößner, J.; Taubmann, J.; et al. Intensity and longevity of SARS-CoV-2 vaccination response in patients with immune-mediated inflammatory disease: A prospective cohort study. *Lancet Rheumatol.* **2022**, *4*, e614–e625. [CrossRef] [PubMed]
4. Moutsopoulos, H.M. A recommended paradigm for vaccination of rheumatic disease patients with the SARS-CoV-2 vaccine. *J. Autoimmun.* **2021**, *121*, 102649. [CrossRef] [PubMed]
5. Rodríguez, Y.; Novelli, L.; Rojas, M.; De Santis, M.; Acosta-Ampudia, Y.; Monsalve, D.M.; Ramírez-Santana, C.; Costanzo, A.; Ridgway, W.M.; Ansari, A.A.; et al. Autoinflammatory and autoimmune conditions at the crossroad of COVID-19. *J Autoimmun.* **2020**, *114*, 102506. [CrossRef] [PubMed]
6. Dahms, K.; Mikolajewska, A.; Ansems, K.; Metzendorf, M.I.; Benstoem, C.; Stegemann, M. Anakinra for the treatment of COVID-19 patients: A systematic review and meta-analysis. *Eur. J. Med. Res.* **2023**, *28*, 100. [CrossRef] [PubMed]
7. Mikolajewska, A.; Fischer, A.L.; Piechotta, V.; Mueller, A.; Metzendorf, M.I.; Becker, M.; Dorando, E.; Pacheco, R.L.; Martimbianco, A.L.C.; Riera, R.; et al. Colchicine for the treatment of COVID-19. *Emergencias* **2023**, *35*, 300–302. [PubMed]
8. Bourguiba, R.; Kyheng, M.; Koné-Paut, I.; Rouzaud, D.; Avouac, J.; Devaux, M.; Abdallah, N.A.; Fautrel, B.; Ferreira-Maldent, N.; Langlois, V.; et al. COVID-19 infection among patients with autoinflammatory diseases: A study on 117 French patients compared with 1545 from the French RMD COVID-19 cohort: COVIMAI—The French cohort study of SARS-CoV-2 infection in patient with systemic autoinflammatory diseases. *RMD Open* **2022**, *8*, e002063. [PubMed]
9. Bindoli, S.; Baggio, C.; Galozzi, P.; Vesentini, F.; Doria, A.; Cosma, C.; Padoan, A.; Sfriso, P. Autoinflammatory Diseases and COVID-19 Vaccination: Analysis of SARS-CoV-2 Anti-S-RBD IgG Levels in a Cohort of Patients Receiving IL-1 Inhibitors. *J. Clin. Med.* **2023**, *12*, 4741. [CrossRef] [PubMed]
10. Ruddy, J.A.; Connolly, C.M.; Boyarsky, B.J.; Werbel, W.A.; Christopher-Stine, L.; Garonzik-Wang, J.; Segev, D.L.; Paik, J.J. High antibody response to two-dose SARS-CoV-2 messenger RNA vaccination in patients with rheumatic and musculoskeletal diseases. *Ann. Rheum. Dis.* **2021**, *80*, 1351–1352. [CrossRef] [PubMed]
11. Shechtman, L.; Lahad, K.; Livneh, A.; Grossman, C.; Druyan, A.; Giat, E.; Lidar, M.; Freund, S.; Manor, U.; Pomerantz, A.; et al. Safety of the BNT162b2 mRNA COVID-19 vaccine in patients with familial Mediterranean fever. *Rheumatology* **2022**, *61*, SI129–SI135. [CrossRef] [PubMed]

Journal of
Clinical Medicine

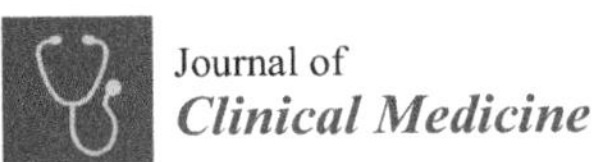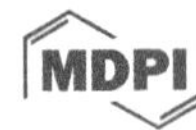

Case Report

Intracardiac Thrombi in Morbus Adamantiades–Behçet in Two Swedish Patients

Raffaele Da Mutten [1], Alexander Borg [1,2], Katerina Chatzidionysiou [1,2] and Ioannis Parodis [1,2,3,*]

[1] Division of Rheumatology, Department of Medicine Solna, Karolinska Institutet, 17176 Stockholm, Sweden; raffaele.damutten@uzh.ch (R.D.M.); alexander.borg@ki.se (A.B.); aikaterini.chatzidionysiou@ki.se (K.C.)

[2] Department of Gastroenterology, Dermatology and Rheumatology, Karolinska University Hospital, 17176 Stockholm, Sweden

[3] Department of Rheumatology, Faculty of Medicine and Health, Örebro University, 70182 Örebro, Sweden

* Correspondence: ioannis.parodis@ki.se; Tel.: +46-722321322

Abstract: Morbus Adamantiades–Behçet (MAB) is an inflammatory disease typically manifesting with oral and genital aphthosis, erythema nodosum, and vasculopathy, and in only around 2%, cardiac involvement. Its prevalence is usually higher along the historic Silk Road, but rarer in Scandinavia where 0.64–4.9 in 100,000 people are affected. We herein present two Swedish patients with cardiac manifestations of Morbus Adamantiades–Behçet. Along with the intracardial thrombi, which both patients presented with, one patient also had cerebrovascular insults leading to visual field deficits as well as involvement of peripheral nerves. Being of Scandinavian origin and showing uncommon symptoms as their initial manifestations of MAB, the 62- and 35-year-old patients presenting herein constitute rare cases.

Keywords: Morbus Adamantiades–Behçet; intracardiac thrombus; rheumatology; autoinflammation

Citation: Da Mutten, R.; Borg, A.; Chatzidionysiou, K.; Parodis, I. Intracardiac Thrombi in Morbus Adamantiades–Behçet in Two Swedish Patients. *J. Clin. Med.* **2023**, *12*, 5377. https://doi.org/10.3390/jcm12165377

Academic Editor: Eugen Feist

Received: 31 July 2023
Revised: 17 August 2023
Accepted: 17 August 2023
Published: 18 August 2023

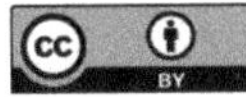

1. Introduction

Morbus Behçet, also known as Morbus Adamantiades–Behçet (MAB), is an inflammatory disease classified as systemic vasculitis [1]. Pathogenetic models that have been proposed include a genetic predisposition that is triggered by infections [1]. Mainly, the Human Leukocyte Antigen (HLA)-B51 allele in the major histocompatibility complex (MHC) is associated with MAB. Also, the prevalence of the disease is considerably more prominent in regions along the historic Silk Road compared with the rest of the world [2,3]. Hence, the occurrence in Scandinavia is rather low with a prevalence ranging from 0.64 to 4.9 in 100,000 people [1,4]. Two relevant sets of criteria have mainly been used. First, the International Study Group criteria were introduced in 1990, showing 91% sensitivity and 96% specificity [5]. In 2014, the International Criteria for Adamantiades–Behçet's Disease were established [3]. None of these criteria sets include cardiac manifestations as the latter are atypical. Only 2.1% of patients have cardiac symptoms as a first sign [6]. The occurrence of symptoms usually includes oral aphthosis, genital aphthosis, erythema nodosum, and, in 19%, vascular manifestations [3,7,8]. Peripheral nerves may be involved over the course of the disease in only 4.9% of the patients, and the heart in roughly 6% [3,6].

Owing to the rarity of the disease in northern Europe and the even more uncommon presentation with heart involvement at the initial encounter with healthcare, we herein present two Swedish patients diagnosed with MAB who presented with heart involvement among the initial symptoms.

2. Case One

We present a 62-year-old man from central Sweden who sought care due to general muscular weakness, weight loss, and increased sweating. The patient had been a smoker for fifteen years but had quit a decade ago, and his medical history was unremarkable apart from asthma, benign prostatic hyperplasia, and surgically treated bilateral carpal tunnel syndrome. After the initial workup showing no signs of malignancy and excluding an infection but showing a significantly elevated erythrocyte sedimentation rate (ESR) and C-reactive protein (CRP), he was treated with prednisolone at a daily dose of 40 mg initially which was later tapered to 20 mg daily. Consequently, the inflammatory markers dropped. One month later, he presented again with a cough and dyspnea on slight exertion. Referred to expert care, he presented with white sputum, Raynaud's phenomenon, muscle weakness, and a loss of vision of the right eye. His legs and feet showed red-purple erythema, indicating a vasculopathy, as illustrated in Figure 1. He also complained of pain in both feet combined with a dorsal extension deficit of the left foot.

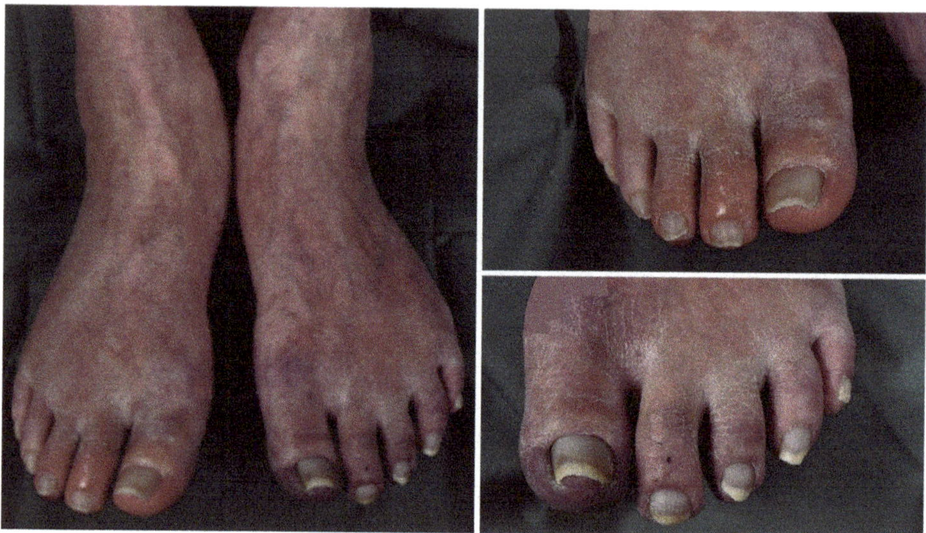

Figure 1. Photographs of case one illustrating signs of vasculopathy.

The neurological evaluation showed no signs of amyotrophic lateral sclerosis and the examination of the cerebrospinal fluid obtained by lumbar puncture was unremarkable. An electroneurography showed a pronounced sensorimotor axonal polyneuropathy. Electromyographically, myopathic changes were detected at multiple sites and the palsy of the left foot was confirmed. A biopsy of the muscle showed no inflammatory cell infiltrates or vasculitis in the small vessels but hints of neurogenic damage. Computed tomography (CT) and later 18F-fluorodesoxyglucose-Positron Emission Tomography-CT (PET-CT) of the thorax as well as a bronchoscopy showed a $CD4^+/CD8^+$ ratio of 1.5 and no signs of malignancy. Hence, pneumonia and sarcoidosis were deemed unlikely. Further, echocardiography showed an ejection fraction of 11%, general hypokinesia, and a thrombus near the apex measuring 10×15 mm.

Ocular diagnostics showed a homonymous right-sided hemianopsia with no signs of intraocular inflammation; it is worth noting that the patient had been under glucocorticoid treatment for several months. The criteria for MAB describe ocular lesions as either anterior uveitis, posterior uveitis, or retinal vasculitis [3]. To this end, it is important to mention that it remains highly unclear what the initial ocular involvement might have been. Possibly, before the treatment with glucocorticoids, there might have been an inflammatory component in the patient's visual impairment, consistent with the ocular items described in the criteria for MAB. A CT and magnetic resonance imaging (MRI) of the head and neck showed multiple relatively recent left occipital infarctions explaining the loss of vision. Medial and posterior territories showed narrowed lumens, likely due to inflammatory or atherosclerotic factors. To prevent further cerebrovascular insults, dalteparin, which was later substituted with a vitamin K antagonist, and acetylsalicylic acid were initiated.

Antinuclear antibodies (ANA), anti-neutrophil cytoplasmatic antibodies (ANCA), cryoglobulins, antiphospholipid antibodies, autoantibodies related to neurological disease, autoantibodies for myositis diagnostics, complement levels, and creatin kinase were unremarkable. Hence, various common rheumatic diseases including systemic lupus erythematosus were deemed unlikely. Hepatitis and tuberculosis were also ruled out by serology and quantiferon testing.

The clinical picture initially brought to mind a vasculitis, and differential diagnoses included polyarteritis nodosa (PAN). On average, 74% of patients with PAN show peripheral neuropathy and 4–30% show cardiac involvement [9]. After the full diagnostic workup and during the patient's stay in the inpatient ward, aphthous ulcers in the oral cavity were observed; this was a new symptom for the patient. Later, genetic diagnostics revealed that the patient had the human leukocyte antigen (HLA)-B51 allele. Together with neurological manifestations as well as vascular involvement, resulting in four points in the International Criteria for Behçet's Disease, the diagnosis MAB with neurological involvement was made [3]. Assuming that ocular involvement might have been a part of the patient's MAB, accounting for this would yield six points in the criteria set. The patient was subsequently initiated on colchicine and methotrexate, and the anticoagulant therapy was continued.

3. Case Two

The second patient was a 35-year-old male, also from central Sweden, who presented with fever, cough, sweating at night, a 3 kg weight loss over the past weeks, and fatigue. Three years before, he had been investigated for erythema nodosum. Yet, no clear etiology was found. One year before, he had repeated episodes of epididymitis, with negative cultures. During the previous winter, the patient had experienced repeated febrile episodes that had been evaluated to be tonsillitides.

At the infectious diseases department, a chest X-ray showed basal infiltrates in the left lung. Inflammatory markers were elevated with a CRP of 110 mg/L and leukocytes of 12×10^9 cells/L. Since urinalysis, virological testing, and four blood cultures did not reveal a pathogen, and antibiotic treatment over the past month had not improved the patient's condition, infectious etiology was becoming unlikely. As the clinical picture did not resemble sarcoidosis, the working diagnosis was an undifferentiated yet systemic inflammatory disease.

During investigation, a murmur was heard during heart auscultation, and echocardiography showed vegetations on the mitral and bicuspid valves. Further, an MRI and transesophageal echocardiography were performed. These revealed a pulmonary embolism as well as an intracardiac thrombus of 4.7 mm in diameter (Figure 2). Using computer tomography, splenomegaly and suspected infarction of the right kidney were ascertained.

Upon suspicion of autoimmune endocarditis, oral treatment with prednisolone was initiated, with good results. Moreover, subcutaneous dalteparin was initiated for the thrombi.

Upon further investigation, oral and genital ulcers were described by the patient since childhood, at least six times a year. Genetic testing revealed the presence of HLA-B51. Together with history of pulmonary embolism, renal infarction, intracardial thrombosis, and erythema nodosum, the diagnosis of MAB was ascertained. The high and acute inflammatory activity at presentation and the recurrent epididymitis strengthened the suspicion. Oral and genital ulcers, vascular manifestations, and skin lesions, together give six points in the International Criteria for Behçet's disease [3].

The glucocorticoids were gradually reduced and discontinued after eight months, while azathioprine and an anti-TNF agent were initiated. Dalteparin was also changed to a vitamin K antagonist, i.e., warfarin. After one year, warfarin was discontinued since a follow-up MRI of the heart showed that the vegetations had resolved. After two years, the anti-TNF agent was also discontinued due to clinical remission.

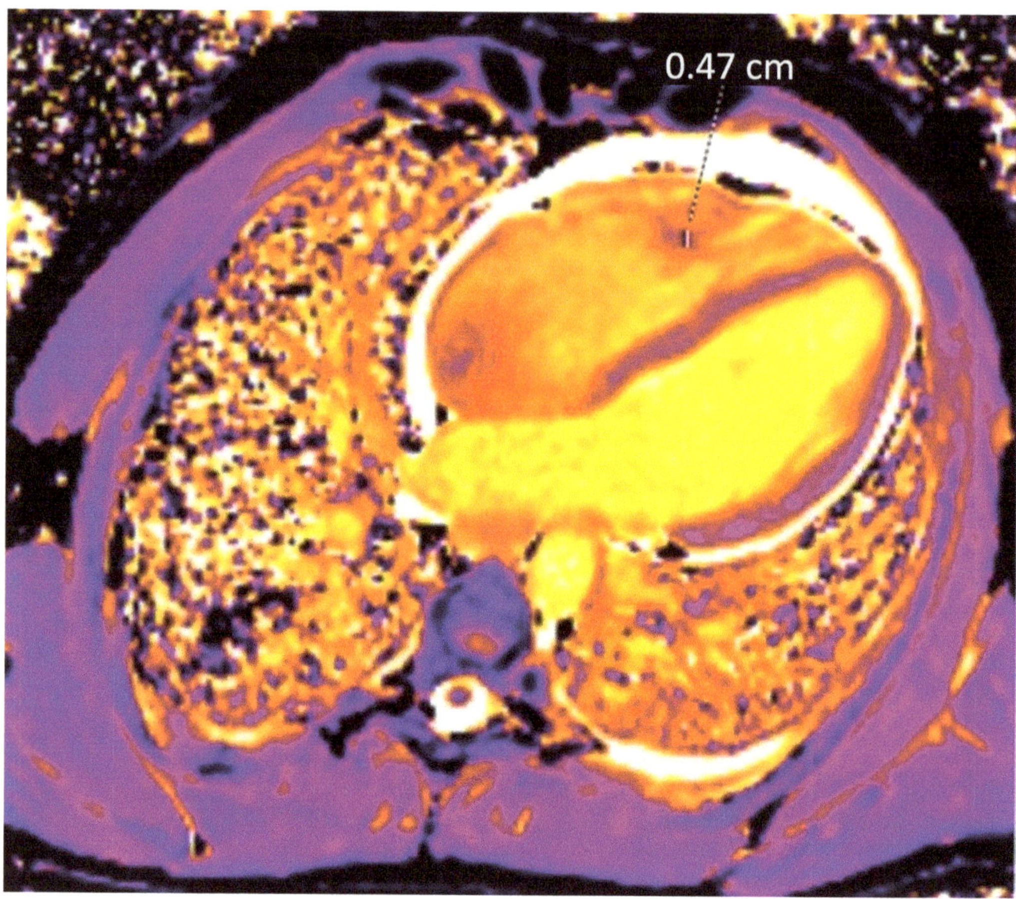

Figure 2. MRI of the heart visualizing a thrombus in the right ventricle.

4. Discussion

4.1. Clinical Presentation

We herein presented two cases of MAB with uncommon initial presentations. The starting point was, in both cases, an unclear inflammatory condition that was treated with glucocorticoids and later referred to the Rheumatology Department. Yet, it took time to arrive at a clear diagnosis. Partially, this could be due to the low probability of MAB since both patients were not from the Silk Road territory [2]. Also, the presentation with coagulopathy and cardiac involvement is not common. Altogether, this made for a very rare constellation.

Usually, symptoms leading to diagnosis are oral (98%) and genital (74%) aphthosis, as well as erythema nodosum (32%) [3]. Large vein thrombosis, epididymitis, and cardiac manifestations constitute less common complications. However, they still are accounted for more often compared to control patients having at least one major MAB sign of a MAB-mimicking disease. The distribution of cardiac involvement in MAB based on a previously reported series of 52 cases [6] is summarized in Table 1.

Table 1. Cardiac involvement in MAB, based on a series of 52 patients [6].

Type of Cardiac Involvement	Frequency, No. (%)
Pericarditis	20 (38.5)
Valvular pathology *	14 (26.9)
Intracardiac thrombosis	10 (19.2)
Myocardial infarction	9 (17.3)
Endomyocardial fibrosis	4 (7.7)
Abnormal ECG findings	31 (59.6)

Data based on a series of 52 patients, reported elsewhere [6]. * Including aortic valve insufficiency, mitral valve insufficiency, tricuspid valve insufficiency, mitral valve prolapse, pulmonary valve prolapse, and multiple endocardial involvement. ECG: electrocardiogram; MAB: Morbus Adamantiades–Behçet.

The first patient showed oral aphthosis, neurological manifestations, and vascular involvement, resulting in four points in the International Criteria for Behçet's Disease, or six points if the ocular lesions are accounted for [3]. The second patient presented with oral and genital aphthosis, vascular manifestations, and skin lesions, which sums up to six points [3]. Hence, in both cases, the diagnostic criteria were met. Importantly, extensive investigations were carried out in both cases, during which multiple alternative explanations and mimickers were ruled out, including infectious diseases. Non-bacterial endocarditis, which upon deposition of sterile fibrin and platelets, can result in non-bacterial thrombotic endocarditis, which may be considered a manifestation of MAB, and could have may have been part of the problem in the second case [10–13].

In a meta-analysis, HLA-B51-positive individuals had a 6-fold higher chance of developing MAB compared with HLA-B51-negative individuals, whereas HLA-B27 positivity also increased the probability of being diagnosed with the disease by almost 2 times [14]. In northern Sweden, the prevalence of HLA-B27-positive individuals is estimated to be 16.6% [15]. Ek et al. [16] stated in a case series of twelve patients in 1993 that only one patient with the HLA-B5 genotype, of which HLA-B51 is a subclass, was not an immigrant [17]. Importantly, the two patients presented herein had no immigration background.

While the Swedish heritage of our patients delayed the diagnostic procedure, these cases emphasize that the disease can also occur in people outside the Silk Road territory, which should not be neglected when patients present with fitting symptoms. Apart from genetic polymorphisms in HLA-B51, interleukin (IL)-10 and IL-10 receptor (IL-10R) have been discussed as factors that may have a role in the pathogenesis of the disease, as have viral and bacterial infections, molecular mimicry, Th1 and Th17 regulation, IL-17, IL-21, IL-23, and endothelial dysfunction [18]. Whether these factors contribute to the disorder that is more or less dependent on heritage or environmental factors has yet to be elucidated.

4.2. Therapy

The 2018 EULAR treatment recommendations suggest both anticoagulant and anti-inflammatory treatment in the case of recurrent deep vein thrombosis, provided that the risk for bleeding is low and pulmonary artery aneurysm is ruled out. However, there is no particular mention of intracardiac thrombosis [19].

Inflammation and coagulopathy are likely linked in MAB [20,21]. An important mechanism seems to be the perivascular neutrophils that facilitate inflammation. Hence, anti-inflammatory treatment is at least equally important as anticoagulation therapy. In fact, a retrospective study of 37 patients has shown that anti-inflammation and anticoagulation treatment combined showed no additional benefit compared with anti-inflammation treatment alone [22]. Furthermore, anticoagulation treatment has, in some cases, been shown to increase the risk of pulmonary artery aneurysm [23].

Eight cases with intracardiac thrombus responded well to glucocorticoids and immunosuppression with either azathioprine or cyclophosphamide, resulting in a resolution of the thrombus and clinical remission in five of those cases [24]. Even though the coagulopathy and cardiac involvement can be treated in many cases, MAB patients with manifestations from the cardiovascular system are characterized by a higher morbidity burden and mortality than those without, and an overall poorer prognosis [6].

In a questionnaire, most American and Israeli rheumatologists as well as about two-thirds of rheumatologists practicing in Turkey, a country among those with the highest prevalence of the disease, stated that they would start immediately with anticoagulation in the case of intracardiac thrombosis [25].

As a matter of fact, with the disease being at the intersections of autoinflammation, autoimmunity, and coagulopathy, therapeutic choices have to be made with caution and desirably by experts.

5. Conclusions

We presented two cases of intracardiac thrombosis in patients with Morbus Adamantiades–Behçet, both of them of a Swedish background. A question that arises is whether the incidence of such cases in Nordic countries is currently underreported due to lack of awareness. Surely, in case of an unclear inflammatory condition along with coagulopathy, MAB should be thought of, especially in the absence of other better fitting diagnoses, and prompt relevant genetic investigation. In terms of therapy, a combination of anti-inflammation and anticoagulation may be needed, with the balance between these two compartments of the therapy being, in several cases, delicate.

Author Contributions: Conceptualization, K.C. and I.P.; methodology, I.P.; software, R.D.M.; resources, I.P.; data curation, R.D.M. and A.B.; writing—original draft preparation, R.D.M.; writing—review and editing, R.D.M., A.B., K.C. and I.P.; visualization, R.D.M.; supervision, K.C. and I.P.; project administration, A.B. and I.P.; funding acquisition, I.P. All authors have read and agreed to the published version of the manuscript.

Funding: This work was funded by the Swedish Rheumatism Association, grant number R-969696; King Gustaf V's 80-year Foundation, grant number FAI-2020-0741; Swedish Society of Medicine, grant number SLS-974449; Nyckelfonden, grant number OLL-974804; Professor Nanna Svartz Foundation, grant number 2021-00436; Ulla and Roland Gustafsson Foundation, grant number 2021-26; Region Stockholm, grant number FoUI-955483; and Karolinska Institutet.

Institutional Review Board Statement: Not applicable.

Informed Consent Statement: Written informed consent has been obtained from the patients to publish this paper.

Data Availability Statement: Not applicable.

Acknowledgments: The authors express gratitude to the patients for allowing us to publish their cases.

Conflicts of Interest: I.P. has received research funding and/or honoraria from Amgen, AstraZeneca, Aurinia Pharmaceuticals, Elli Lilly, Gilead, GlaxoSmithKline, Janssen, Novartis, Otsuka, and Roche. The other authors declare that they have no conflict of interest related to this work. The funders had no role in the design of the study, the analyses or interpretation of data, or the writing of the manuscript.

References

1. Tong, B.; Liu, X.; Xiao, J.; Su, G. Immunopathogenesis of Behcet's Disease. *Front. Immunol.* **2019**, *10*, 665. [CrossRef] [PubMed]
2. Davatchi, F.; Chams-Davatchi, C.; Shams, H.; Shahram, F.; Nadji, A.; Akhlaghi, M.; Faezi, T.; Ghodsi, Z.; Sadeghi Abdollahi, B.; Ashofteh, F.; et al. Behcet's Disease: Epidemiology, Clinical Manifestations, and Diagnosis. *Expert Rev. Clin. Immunol.* **2017**, *13*, 57–65. [CrossRef]
3. International Team for the Revision of the International Criteria for Behçet's Disease (ITR-ICBD); Davatchi, F.; Assaad-Khalil, S.; Calamia, K.T.; Crook, J.E.; Sadeghi-Abdollahi, B.; Schirmer, M.; Tzellos, T.; Zouboulis, C.C.; Akhlagi, M.; et al. The International Criteria for Behçet's Disease (ICBD): A Collaborative Study of 27 Countries on the Sensitivity and Specificity of the New Criteria. *J. Eur. Acad. Dermatol. Venereol.* **2014**, *28*, 338–347. [CrossRef]
4. Mohammad, A.; Mandl, T.; Sturfelt, G.; Segelmark, M. Incidence, Prevalence and Clinical Characteristics of Behcet's Disease in Southern Sweden. *Rheumatology* **2013**, *52*, 304–310. [CrossRef] [PubMed]
5. Criteria for Diagnosis of Behçet's Disease. International Study Group for Behçet's Disease. *Lancet* **1990**, *335*, 1078–1080.

6.   Geri, G.; Wechsler, B.; Thi Huong, D.L.; Isnard, R.; Piette, J.-C.; Amoura, Z.; Resche-Rigon, M.; Cacoub, P.; Saadoun, D. Spectrum of Cardiac Lesions in Behçet Disease: A Series of 52 Patients and Review of the Literature. *Medicine* **2012**, *91*, 25–34. [CrossRef]

7.   Ideguchi, H.; Suda, A.; Takeno, M.; Ueda, A.; Ohno, S.; Ishigatsubo, Y. Characteristics of Vascular Involvement in Behçet's Disease in Japan: A Retrospective Cohort Study. *Clin. Exp. Rheumatol.* **2011**, *29*, S47–S53.

8.   Chen, Y.; Cai, J.-F.; Lin, C.-H.; Guan, J.-L. Demography of Vascular Behcet's Disease with Different Gender and Age: An Investigation with 166 Chinese Patients. *Orphanet J. Rare Dis.* **2019**, *14*, 88. [CrossRef]

9.   Hernández-Rodríguez, J.; Alba, M.A.; Prieto-González, S.; Cid, M.C. Diagnosis and Classification of Polyarteritis Nodosa. *J. Autoimmun.* **2014**, *48–49*, 84–89. [CrossRef]

10.   Mazzoni, C.; Scheggi, V.; Mariani, T. Cardiac Involvement in Behçet Disease Presenting as Non-Bacterial Thrombotic Endocarditis: A Case Report. *J. Cardiol. Cases* **2021**, *24*, 157–160. [CrossRef]

11.   Kang, H.M.; Kim, G.B.; Jang, W.-S.; Kwon, B.S.; Bae, E.J.; Noh, C.I.; Choi, J.Y.; Kim, Y.J. An Adolescent with Aortic Regurgitation Caused by Behçet's Disease Mimicking Endocarditis. *Ann. Thorac. Surg.* **2013**, *95*, e147–e149. [CrossRef] [PubMed]

12.   Lee, H.S.; Choi, W.S.; Kim, K.H.; Kang, J.K.; Kim, N.Y.; Park, S.H.; Park, Y.; Nam, E.J.; Yang, D.H.; Park, H.S.; et al. Aseptic Endocarditis in Behçet's Disease Presenting as Tricuspid Valve Stenosis. *Korean Circ. J.* **2011**, *41*, 399. [CrossRef]

13.   Nassenstein, K.; Deluigi, C.C.; Afube, T.; Schaaf, B.; Lorenzen, J.; Bruder, O. Nonbacterial Endocarditis Presenting as a Right Ventricular Tumor in Assumed Behçet's Disease. *Herz* **2015**, *40*, 225–227. [CrossRef] [PubMed]

14.   Khabbazi, A.; Vahedi, L.; Ghojazadeh, M.; Pashazadeh, F.; Khameneh, A. Association of HLA-B27 and Behcet's Disease: A Systematic Review and Meta-Analysis. *Autoimmun. Highlights* **2019**, *10*, 2. [CrossRef] [PubMed]

15.   Bjelle, A.; Cedergren, B.; Rantapää Dahlqvist, S. HLA B 27 in the Population of Northern Sweden. *Scand. J. Rheumatol.* **1982**, *11*, 23–26. [CrossRef] [PubMed]

16.   Ek, L.; Hedfors, E. Behçet's Disease: A Review and a Report of 12 Cases from Sweden. *Acta Derm. Venereol.* **1993**, *73*, 251–254. [CrossRef]

17.   Shenavandeh, S.; Jahanshahi, K.A.; Aflaki, E.; Tavassoli, A. Frequency of HLA-B5, HLA-B51 and HLA-B27 in Patients with Idiopathic Uveitis and Behçet's Disease: A Case-Control Study. *Rheumatology* **2018**, *56*, 67–72. [CrossRef]

18.   Pineton de Chambrun, M.; Wechsler, B.; Geri, G.; Cacoub, P.; Saadoun, D. New Insights into the Pathogenesis of Behçet's Disease. *Autoimmun. Rev.* **2012**, *11*, 687–698. [CrossRef]

19.   Hatemi, G.; Christensen, R.; Bang, D.; Bodaghi, B.; Celik, A.F.; Fortune, F.; Gaudric, J.; Gul, A.; Kötter, I.; Leccese, P.; et al. 2018 Update of the EULAR Recommendations for the Management of Behçet's Syndrome. *Ann. Rheum. Dis.* **2018**, *77*, 808–818. [CrossRef]

20.   Keser, G. Inflammation-Induced Thrombosis: Mechanisms, Disease Associations and Management. *Curr. Pharm. Des.* **2012**, *18*, 1478–1493. [CrossRef]

21.   Emmi, G.; Silvestri, E.; Squatrito, D.; Amedei, A.; Niccolai, E.; D'Elios, M.M.; Della Bella, C.; Grassi, A.; Becatti, M.; Fiorillo, C.; et al. Thrombosis in Vasculitis: From Pathogenesis to Treatment. *Thromb. J.* **2015**, *13*, 15. [CrossRef] [PubMed]

22.   Ahn, J.K.; Lee, Y.S.; Jeon, C.H.; Koh, E.-M.; Cha, H.-S. Treatment of Venous Thrombosis Associated with Behcet's Disease: Immunosuppressive Therapy Alone versus Immunosuppressive Therapy plus Anticoagulation. *Clin. Rheumatol.* **2008**, *27*, 201–205. [CrossRef] [PubMed]

23.   Uzun, O.; Akpolat, T.; Erkan, L. Pulmonary Vasculitis in Behçet Disease. *Chest* **2005**, *127*, 2243–2253. [CrossRef] [PubMed]

24.   Ben Ghorbel, I.; Belfeki, N.; Houman, M.H. Intracardiac Thrombus in Behçet's Disease. *Reumatismo* **2016**, *68*, 148–153. [CrossRef] [PubMed]

25.   Tayer-Shifman, O.E.; Seyahi, E.; Nowatzky, J.; Ben-Chetrit, E. Major Vessel Thrombosis in Behçet's Disease: The Dilemma of Anticoagulant Therapy—The Approach of Rheumatologists from Different Countries. *Clin. Exp. Rheumatol.* **2012**, *30*, 735–740.

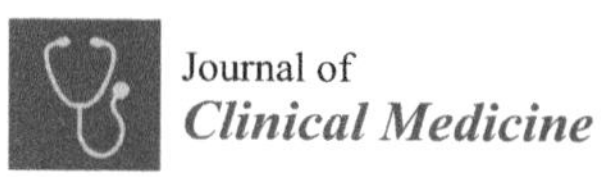

Journal of
Clinical Medicine

MDPI

Article

Optimized Treatment of Interleukin (IL-1)-Mediated Autoinflammatory Diseases: Impact of Disease Activity-Based Treatment Adjustments

Tatjana Welzel [1,2,3,†], Beate Zapf [3,†], Jens Klotsche [4], Özlem Satirer [3], Susanne M. Benseler [5,6,‡] and Jasmin B. Kuemmerle-Deschner [3,*,‡]

[1] Pediatric Rheumatology, University Children's Hospital Basel, University of Basel, 4031 Basel, Switzerland
[2] Pediatric Research Centre, University Children's Hospital Basel, University of Basel, 4031 Basel, Switzerland
[3] Division of Pediatric Rheumatology, Department of Pediatrics, autoinflammatory reference centre Tuebingen, University Hospital Tuebingen, 72076 Tuebingen, Germany
[4] German Rheumatism Research Centre Berlin, 10117 Berlin, Germany
[5] Pediatric Rheumatology, Department of Paediatrics, Alberta Children's Hospital, Cumming School of Medicine, University of Calgary, Calgary, AB T2N 4N1, Canada; susanne.benseler@ahs.ca
[6] Children's Health Ireland (CHI), D01 R5P3 Dublin, Ireland
*   Correspondence: kuemmerle.deschner@uni-tuebingen.de
[†] These authors contributed equally to this work and should therefore be considered co-first authors.
[‡] These authors contributed equally to this work and should therefore be considered co-senior authors.

Abstract: Background: Effective control of disease activity in Interleukin-1 autoinflammatory diseases (IL-1 AID) is crucial to prevent damage. The aim was to longitudinally analyze the impact of protocolized disease activity-based treatment adjustments in a real-life cohort. **Methods:** A single-center study of consecutive children with IL-1 AID followed between January 2016 and December 2019 was performed. Demographics, phenotypes, genotypes, inflammatory markers, physician (PGA), and patient/parent (PPGA) global assessment were captured. Disease activity and treatment changes were assessed. The impact of distinct parameters on disease activity trajectories was analyzed. **Results:** A total of 56 children were included, median follow-up was 2.1 years reflecting 361 visits. Familial Mediterranean Fever was the most common IL-1 AID. At the first visit, 68% of the patients had moderate/severe disease activity. Disease activity-based treatment adjustments were required in 28/56 children (50%). At last follow-up, 79% had a well-controlled disease. Both PGA and PPGA decreased significantly over time ($p < 0.001$; $p < 0.017$, respectively), however, both differed statistically at last visit ($p < 0.001$). Only PGA showed a significant estimated mean decrease across all IL-1 AID over time. **Conclusions:** Disease activity-based treatment adjustments can effectively refine treat-to-target strategies, enable personalized precision health approaches, and improve outcomes in children with IL-1 AID.

Keywords: autoinflammatory disease; FMF; CAPS; TRAPS; remission; personalized medicine; effectiveness; exposure–response; outcome; monitoring

Citation: Welzel, T.; Zapf, B.; Klotsche, J.; Satirer, Ö.; Benseler, S.M.; Kuemmerle-Deschner, J.B. Optimized Treatment of Interleukin (IL-1)-Mediated Autoinflammatory Diseases: Impact of Disease Activity-Based Treatment Adjustments. *J. Clin. Med.* **2024**, *13*, 2319. https://doi.org/10.3390/jcm13082319

Academic Editor: Eugen Feist

Received: 16 March 2024
Revised: 7 April 2024
Accepted: 8 April 2024
Published: 17 April 2024

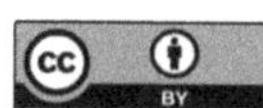

1. Introduction

Interleukin-1-mediated autoinflammatory diseases (IL-1 AID) are caused by pathogenic gene variants encoding the inflammasome, resulting in excessive release of (pro-) inflammatory cytokines [1]. Clinical characteristics of active IL-1 AID include recurrent fever, inflammation of the central nervous system, eyes, skin, serous membrane, and the musculoskeletal system, typically paired with elevated laboratory inflammatory parameters [2]. Although awareness has increased in the past years, several patients face a long journey until being diagnosed or treated [3,4]. Uncontrolled disease activity can result in organ damage, disability, reduced health-related quality of life (HRQoL), school and work absenteeism, and increased risk of mortality [5–7]. Furthermore, both the patient and the entire family carry a significant psychological burden. Therefore, effective treatment with the achievement of no or as mild as possible disease activity is essential after diagnosis is made.

The approval of effective treatment for IL-1 AID and treatment recommendations, along with the availability of disease activity monitoring parameters, such as the autoinflammatory disease activity index (AIDAI), autoinflammatory disease damage index (ADDI), the physician global assessment (PGA), and the patient/parent global assessment (PPGA), as well as specific laboratory inflammatory makers have significantly improved the patients' management [8–13]. Based on the growing evidence of a relationship between disease activity, drug exposure, and treatment response in inflammatory diseases, the AID management should take personalized treatment approaches and disease activity-based treatment adjustments into account.

Disease activity-based treatment adjustments, also known as the treat-to-target (T2T) strategy, contain regular disease activity monitoring in a patient and disease activity-based treatment adjustments to achieve the desired target of no or mild disease activity [14]. T2T strategies were originally developed for optimized treatment in patients with rheumatoid arthritis and have been adopted for the management of several other chronic diseases [15].

Recently, T2T strategies for IL-1 AID were published [16–18]. However, longitudinal real-life data of disease activity-based treatment adjustments and their impact on IL-1 AID in childhood is scarce. In addition, data on disease activity parameters or the most promising composite measures after established treatment to monitor disease activity in IL-1 AID are needed.

Therefore, the objectives of this study were (i) to longitudinally assess the disease activity of children and adolescents with different IL-1 AID diagnoses, (ii) to analyze the individually performed disease activity-based treatment adjustments and their response, and (iii) to evaluate the impact of distinct parameters on disease activity trajectories/changes.

2. Materials and Methods

This was a single-center study assessing disease activity and disease activity-based treatment adjustments in children and adolescents with IL-1 AID between 1 January 2016 and 31 December 2019. Pediatric patients aged ≤18 years diagnosed with cryopyrin-associated periodic syndromes (CAPS), tumor necrosis factor-associated periodic syndrome (TRAPS), the mevalonate kinase deficiency (MKD), and the Familial Mediterranean Fever (FMF) were included if they fulfilled AID classification criteria [19], or in the case of FMF and CAPS, met either the classification and/or the diagnostic criteria [19–21]. Children and adolescents cared for less than one year or those with fewer than three routine visits during the study period were excluded. Data were captured in the designated, institutional web-based Arthritis and Rheumatism Database and Information System (ARDIS, ARDIS2, axaris software & systeme GmbH, 89160 Dornstadt, Germany). Data analysis was performed pseudonymized. Ethics approval was obtained from the ethics committee of Karl Eberhard University Tuebingen (050/2021BO2).

2.1. Patient Related Data

Demographic data included clinical AID diagnosis, sex, age at symptom onset, and diagnosis, as well as follow-up time. Furthermore, for those patients with genetic testing, the genotype was recorded. The genotypes were classified as pathogenic, likely pathogenic, variants of unknown significance (VUS), likely benign, or benign according to the American College of Medical Genetics and Genomics and Infevers [22–24]. In addition, the treatment of interest was recorded and included colchicine or one of the following biological Disease-Modifying AntiRheumatic Drugs (bDMARD): IL-1 inhibition, IL-6 inhibition, and/or TNF-α inhibition. In each visit, disease activity and information on the treatment regimen (absolute dose and body weight-based dose, frequency/administration interval, and admission route) were captured. Data collection was performed for each patient at the following visits: (i) the first visit in the study period, (ii) follow-up visits, defined as routine visits every 3 to 6 months during the study period, and (iii) the last study visit, defined as the last documented routine visit before study end.

2.2. Treatment Regimen and Definitions

The treatment regimen was compared intra-individually between the visits. Treatment escalations were categorized as (i) treatment start, (ii) treatment switch, (iii) dose increase, and (iv) administration frequency increase. Treatment start was defined as treatment initiation of colchicine or bDMARDs in a former treatment-naïve IL-1 AID patient. Treatment switch was defined as a switch from colchicine to a bDMARD, switch between different bDMARDs or an add-on drug, e.g., bDMARD treatment added on colchicine maintenance treatment between study visits. Dose increase was defined as an increase in absolute colchicine dose (mg) or an increase in mg/kg bDMARDs dosages in children between study visits. Administration frequency increase was defined as a shortening of the administration interval for bDMARDs between study visits, e.g., anakinra administration twice daily instead of once daily or canakinumab administration switching from eight weekly (q8w) to four weekly (q4w).

2.3. Definition of Disease Activity

In accordance with published studies, the physician global assessment (PGA) was used for the physician's perspective recorded on a 10 cm visual analog scale (VAS), with 0 representing no and 10 maximum disease activity. The patient/parent perspective was captured through the patient/parent global assessment (PPGA) and was recorded on the 10 cm VAS, with 0 representing no and 10 maximum disease activity. Furthermore, inflammatory markers were captured, including C-reactive Protein (CRP) and Serum Amyloid A (SAA) [16,25–27]. Disease activity categories were: (i) mild, if PGA $\leq$ 2 cm plus CRP < 1.5 mg/dL and/or SAA levels < 30 mg/L; (ii) moderate, if PGA > 2–5 cm plus CRP 1.5 < 2.5 mg/dL and/or SAA $\geq$ 30 < 50 mg/L; and (iii) severe, if PGA > 5 cm plus CRP $\geq$ 2.5 mg/dL and/or SAA $\geq$ 50 mg/L. An increase in disease activity was defined as a switch of category from mild to moderate, mild to severe, or moderate to severe.

2.4. Outcome

The primary outcome was disease activity at last study visit. Secondary outcomes included the number of episodes with increased disease activity over time, the number and characteristics of performed treatment adjustments, applied dosing regimens, treatment responses, and disease activity trajectories/changes.

2.5. Analysis

Patients' characteristics were summarized using descriptive statistics. Categorical variables were presented as numbers (%) and continuous variables were shown as mean (SD) or as median (interquartile range, IQR 25. and 75. percentile). The proportion of patients with mild disease activity at first and last study visit was compared using the McNemar sign rank test. The change in disease activity category was analyzed using generalized linear mixed models, adjusting the baseline value to the previous study visit. The significance level in this study was defined as $p < 0.05$. A paired *t*-test was used to examine whether there was a significant difference in the means of the PGA or PPGA. For the exploratory analysis of the influence of genotype on disease activity, pathogenic and likely pathogenic variants were combined. Mean PGA and PPGA over time in different IL-1 AID was estimated by non-parametric local polynomial approximation. The Statistical analyses were conducted by SPSS 28.0.1.1 (IBM Corporation, Statistics for Windows, 2021, Armonk, NY, USA) and STATA 12.1 (StataCorp. LLC., College Station, TX, USA).

3. Results

In total, 56 children and adolescents with IL-1 AID were included, with 19 (34%) being girls. The median age at symptom onset for the entire cohort was 2.5 years (IQR

0.5; 4.1). Children with CAPS showed the first disease symptoms early in infancy (median 0.3 years [IQR 0.2; 0.5]). The median age at diagnosis for the entire cohort was 4.9 years (IQR 3.0; 7.7). At the first study visit, the median age was 4.9 years (IQR 3.3; 8.1). FMF was the most common diagnosis, seen in 46/56 (82%) patients, followed by CAPS diagnosed in 9/56 (16%), and 1 child was diagnosed with TRAPS. Eight out of nine children with CAPS had a moderate and one had a mild phenotype. In 63% of the FMF patients, at least one (likely) pathogenic variant or one VUS was detected; the remaining FMF patients were diagnosed clinically. The median follow-up time for the whole cohort was 2.1 years (IQR 1.4; 2.7) corresponding to a total of 361 visits. At the first visit, 15/56 children (27%) had already received colchicine. Of these, 14 children were diagnosed with FMF and one with CAPS. Only one FMF patient had been started on a combination treatment of anakinra and colchicine at enrolment (Table 1 and Supplementary Tables S1 and S2).

Table 1. Demographic and genetic characteristics of children with IL-1 AID.

	Total *n* = 56 (100%)	FMF *n* = 46 (82%)	CAPS *n* = 9 (16%)	TRAPS *n* = 1 (2%)
Demographic characteristics				
Female [1]	19 (34)	17 (37)	2 (22)	0
Symptom onset, age in years [2]	2.5 (0.5; 4.1)	2.9 (1.6; 4.7)	0.3 (0.2; 0.5)	2.7
Diagnosis, age in years [2]	4.9 (3.0; 7.7)	5.1 (3.6; 7.5)	2.8 (1.9; 4.5)	12.9
First study visit, age in years [2]	4.9 (3.3; 8.1)	5.1 (3.7; 8.0)	3.2 (1.9; 4.5)	13.0
Follow-up, years [2]	2.1 (1.4; 2.7)	1.9 (1.4; 2.5)	2.5 (2.3; 2.9)	3.0
Genetic variants				
Pathogenic/likely pathogenic [1]	28 (50)	25 (54)	2 (22)	1 (100)
VUS [1]	11 (20)	4 (9)	7 (78)	0

[1] *n* (%); [2] median (IQR). Abbreviations: *n*: Number of patients, IQR: Interquartile range, FMF: Familial Mediterranean Fever, CAPS: Cryopyrin-associated periodic syndromes, TRAPS: Tumor necrosis factor receptor-1-associated periodic syndrome, VUS: Variant of unknown significance.

3.1. Disease Activity over Time

At the first visit, 18/56 (32%) children presented with mild disease activity, 28 (50%) had moderate, and 10 (18%) severe disease activity. In contrast, at the last study visit, 44/56 (79%) children had mild disease activity, 10/56 (18%) moderate, and 2/56 (4%) severe disease activity. Over time, 36/56 (64%) children experienced at least one episode of increased disease activity. Changes were observed from mild to moderate in 17/36 (47%) children, from mild to severe in 12/36 (33%), and from moderate to severe in 7/36 (20%) children. A subsequent episode of increased disease activity was documented in 17/56 (30%), including mild to moderate in 13/17 (77%) and mild to severe in 4/17 (24%) (Figure 1 and Table 2).

Table 2. First and subsequent episodes of disease activity increase and performed treatment adjustments in children with IL-1 AID.

	Total *n* = 56	FMF *n* = 46	CAPS *n* = 9	TRAPS *n* = 1
First episode of increased disease activity, *n* (%)	36 (64)	30 (65)	5 (56)	1 (100)
Treatment adjustment in 28 out of 36 children *				
New treatment start, *n* (%)	19 (34)	15 (33)	3 (33)	1(100)
Treatment switch *n*, (%)	4 (7)	3 (7)	1 (11)	0 (0)
Dose increase *n*, (%)	8 (14)	7 (15)	1 (11)	0 (0)
Administration frequency increase, *n* (%)	0 (0)	0 (0)	0 (0)	0 (0)

Table 2. *Cont.*

	Total $n = 56$	FMF $n = 46$	CAPS $n = 9$	TRAPS $n = 1$
Subsequent episode of increased disease activity, *n* (%)	17 (30)	13 (28)	4 (44)	0 (0)
Treatment adjustments in 7 out of 17 children *				
New treatment start, *n* (%)	2 (4)	2 (4)	0 (0)	0 (0)
Treatment switch, *n* (%)	1 (2)	1 (2)	0 (0)	0 (0)
Dose increase, *n* (%)	3 (5)	1 (2)	2 (22)	0 (0)
Administration frequency increase, *n* (%)	1 (2)	0 (0)	1 (11)	0 (0)

n: Number of patients, % percentage, * One patient might have received multiple treatment adjustments. Abbreviations FMF: Familial Mediterranean Fever, CAPS: Cryopyrin-associated periodic syndromes, TRAPS: Tumor necrosis factor receptor-1-associated periodic syndrome.

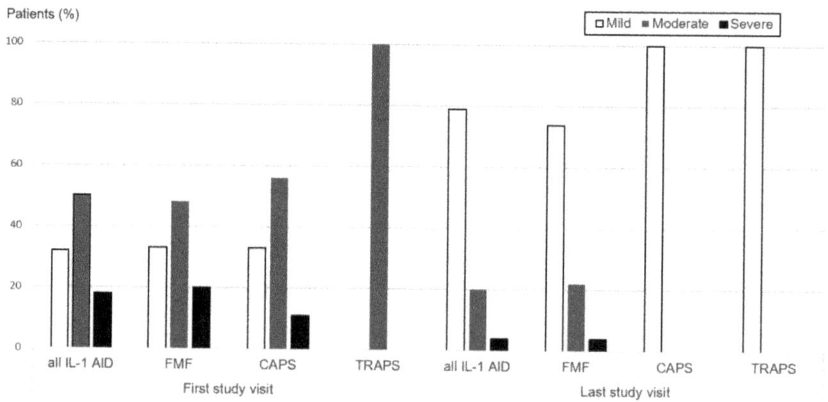

Figure 1. Disease activity in 56 children and adolescents with IL-1 AID at first and last study visit. Legend: Disease activity assessed at first and last study visit in children with IL-1 AID (all IL-1 AID; $n = 56$) and for IL-1 AID subgroups (FMF = 46, CAPS = 9, TRAPS = 1). Disease activity categories were defined as mild, moderate, and severe. A significant increase in mild disease activity category was shown between first and last study visit (McNemars sign rank test; all IL-1 AID $p < 0.001$, FMF $p < 0.001$, and CAPS $p = 0.031$). Abbreviations: IL: Interleukin, AID: Autoinflammatory disease, FMF: Familial Mediterranean Fever, CAPS: Cryopyrin-associated periodic syndromes, TRAPS: Tumor necrosis factor receptor-1-associated periodic syndrome.

3.2. Treatment Adjustments

3.2.1. Disease Activity-Based Treatment Adjustments

The first episode of increased disease activity resulted in treatment adjustments in 28/36 (78%) children with disease activity increase. In 19/28 children, a new treatment was started, a treatment switch was performed in four and a dose increase was performed in eight children. Treatment adjustments were distributed similarly between groups of children diagnosed with FMF and CAPS. A subsequent episode of increased disease activity was seen in 17/56 (30%) children during follow-up. Treatment was adjusted in seven (41%) out of the 17 children. Adjustments included new treatment start in two children, switch in one, dose increase in three, and increase in administration frequency in one. CAPS patients experiencing a subsequent disease activity increase typically received a dose adjustment (Table 2).

3.2.2. Specific Dosing Regimen

Median colchicine dose captured during the study for CAPS and FMF patients was 1 mg/day (maximum dose 1.5 mg/day) and 0.75 mg/day (maximum dose 1 mg/day), respectively. However, in those children with FMF carrying homozygous pathogenic/likely pathogenic *MEFV* variants, the median colchicine dose (1.13 mg/day) and the maximum colchicine dose (1.75 mg/day) were higher compared to FMF patients carrying heterozygous (likely) pathogenic variants (median dose 0.75 mg/day, maximum dose 1 mg/day). Four patients with FMF received anakinra; the median dose was 1.55 mg/kg once daily with a maximum dose of 1.62 mg/kg once daily. For canakinumab in CAPS, the median dose and the maximum dose was 3.93 mg/kg and 6.13 mg/kg, respectively. The administration frequency ranged from q4w (n = 17 visits) to q8w (n = 8 visits). The maximum canakinumab dose for the TRAPS patient was 2.78 mg/kg q4w. The two FMF patients treated with canakinumab had a median dose of 3.2 mg/kg and a maximum dose of 4.2 mg/kg q4w.

3.3. Impact on Disease Activity Trajectories

3.3.1. PGA and PPGA

Overall, patient/parent-derived global assessments (PPGA) of disease activity tended to be higher than physician-derived assessment (PGA) values. In 48/56 patients, both the PGA and the PPGA were available at the first and the last study visit. At the first visit, PGA and PPGA were comparable (p = 0.317). Within the study period, both measures decreased significantly ($p < 0.001$ and $p < 0.017$, respectively). PGA and PPGA differed statistically significantly ($p < 0.001$) at the last study visit (Figure 2). CAPS and FMF patients showed comparable mean PGA and PPGA over the first 12 months when assessed by non-parametric regression analysis (Figure 3).

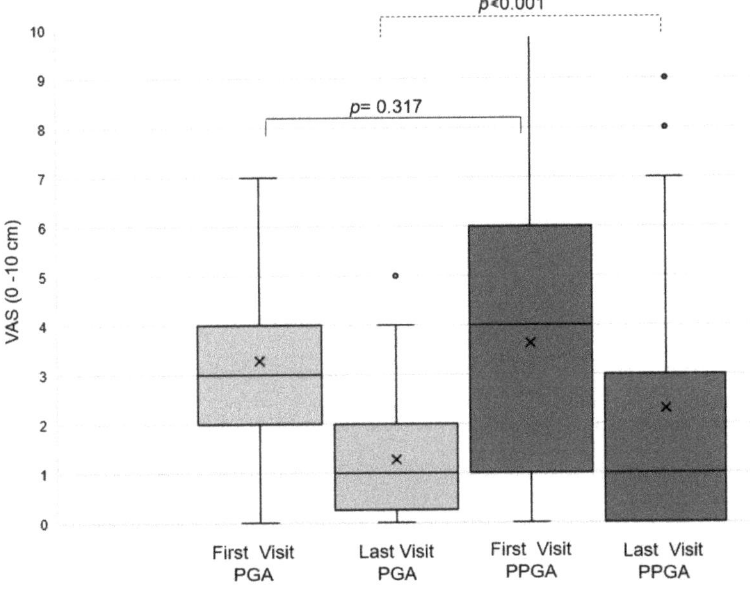

Figure 2. The association of treatment and disease activity-based treatment adjustments with the physician global assessment (PGA) and patient/parent global assessment (PPGA) at the first and last visit. Legend: Boxplot of the physician-derived global assessment (PGA) and the patient/parent-derived global assessment (PPGA) assessed with the visual analog scale (VAS) at the first and last visit. At the first visit, the median PGA was 3 (mean 3.1 ± 1.6) and the median PPGA was 4 (mean 3.6 ± 2.9). At the last visit, the median PGA was 1 (mean 1.2 ± 1.1) and the median PPGA was 1 (mean 2.2 ± 2.6). The paired t-test indicated statistical differences between the PPGA and PGA at the last visit. Legend: mean value (x), median (-).

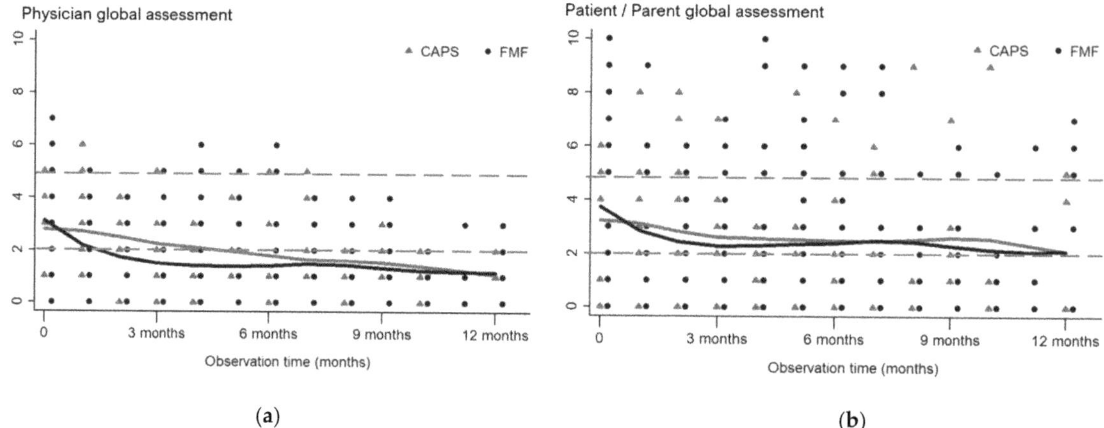

Figure 3. Longitudinal disease activity changes derived by the physician (PGA) and patient/parent (PPGA) in pediatric CAPS and FMF patients for 12 months after the first study visit. Legend: Course of (**a**) physician global assessment (PGA) and (**b**) patient/parent global assessment (PPGA) in children and adolescents with CAPS (grey triangle) and FMF (black dot) over the first 12 months after the first study visit estimated by local polynomial approximation. The PGA and PPGA are represented on the visual analog scale. Grey line: Local polynomial approximation for CAPS. Black line: Local polynomial approximation for FMF. Dashed gray line: Cut of PGA/PPGA > 2 cm and PGA > 5 cm. Abbreviations: FMF: Familial Mediterranean Fever, CAPS: Cryopyrin-associated periodic syndromes.

3.3.2. Parameter Trajectories/Changes

The mean change of PGA, PPGA, CRP, and SAA adjusted for baseline values was determined over observation time in all three IL-1 AID subgroups. The decrease in PGA over time reached statistical significance in all subgroups with an estimated mean decrease of -0.12 ($p < 0.001$) for CAPS, -0.15 ($p = 0.001$) for FMF, and -0.11 ($p < 0.001$) for TRAPS. Additionally, a significant estimated mean decrease for the CRP (-0.05; $p = 0.026$) was detected in CAPS only. The six-monthly change in PGA adjusted for baseline values showed a significant estimated mean decrease, irrespective of pathogenic/likely pathogenic variants, VUS, or clinically diagnosed IL-1 AID (Table 3).

Table 3. Mean change of disease activity parameters adjusted for baseline values between IL-1 AID and genotypes.

IL-1 AID Subgroups

	CAPS			FMF			TRAPS		
	beta [1]	95%CI	*p* Value	beta [1]	95%CI	*p* Value	beta [1]	95%CI	*p* Value
PGA	-0.12	-0.16; -0.08	<0.001	-0.15	-0.24; -0.06	0.001	-0.11	-0.17; -0.06	<0.001
PPGA	-0.09	-0.19; 0.02	0.100	-0.11	-0.32; 0.10	0.304	-0.08	-0.21; 0.05	0.247
CRP	-0.05	-0.10; -0.01	0.026	-0.10	-0.23; 0.03	0.130	-0.04	-0.09; 0.01	0.093
SAA	-2.49	-5.68; 0.71	0.127	-4.21	-10.62; 2.21	0.199	-2.26	-5.99; 1.47	0.236

Table 3. *Cont.*

Genotypes								
	Pathogenic/likely pathogenic variants			VUS			No genetic testing/no VUS or (likely) pathogenic variants detected		
	beta [1]	95%CI	*p* value	beta [1]	95%CI	*p* value	beta [1]	95%CI	*p* value
PGA	−0.13	−0.19; −0.08	<0.001	−0.09	−0.17; −0.01	0.020	−0.15	−0.26; −0.05	0.004
PPGA	−0.09	−0.23; 0.06	0.225	−0.08	−0.22; 0.06	0.280	−0.07	−0.28; 0.14	0.526
CRP	−0.07	−0.16; 0.01	0.073	−0.05	−0.12; 0.01	0.111	−0.04	−0.13; 0.05	0.444
SAA	−3.18	−8.97; 2.62	0.283	−2.67	−6.15; 0.80	0.132	−1.73	−10.25; 6.79	0.691

[1] Changes per six months adjusted for values at first study visit. FMF: Familial Mediterranean Fever, CAPS: Cryopyrin-associated periodic syndromes, TRAPS: Tumor necrosis factor receptor-1-associated periodic syndrome, VUS: Variant of unknown significance, physician global assessment (PGA), patient/parent global assessment (PPGA), CRP: C-reactive Protein, SAA: Serum Amyloid A, CI: Confidence Interval.

4. Discussion

This is the first comprehensive study analyzing the impact of disease activity-based treatment adjustments longitudinally in children and adolescents with different IL-1 AID in a real-life cohort. At the first study visit, 68% had moderate to severe disease activity, two-thirds (64%) experienced at least one flare episode, and one-third had subsequent episodes over the study's duration. Overall, the approach of iterative disease activity-based treatment adjustments resulted in significant clinical improvements; most patients (79%) were asymptomatic and met the criteria for the mild disease activity category at the last study visit. Importantly, PGA and PPGA were similar at the first visit but differed significantly at the last follow-up ($p < 0.001$). The mean change of the PGA adjusted for baseline values over time revealed a significant decrease independent of genotype, clinical diagnosis, or IL-1 AID subgroup. These results highlight the importance of disease activity-based treatment adjustments and emphasize the need to further investigate the impact of distinct disease activity parameters.

Disease activity-based treatment adjustments can improve the outcome of patients with IL-1 AID including achieving remission/mild disease activity, improving HrQoL, and reducing the risk of organ damage. A rationale for disease activity-based treatment adjustments is the interplay of patient-related (e.g., age, living circumstances), disease-related (e.g., genotype, organ damage), and treatment-related (e.g., pharmacokinetics, side effects) factors [28–30]. The integration of these factors results in individual disease activity trajectories, as demonstrated in this study. In IL-1 AID, the genotype has been shown to influence the clinical phenotype, disease activity, and risk of organ damage [31–35]. External triggers including stress, lack of sleep, infections, and exercise as well as comorbidities can impact individual disease activity [36,37]. This complex interplay mandates the need for personalized treatment adjustments. Consequently, standardized disease activity monitoring and disease activity-based treatment adjustments are crucial to optimize care [14]. Drug exposure–response relationships have been reported for some inflammatory diseases in the past, indicating the need for higher drug exposure to control high disease activity [38,39]. This study emphasizes the drug exposure–response relationship across different IL-1 AID. The performed individual adjustments resulted in well-controlled disease in the majority of children (79%). In addition, a trend towards higher drug dosing in children with homozygous pathogenic/likely pathogenic *MEFV* gene variants compared to heterozygous carriers was observed. The exposure–response relationship in IL-1 AID aligns with the published data: patients with severe CAPS phenotypes needed higher drug exposure to control disease activity in contrast to mild phenotypes [10,40]; FMF patients with homozygous pathogenic gene variants (*M694V, M680I*) or compound heterozygous gene variants (*M694V/M680I, M694/V726A*) required higher colchicine doses (mean average range 1.19 mg/day to 1.09 mg/day) compared to those with any heterozygous genotype (average dose 0.81 mg/day) [41]. Based on the drug exposure–response relationship in IL-1 AID, T2T strategies can help to avoid drug underexposure and associated treatment failure. Additionally, they may guide treatment tapering decisions [17,28,42,43]. Individualized disease activity-based treatments and the application of T2T recommendations in IL-1 AID can, therefore, reduce the risk of suboptimal disease management, associated morbidity, and long-term organ damage [10,16,17,44]. Furthermore, it can avoid drug overexposure with increased risk of adverse events and higher drug costs than needed [43,45–48]. The drug exposure–response relationship and individual factors need to be considered as they help to further refine and optimize the management of children and adolescents with IL-1 AID.

Iterative, standardized disease activity monitoring over the disease course is crucial in IL-1 AID management. It is the cornerstone for T2T approaches. In the past, the development of valid disease activity assessment tools, standardized outcome measures, and HrQoL instruments in pediatric rheumatology have been important milestones for enabling optimal patient care [49]. The disease activity and disease burden are commonly assessed and quantified by the physician (e.g., PGA) and the patient/parent (e.g., PPGA), by HrQoL tools and missed school/working days, measurement of inflammatory markers, assessment of systemic and organ-specific signs of active disease, and evaluation of disease damage [10,18]. Important milestones for disease activity monitoring in IL-1 AID included the validation of the AIDAI and the development of the ADDI [8,9]. Furthermore, the identification of advanced inflammatory markers such as SAA, S100A8/A9, and S100A12 facilitated the recognition of subclinical inflammation [50–52]. In this study, we used a composite score for the assessment of disease activity, combining inflammatory markers and PGA. In addition, the PPGA was captured iteratively. The six-monthly mean changes in PGA, PPGA, SAA, and CRP adjusted for baseline values revealed a decrease in all disease activity parameters. Importantly, only PGA changes were found to be significant across all IL-1 subgroups. The estimated mean CRP decrease over time was only significant for CAPS. Mean PGA and PPGA values were similar at the first study visit; however, they differed significantly at the last visit. In line with the published evidence, patient/parent-derived values (PPGA) in this study tended to be higher than those of the physician (PGA) [53,54]. This might reflect the different concepts physicians and families consider when scoring. PPGA may also capture levels of fatigue, pain, psychological co-morbidities, and impaired social participation experienced by the patient and family [55,56]. This highlights the importance of clarity on measuring constructs of disease activity, disease damage, burden of illness, and objective assessment of fatigue/sleep quality [57]. Recently, the *Protokolle in der Kinderrheumatologie* (PRO-KIND) initiative of the German Society for Pediatric Rheumatology (GKJR) has proposed a new composite tool for FMF [17]. This multidimensional instrument combines the assessment of flare frequency, missed school/working days, inflammatory markers, chronic sequelae/disease damage, the PGA, and the PPGA [17]. However, this tool has not been evaluated so far. Our results confirm that T2T approaches to IL-1 AID can effectively control disease activity and guide treatment adjustments. However, the overall burden of autoinflammation exceeds the concepts of disease activity and requires a multidimensional approach including capturing the disease impact on participation and mental health.

This study has several limitations. The sample size was small (n = 56); however, IL-1 AID are orphan diseases. The analysis was comprehensive, as the study population was well defined and the median follow-up of 2.1 years resulted in 361 visits. The study was conducted at a national reference center for patients with AID potentially biasing the sample towards children and adolescents with more severe, potentially difficult to treat disease courses. This may raise concerns about the limited generalizability of our results. However, the cohort included the entire disease severity spectrum across different IL-1 AID and analyzed the impact of disease activity-based treatment adjustments. Lastly, disease activity was assessed by commonly used composite scores, combining laboratory parameters and physician global assessments [16,25–27], neither AIDAI nor ADDI were formally integrated. However, both instruments are regularly reviewed at clinical routine visits, and, therefore, inform the global assessments.

5. Conclusions

This study demonstrates the importance of personalized disease activity-based treatment adjustments in IL-1 AID to optimize care and improve outcomes. It can help in preventing drug over- and underexposure. Prospective data collection and outcome assessments to further refine recently published T2T strategies and disease activity monitoring is critical. These insights will help to further optimize disease activity-based step-up but also step-down treatment in IL-1 AID.

Supplementary Materials: The following supporting information can be downloaded at https://www.mdpi.com/article/10.3390/jcm13082319/s1, Supplementary Table S1: Detected gene variants. Supplementary Table S2: Treatment at first study visit in children with IL-1 AID.

Author Contributions: Conceptualization: T.W., S.M.B., J.B.K.-D., B.Z. and J.K. Methodology: T.W., B.Z., J.K., S.M.B. and J.B.K.-D. Formal analysis: B.Z. and J.K. Writing—original draft preparation: T.W. and B.Z. Review and Editing: Ö.S., J.B.K.-D., S.M.B. and J.K. Each author made substantial contributions to the manuscript and has approved the submitted version. All authors have read and agreed to the published version of the manuscript.

Funding: We received financial support for publication fees by the Open Access Publication Fund of the University of Tübingen.

Institutional Review Board Statement: Ethics approval was obtained from the ethics committee of Karl Eberhard University Tuebingen (050/2021BO2, date of first approval: 23 February 2021).

Informed Consent Statement: Patient consent was waived by the local ethics committee.

Data Availability Statement: All relevant data are shown in the manuscript and Supplementary Material. Upon reasonable request and with obtained ethical approval, the dataset can be made available by the corresponding author.

Acknowledgments: We acknowledge support from the Open Access Publication Fund of the University of Tübingen.

Conflicts of Interest: T.W. has given invited talks for Novartis without a personal honorarium. B.Z., Ö.S., J.K. and S.M.B. have no conflicts of interest; J.B.K.-D. has received grants and speaker fees from Novartis and SOBI.

References

1. Broderick, L.; De Nardo, D.; Franklin, B.S.; Hoffman, H.M.; Latz, E. The inflammasomes and autoinflammatory syndromes. *Annu. Rev. Pathol.* **2015**, *10*, 395–424. [CrossRef] [PubMed]
2. Lachmann, H.J. Periodic fever syndromes. *Best. Pract. Res. Clin. Rheumatol.* **2017**, *31*, 596–609. [CrossRef] [PubMed]
3. Toplak, N.; Frenkel, J.; Ozen, S.; Lachmann, H.J.; Woo, P.; Koné-Paut, I.; De Benedetti, F.; Neven, B.; Hofer, M.; Dolezalova, P.; et al. An International registry on Autoinflammatory diseases: The Eurofever experience. *Ann. Rheum. Dis.* **2012**, *71*, 1177–1182. [CrossRef] [PubMed]
4. Blank, N.; Kotter, I.; Schmalzing, M.; Rech, J.; Krause, K.; Kohler, B.; Kaudewitz, D.; Nitschke, M.; Haas, C.S.; Lorenz, H.M.; et al. Clinical presentation and genetic variants in patients with autoinflammatory diseases: Results from the German GARROD registry. *Rheumatol. Int.* **2024**, *44*, 263–271. [CrossRef] [PubMed]
5. Cipolletta, S.; Giudici, L.; Punzi, L.; Galozzi, P.; Sfriso, P. Health-related quality of life, illness perception, coping strategies and the distribution of dependency in autoinflammatory diseases. *Clin. Exp. Rheumatol.* **2019**, *37* (Suppl. S121), 156–157. [PubMed]
6. Erbis, G.; Schmidt, K.; Hansmann, S.; Sergiichuk, T.; Michler, C.; Kuemmerle-Deschner, J.B.; Benseler, S.M. Living with autoinflammatory diseases: Identifying unmet needs of children, adolescents and adults. *Pediatr. Rheumatol. Online J.* **2018**, *16*, 81. [CrossRef] [PubMed]
7. Vasse, M.; Reumaux, H.; Kone-Paut, I.; Quartier, P.; Hachulla, E. Socio-professional impact and quality of life of cryopyrin-associated periodic syndromes in 54 patients in adulthood. *Clin. Exp. Rheumatol.* **2023**, *41*, 2039–2043. [CrossRef] [PubMed]

8. Piram, M.; Kone-Paut, I.; Lachmann, H.J.; Frenkel, J.; Ozen, S.; Kuemmerle-Deschner, J.; Stojanov, S.; Simon, A.; Finetti, M.; Sormani, M.P.; et al. Validation of the auto-inflammatory diseases activity index (AIDAI) for hereditary recurrent fever syndromes. *Ann. Rheum. Dis.* **2014**, *73*, 2168–2173. [CrossRef] [PubMed]

9. Ter Haar, N.M.; van Delft, A.L.J.; Annink, K.V.; van Stel, H.; Al-Mayouf, S.M.; Amaryan, G.; Anton, J.; Barron, K.S.; Benseler, S.; Brogan, P.A.; et al. In silico validation of the Autoinflammatory Disease Damage Index. *Ann. Rheum. Dis.* **2018**, *77*, 1599–1605. [CrossRef]

10. Romano, M.; Arici, Z.S.; Piskin, D.; Alehashemi, S.; Aletaha, D.; Barron, K.S.; Benseler, S.; Berard, R.; Broderick, L.; Dedeoglu, F.; et al. The 2021 EULAR/American College of Rheumatology points to consider for diagnosis, management and monitoring of the interleukin-1 mediated autoinflammatory diseases: Cryopyrin-associated periodic syndromes, tumour necrosis factor receptor-associated periodic syndrome, mevalonate kinase deficiency, and deficiency of the interleukin-1 receptor antagonist. *Ann. Rheum. Dis.* **2022**, *81*, 907–921. [CrossRef]

11. Ozen, S.; Demirkaya, E.; Erer, B.; Livneh, A.; Ben-Chetrit, E.; Giancane, G.; Ozdogan, H.; Abu, I.; Gattorno, M.; Hawkins, P.N.; et al. EULAR recommendations for the management of familial Mediterranean fever. *Ann. Rheum. Dis.* **2016**, *75*, 644–651. [CrossRef] [PubMed]

12. De Benedetti, F.; Gattorno, M.; Anton, J.; Ben-Chetrit, E.; Frenkel, J.; Hoffman, H.M.; Kone-Paut, I.; Lachmann, H.J.; Ozen, S.; Simon, A.; et al. Canakinumab for the Treatment of Autoinflammatory Recurrent Fever Syndromes. *N. Engl. J. Med.* **2018**, *378*, 1908–1919. [CrossRef] [PubMed]

13. Hentgen, V.; Vinit, C.; Fayand, A.; Georgin-Lavialle, S. The Use of Interleukine-1 Inhibitors in Familial Mediterranean Fever Patients: A Narrative Review. *Front. Immunol.* **2020**, *11*, 971. [CrossRef] [PubMed]

14. Smolen, J.S. Treat-to-target: Rationale and strategies. *Clin. Exp. Rheumatol.* **2012**, *30*, S2–S6. [PubMed]

15. Solomon, D.H.; Bitton, A.; Katz, J.N.; Radner, H.; Brown, E.M.; Fraenkel, L. Review: Treat to target in rheumatoid arthritis: Fact, fiction, or hypothesis? *Arthritis Rheumatol.* **2014**, *66*, 775–782. [CrossRef] [PubMed]

16. Hansmann, S.; Lainka, E.; Horneff, G.; Holzinger, D.; Rieber, N.; Jansson, A.F.; Rosen-Wolff, A.; Erbis, G.; Prelog, M.; Brunner, J.; et al. Consensus protocols for the diagnosis and management of the hereditary autoinflammatory syndromes CAPS, TRAPS and MKD/HIDS: A German PRO-KIND initiative. *Pediatr. Rheumatol. Online J.* **2020**, *18*, 17. [CrossRef] [PubMed]

17. Ehlers, L.; Rolfes, E.; Lieber, M.; Muller, D.; Lainka, E.; Gohar, F.; Klaus, G.; Girschick, H.; Horstermann, J.; Kummerle-Deschner, J.; et al. Treat-to-target strategies for the management of familial Mediterranean Fever in children. *Pediatr. Rheumatol. Online J.* **2023**, *21*, 108. [CrossRef]

18. Georgin-Lavialle, S.; Savey, L.; Cuisset, L.; Boursier, G.; Boffa, J.J.; Delplanque, M.; Bourguiba, R.; Monfort, J.B.; Touitou, I.; Grateau, G.; et al. French protocol for the diagnosis and management of familial Mediterranean fever. *Rev. Med. Interne* **2023**, *44*, 602–616. [CrossRef] [PubMed]

19. Gattorno, M.; Hofer, M.; Federici, S.; Vanoni, F.; Bovis, F.; Aksentijevich, I.; Anton, J.; Arostegui, J.I.; Barron, K.; Ben-Cherit, E.; et al. Classification criteria for autoinflammatory recurrent fevers. *Ann. Rheum. Dis.* **2019**, *78*, 1025–1032. [CrossRef]

20. Kuemmerle-Deschner, J.B.; Ozen, S.; Tyrrell, P.N.; Kone-Paut, I.; Goldbach-Mansky, R.; Lachmann, H.; Blank, N.; Hoffman, H.M.; Weissbarth-Riedel, E.; Hugle, B.; et al. Diagnostic criteria for cryopyrin-associated periodic syndrome (CAPS). *Ann. Rheum. Dis.* **2017**, *76*, 942–947. [CrossRef]

21. Yalcinkaya, F.; Ozen, S.; Ozcakar, Z.B.; Aktay, N.; Cakar, N.; Duzova, A.; Kasapcopur, O.; Elhan, A.H.; Doganay, B.; Ekim, M.; et al. A new set of criteria for the diagnosis of familial Mediterranean fever in childhood. *Rheumatology* **2009**, *48*, 395–398. [CrossRef] [PubMed]

22. Richards, S.; Aziz, N.; Bale, S.; Bick, D.; Das, S.; Gastier-Foster, J.; Grody, W.W.; Hegde, M.; Lyon, E.; Spector, E.; et al. Standards and guidelines for the interpretation of sequence variants: A joint consensus recommendation of the American College of Medical Genetics and Genomics and the Association for Molecular Pathology. *Genet. Med.* **2015**, *17*, 405–424. [CrossRef] [PubMed]

23. Milhavet, F.; Cuisset, L.; Hoffman, H.M.; Slim, R.; El-Shanti, H.; Aksentijevich, I.; Lesage, S.; Waterham, H.; Wise, C.; Sarrauste de Menthiere, C.; et al. The infevers autoinflammatory mutation online registry: Update with new genes and functions. *Hum. Mutat.* **2008**, *29*, 803–808. [CrossRef] [PubMed]

24. Infevers: An Online Database for Autoinflammatory Mutations. Copyright. Available online: https://infevers.umai-montpellier.fr (accessed on 1 November 2023).

25. Kuemmerle-Deschner, J.B.; Hofer, F.; Endres, T.; Kortus-Goetze, B.; Blank, N.; Weissbarth-Riedel, E.; Schuetz, C.; Kallinich, T.; Krause, K.; Rietschel, C.; et al. Real-life effectiveness of canakinumab in cryopyrin-associated periodic syndrome. *Rheumatology* **2016**, *55*, 689–696. [CrossRef] [PubMed]

26. Kuemmerle-Deschner, J.B.; Ramos, E.; Blank, N.; Roesler, J.; Felix, S.D.; Jung, T.; Stricker, K.; Chakraborty, A.; Tannenbaum, S.; Wright, A.M.; et al. Canakinumab (ACZ885, a fully human IgG1 anti-IL-1beta mAb) induces sustained remission in pediatric patients with cryopyrin-associated periodic syndrome (CAPS). *Arthritis Res. Ther.* **2011**, *13*, R34. [CrossRef] [PubMed]

27. Welzel, T.; Wildermuth, A.L.; Deschner, N.; Benseler, S.M.; Kuemmerle-Deschner, J.B. Colchicine—An effective treatment for children with a clinical diagnosis of autoinflammatory diseases without pathogenic gene variants. *Pediatr. Rheumatol. Online J.* **2021**, *19*, 142. [CrossRef] [PubMed]

28. Welzel, T.; Oefelein, L.; Twilt, M.; Pfister, M.; Kuemmerle-Deschner, J.B.; Benseler, S.M. Tapering of biological treatment in autoinflammatory diseases: A scoping review. *Pediatr. Rheumatol. Online J.* **2022**, *20*, 67. [CrossRef]

29. Parlar, K.; Ates, M.B.; Onal, M.E.; Bostanci, E.; Azman, F.N.; Ugurlu, S. Factors triggering familial mediterranean fever attacks, do they really exist? *Intern. Emerg. Med.* **2024**. [CrossRef] [PubMed]

30. Kharouf, F.; Tsemach-Toren, T.; Ben-Chetrit, E. IL-1 inhibition in familial Mediterranean fever: Clinical outcomes and expectations. *Clin. Exp. Rheumatol.* **2022**, *40*, 1567–1574. [CrossRef]

31. Levy, R.; Gerard, L.; Kuemmerle-Deschner, J.; Lachmann, H.J.; Kone-Paut, I.; Cantarini, L.; Woo, P.; Naselli, A.; Bader-Meunier, B.; Insalaco, A.; et al. Phenotypic and genotypic characteristics of cryopyrin-associated periodic syndrome: A series of 136 patients from the Eurofever Registry. *Ann. Rheum. Dis.* **2015**, *74*, 2043–2049. [CrossRef]

32. Ter Haar, N.M.; Jeyaratnam, J.; Lachmann, H.J.; Simon, A.; Brogan, P.A.; Doglio, M.; Cattalini, M.; Anton, J.; Modesto, C.; Quartier, P.; et al. The Phenotype and Genotype of Mevalonate Kinase Deficiency: A Series of 114 Cases From the Eurofever Registry. *Arthritis Rheumatol.* **2016**, *68*, 2795–2805. [CrossRef] [PubMed]

33. Ben-Zvi, I.; Danilesko, I.; Yahalom, G.; Kukuy, O.; Rahamimov, R.; Livneh, A.; Kivity, S. Risk factors for amyloidosis and impact of kidney transplantation on the course of familial Mediterranean fever. *Isr. Med. Assoc. J.* **2012**, *14*, 221–224. [PubMed]

34. Labrousse, M.; Kevorkian-Verguet, C.; Boursier, G.; Rowczenio, D.; Maurier, F.; Lazaro, E.; Aggarwal, M.; Lemelle, I.; Mura, T.; Belot, A.; et al. Mosaicism in autoinflammatory diseases: Cryopyrin-associated periodic syndromes (CAPS) and beyond. A systematic review. *Crit. Rev. Clin. Lab. Sci.* **2018**, *55*, 432–442. [CrossRef] [PubMed]

35. Bas, B.; Sayarlioglu, H.; Yarar, Z.; Dilek, M.; Arik, N.; Sayarlioglu, M. Investigation of the relationship between disease severity and development of amyloidosis and genetic mutation in FMF disease. *Ir. J. Med. Sci.* **2023**, *192*, 1497–1503. [CrossRef] [PubMed]

36. Lachmann, H.J.; Papa, R.; Gerhold, K.; Obici, L.; Touitou, I.; Cantarini, L.; Frenkel, J.; Anton, J.; Kone-Paut, I.; Cattalini, M.; et al. The phenotype of TNF receptor-associated autoinflammatory syndrome (TRAPS) at presentation: A series of 158 cases from the Eurofever/EUROTRAPS international registry. *Ann. Rheum. Dis.* **2014**, *73*, 2160–2167. [CrossRef] [PubMed]

37. Vitale, A.; Lucherini, O.M.; Galeazzi, M.; Frediani, B.; Cantarini, L. Long-term clinical course of patients carrying the Q703K mutation in the NLRP3 gene: A case series. *Clin. Exp. Rheumatol.* **2012**, *30*, 943–946. [PubMed]

38. Paul, S.; Marotte, H.; Kavanaugh, A.; Goupille, P.; Kvien, T.K.; de Longueville, M.; Mulleman, D.; Sandborn, W.J.; Vande Casteele, N. Exposure-Response Relationship of Certolizumab Pegol and Achievement of Low Disease Activity and Remission in Patients with Rheumatoid Arthritis. *Clin. Transl. Sci.* **2020**, *13*, 743–751. [CrossRef]

39. Ternant, D.; Azzopardi, N.; Raoul, W.; Bejan-Angoulvant, T.; Paintaud, G. Influence of Antigen Mass on the Pharmacokinetics of Therapeutic Antibodies in Humans. *Clin. Pharmacokinet.* **2019**, *58*, 169–187. [CrossRef]

40. Caorsi, R.; Lepore, L.; Zulian, F.; Alessio, M.; Stabile, A.; Insalaco, A.; Finetti, M.; Battagliese, A.; Martini, G.; Bibalo, C.; et al. The schedule of administration of canakinumab in cryopyrin associated periodic syndrome is driven by the phenotype severity rather than the age. *Arthritis Res. Ther.* **2013**, *15*, R33. [CrossRef]

41. Knieper, A.M.; Klotsche, J.; Lainka, E.; Berger, T.; Dressler, F.; Jansson, A.F.; Rietschel, C.; Oommen, P.T.; Berendes, R.; Niehues, T.; et al. Familial Mediterranean fever in children and adolescents: Factors for colchicine dosage and predicting parameters for dose increase. *Rheumatology* **2017**, *56*, 1597–1606. [CrossRef]

42. Cohen, K.; Spielman, S.; Semo-Oz, R.; Bitansky, G.; Gerstein, M.; Yacobi, Y.; Vivante, A.; Tirosh, I. Colchicine treatment can be discontinued in a selected group of pediatric FMF patients. *Pediatr. Rheumatol. Online J.* **2023**, *21*, 2. [CrossRef] [PubMed]

43. Shehadeh, K.; Levinsky, Y.; Kagan, S.; Zuabi, T.; Tal, R.; Aviran, N.H.; Butbul Aviel, Y.; Tirosh, I.; Spielman, S.; Miller-Barmak, A.; et al. An "On Demand" canakinumab regimen for treating children with Colchicine-Resistant familial Mediterranean fever—A multicentre study. *Int. Immunopharmacol.* **2024**, *132*, 111967. [CrossRef] [PubMed]

44. Duzova, A.; Bakkaloglu, A.; Besbas, N.; Topaloglu, R.; Ozen, S.; Ozaltin, F.; Bassoy, Y.; Yilmaz, E. Role of A-SAA in monitoring subclinical inflammation and in colchicine dosage in familial Mediterranean fever. *Clin. Exp. Rheumatol.* **2003**, *21*, 509–514. [PubMed]

45. Russell, M.D.; Bukhari, M.; Galloway, J. The price of good health care. *Rheumatology* **2019**, *58*, 931–932. [CrossRef] [PubMed]

46. Singh, J.A.; Cameron, C.; Noorbaloochi, S.; Cullis, T.; Tucker, M.; Christensen, R.; Ghogomu, E.T.; Coyle, D.; Clifford, T.; Tugwell, P.; et al. Risk of serious infection in biological treatment of patients with rheumatoid arthritis: A systematic review and meta-analysis. *Lancet* **2015**, *386*, 258–265. [CrossRef]

47. Welzel, T.; Golhen, K.; Atkinson, A.; Gotta, V.; Ternant, D.; Kuemmerle-Deschner, J.B.; Michler, C.; Koch, G.; van den Anker, J.N.; Pfister, M.; et al. Prospective study to characterize adalimumab exposure in pediatric patients with rheumatic diseases. *Pediatr. Rheumatol. Online J.* **2024**, *22*, 5. [CrossRef] [PubMed]

48. Kavrul Kayaalp, G.; Caglayan, S.; Demirkan, F.G.; Guliyeva, V.; Otar Yener, G.; Ozturk, K.; Demir, F.; Ozdel, S.; Cakan, M.; Sonmez, H.E.; et al. Is it possible to extend the dose interval of canakinumab treatment in children with familial Mediterranean fever? PeRA group experience. *Pediatr. Rheumatol. Online J.* **2023**, *21*, 140. [CrossRef] [PubMed]

49. Ruperto, N.; Martini, A. International research networks in pediatric rheumatology: The PRINTO perspective. *Curr. Opin. Rheumatol.* **2004**, *16*, 566–570. [CrossRef] [PubMed]

50. Wittkowski, H.; Kuemmerle-Deschner, J.B.; Austermann, J.; Holzinger, D.; Goldbach-Mansky, R.; Gramlich, K.; Lohse, P.; Jung, T.; Roth, J.; Benseler, S.M.; et al. MRP8 and MRP14, phagocyte-specific danger signals, are sensitive biomarkers of disease activity in cryopyrin-associated periodic syndromes. *Ann. Rheum. Dis.* **2011**, *70*, 2075–2081. [CrossRef]

51. Cakan, M.; Karadag, S.G.; Tanatar, A.; Sonmez, H.E.; Ayaz, N.A. The Value of Serum Amyloid A Levels in Familial Mediterranean Fever to Identify Occult Inflammation during Asymptomatic Periods. *J. Clin. Rheumatol.* **2021**, *27*, 1–4. [CrossRef]

52. Lieber, M.; Kallinich, T.; Lohse, P.; Klotsche, J.; Holzinger, D.; Foell, D.; Wittkowski, H. Increased serum concentrations of neutrophil-derived protein S100A12 in heterozygous carriers of MEFV mutations. *Clin. Exp. Rheumatol.* **2015**, *33*, S113–S116. [PubMed]
53. Desthieux, C.; Hermet, A.; Granger, B.; Fautrel, B.; Gossec, L. Patient-Physician Discordance in Global Assessment in Rheumatoid Arthritis: A Systematic Literature Review with Meta-Analysis. *Arthritis Care Res.* **2016**, *68*, 1767–1773. [CrossRef] [PubMed]
54. Floris, A.; Espinosa, G.; Serpa Pinto, L.; Kougkas, N.; Lo Monaco, A.; Lopalco, G.; Orlando, I.; Bertsias, G.; Cantarini, L.; Cervera, R.; et al. Discordance between patient and physician global assessment of disease activity in Behcet's syndrome: A multicenter study cohort. *Arthritis Res. Ther.* **2020**, *22*, 278. [CrossRef] [PubMed]
55. Challa, D.N.V.; Crowson, C.S.; Davis, J.M., 3rd. The Patient Global Assessment of Disease Activity in Rheumatoid Arthritis: Identification of Underlying Latent Factors. *Rheumatol. Ther.* **2017**, *4*, 201–208. [CrossRef]
56. Monti, S.; Delvino, P.; Klersy, C.; Coppa, G.; Milanesi, A.; Montecucco, C. Factors influencing patient-reported outcomes in ANCA-associated vasculitis: Correlates of the Patient Global Assessment. *Semin. Arthritis Rheum.* **2022**, *56*, 152048. [CrossRef]
57. Incesu, C.; Kayaalp, G.K.; Demirkan, F.G.; Koker, O.; Cakmak, F.; Akgun, O.; Ayaz, N.A.; Omeroglu, R.N. The assessment of fatigue and sleep quality among children and adolescents with familial Mediterranean fever: A case-control and correlation study. *Eur. J. Pediatr.* **2024**. [CrossRef]

MDPI

St. Alban-Anlage 66

4052 Basel

Switzerland

www.mdpi.com

Journal of Clinical Medicine Editorial Office

E-mail: jcm@mdpi.com

www.mdpi.com/journal/jcm

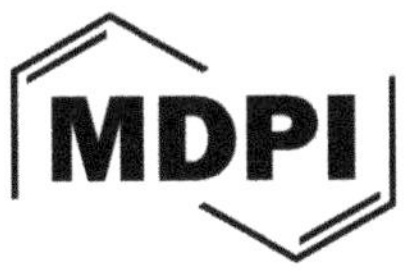